Preventing and Avoiding Complications in Hand Surgery

Editor

KEVIN C. CHUNG

HAND CLINICS

www.hand.theclinics.com

Consulting Editor
KEVIN C. CHUNG

May 2015 • Volume 31 • Number 2

ELSEVIER

1600 John F. Kennedy Boulevard • Suite 1800 • Philadelphia, Pennsylvania, 19103-2899

http://www.theclinics.com

HAND CLINICS Volume 31, Number 2
May 2015 ISSN 0749-0712, ISBN-13: 978-0-323-37599-3

Editor: Jennifer Flynn-Briggs
Developmental Editor: Colleen Viola

Hand Clinics (ISSN 0749-0712) is published quarterly by Elsevier Inc., 360 Park Avenue South, New York, NY 10010-1710. Months of publication are February, May, August, and November. Business and Editorial Offices: 1600 John F. Kennedy Blvd., Ste. 1800, Philadelphia, PA 19103-2899. Customer Service Office: 3251 Riverport Lane, Maryland Heights, MO 63043. Periodicals postage paid at New York, NY and at additional mailing offices. Subscription price is $390.00 per year (domestic individuals), $606.00 per year (domestic institutions), $194.00 per year (domestic students/residents), $445.00 per year (Canadian individuals), $691.00 per year (Canadian institutions), $530.00 per year (international individuals), $691.00 per year (international institutions), and $256.00 per year (international and Canadian students/residents). Foreign air speed delivery is included in all *Clinics* subscription prices. All prices are subject to change without notice. **POSTMASTER:** Send address changes to *Hand Clinics*, Elsevier Health Sciences Division, Subscription Customer Service, 3251 Riverport Lane, Maryland Heights, MO 63043. Customer Service (orders, claims, online, change of address): Elsevier Health Sciences Division, Subscription Customer Service, 3251 Riverport Lane, Maryland Heights, MO 63043. Tel: 1-800-654-2452 (U.S. and Canada); 314-447-8871 (outside U.S. and Canada). Fax: 314-447-8029. E-mail: journalscustomerservice-usa@elsevier.com (for print support); journalsonlinesupport-usa@elsevier.com (for online support).

Reprints. For copies of 100 or more of articles in this publication, please contact the Commercial Reprints Department, Elsevier Inc., 360 Park Avenue South, New York, New York 10010-1710. Tel.: 212-633-3874; Fax: 212-633-3820; E-mail: reprints@elsevier.com.

Hand Clinics is covered in *MEDLINE/PubMed (Index Medicus), Current Contents/Clinical Medicine, EMBASE/Excerpta Medica,* and *ISI/BIOMED.*

Contributors

CONSULTING EDITOR

KEVIN C. CHUNG, MD, MS
Charles B. G. de Nancrede Professor of Surgery; Professor of Plastic Surgery and Orthopaedic Surgery; Chief of Hand Surgery, University of Michigan Health System; Assistant Dean for Faculty Affairs, University of Michigan Medical School, Ann Arbor, Michigan

EDITOR

KEVIN C. CHUNG, MD, MS
Charles B. G. de Nancrede Professor of Surgery; Professor of Plastic Surgery and Orthopaedic Surgery; Chief of Hand Surgery, University of Michigan Health System; Assistant Dean for Faculty Affairs, University of Michigan Medical School, Ann Arbor, Michigan

AUTHORS

HEE-CHAN AHN, MD
Cheon & Woo's Institute for Hand and Reconstructive Microsurgery, W Hospital, Dalseo Gu, Daegu, Korea

DAVID J. BOZENTKA, MD
Chief, Hand Surgery; Associate Professor of Orthopedic Surgery, Department of Orthopedic Surgery, University of Pennsylvania, Philadelphia, Pennsylvania

R. CHRISTOPHER CHADDERDON, MD
OrthoCarolina, Charlotte, North Carolina

HO-JUN CHEON, MD
Cheon & Woo's Institute for Hand and Reconstructive Microsurgery, W Hospital, Dalseo Gu, Daegu, Korea

KEVIN CHEUNG, MSc, MD
Hand and Microsurgery Fellow, Division of Plastic Surgery, Harvard Medical School, Beth Israel Deaconess Medical Center, Boston, Massachusetts

KEVIN C. CHUNG, MD, MS
Charles B. G. de Nancrede Professor of Surgery; Professor of Plastic Surgery and Orthopaedic Surgery; Chief of Hand Surgery, University of Michigan Health System; Assistant Dean for Faculty Affairs, University of Michigan Medical School, Ann Arbor, Michigan

TOD A. CLARK, MD, MSc, FRCSC
Section of Orthopedic Surgery, Panam Clinic, University of Manitoba, Poseidon Bay, Winnipeg, Manitoba, Canada

GARET C. COMER, MD
Fellow, Department of Orthopedic Surgery, Robert A. Chase Hand and Upper Limb Center, Stanford University, Redwood City, California

ALEX G. DUKAS, MD, MA
Resident Physician, Department of Orthopedic Surgery, UConn Health Center, New England Musculoskeletal Institute, Farmington, Connecticut

KYLE R. EBERLIN, MD
Hand Surgery Service, Massachusetts General Hospital; Division of Plastic and Reconstructive Surgery, Massachusetts General Hospital, Harvard Medical School, Boston, Massachusetts

JOEL FERREIRA, MD
Hand and Upper Extremity Fellow, Department of Orthopedics, University of Pittsburgh, Pittsburgh, Pennsylvania

JOHN R. FOWLER, MD
Assistant Professor, Department of Orthopedics, University of Pittsburgh, Pittsburgh, Pennsylvania

VARUN K. GAJENDRAN, MD
Department of Orthopedic Surgery, MetroHealth Medical Center, Cleveland, Ohio

VISHAL K. GAJENDRAN, BS
University of Toledo College of Medicine, Toledo, Ohio

MICHAEL P. GASPAR, MD
Clinical Research Fellow in Hand and Upper Extremity Surgery, The Philadelphia Hand Center, Philadelphia, Pennsylvania

R. GLENN GASTON, MD
Hand Fellowship Director, OrthoCarolina, Chief of Hand Surgery, Carolinas Medical Center, Charlotte, North Carolina

SREENADH GELLA, MBBS, MS (Orth), FRCS (T&O)
Section of Orthopedic Surgery, Panam Clinic, University of Manitoba, Poseidon Bay, Winnipeg, Manitoba, Canada

ALBERT V. GEORGE, MD
Department of Orthopedic Surgery, University of Michigan Hospital, University of Michigan, Ann Arbor, Michigan

JENNIFER L. GIUFFRE, MD, FRCSC
Section of Plastic Surgery, Panam Clinic, University of Manitoba, Poseidon Bay, Winnipeg, Manitoba, Canada

RUBY GREWAL, MSc, MD, FRCSC
Associate Professor, Division of Orthopedic Surgery, Roth|McFarlane Hand and Upper Limb Centre, St. Joseph's Health Care, Western University, London, Ontario, Canada

MATTHEW T. HOUDEK, MD
Division of Hand and Microvascular Surgery, Department of Orthopedic Surgery, Mayo Clinic, Rochester, Minnesota

PATRICK M. KANE, MD
Fellow in Hand and Upper Extremity Surgery, The Philadelphia Hand Center, Philadelphia, Pennsylvania

DONG-HO KANG, MD
Cheon & Woo's Institute for Hand and Reconstructive Microsurgery, W Hospital, Dalseo Gu, Daegu, Korea

JONG-MIN KIM, MD
Cheon & Woo's Institute for Hand and Reconstructive Microsurgery, W Hospital, Dalseo Gu, Daegu, Korea

YOUNG-WOO KIM, MD, PhD
Cheon & Woo's Institute for Hand and Reconstructive Microsurgery, W Hospital, Dalseo Gu, Daegu, Korea

AMY L. LADD, MD
Professor, Department of Orthopedic Surgery; Chief, Robert A. Chase Hand and Upper Limb Center, Stanford University, Palo Alto, California

MATTHEW A. LANGFORD, MD
LCDR/MC/USN, Hand Fellow, Department of Orthopedic Surgery, Wake Forest School of Medicine, Winston-Salem, North Carolina

JEFFREY N. LAWTON, MD
Associate Professor and Chief Elbow, Hand and Microsurgery, Department of Orthopedic Surgery, University of Michigan, Ann Arbor, Michigan

ZHONGYU LI, MD, PhD
Associate Professor, Department of Orthopedic Surgery, Wake Forest School of Medicine, Winston-Salem, North Carolina

KRISTINA LUTZ, MD
Chief Resident, Division of Plastic Surgery, Department of Surgery, Roth|McFarlane Hand and Upper Limb Centre, St. Joseph's Health Care, Western University, London, Ontario, Canada

KEVIN J. MALONE, MD
Department of Orthopedic Surgery, MetroHealth Medical Center, Cleveland, Ohio

ALEXANDRA L. MATHEWS, BS
Research Assistant, Section of Plastic Surgery, Department of Surgery, University of Michigan Health System, Ann Arbor, Michigan

HYUN-JE NAM, MD
Cheon & Woo's Institute for Hand and Reconstructive Microsurgery, W Hospital, Dalseo Gu, Daegu, Korea

KAGAN OZER, MD
Associate Professor, Department of Orthopedic Surgery, University of Michigan, Ann Arbor, Michigan

JOEY PIPICELLI, MScOT, CHT, OT Reg (Ont)
PhD Student; Occupational Therapist; Certified Hand Therapist, Division of Hand Therapy, Faculty of Rehabilitation Sciences, Roth|McFarlane Hand and Upper Limb Centre, St. Joseph's Health Care, Western University, London, Ontario, Canada

NICHOLAS PULOS, MD
Resident, Department of Orthopedic Surgery, University of Pennsylvania, Philadelphia, Pennsylvania

DAVID RING, MD, PhD
Hand Surgery Service, Professor, Department of Orthopedic Surgery, Massachusetts General Hospital, Harvard Medical School, Boston, Massachusetts

TAMARA D. ROZENTAL, MD
Associate Professor, Department of Orthopedics, Harvard Medical School, Beth Israel Deaconess Medical Center, Boston, Massachusetts

DOUGLAS M. SAMMER, MD
Associate Professor, Departments of Plastic and Orthopedic Surgery, Program Director Hand Surgery Fellowship, University of Texas Southwestern Medical Center, Dallas, Texas

KATHERINE B. SANTOSA, MD
House Officer, Section of Plastic Surgery, Department of Surgery, University of Michigan Health System, Ann Arbor, Michigan

ELLEN S. SATTESON, MD
Department of Orthopedic Surgery; Resident, PGY III, Department of Plastic Surgery, Wake Forest School of Medicine, Winston-Salem, North Carolina

ALEXANDER Y. SHIN, MD
Division of Hand and Microvascular Surgery, Department of Orthopedic Surgery, Mayo Clinic, Rochester, Minnesota

EON K. SHIN, MD
Assistant Professor of Orthopedic Surgery, Department of Orthopedic Surgery, Thomas Jefferson University Hospital; The Philadelphia Hand Center, Philadelphia, Pennsylvania

JENNIFER F. WALJEE, MD, MPH, MS
Assistant Professor, Section of Plastic Surgery, Department of Surgery, University of Michigan Health System, Ann Arbor, Michigan

KEMPLAND C. WALLEY, BSc
Department of Orthopedics, Harvard Medical School, Beth Israel Deaconess Medical Center, Boston, Massachusetts

JENNIFER MORIATIS WOLF, MD
Associate Professor, Department of Orthopedic Surgery, UConn Health Center, New England Musculoskeletal Institute, Farmington, Connecticut

SANG-HYUN WOO, MD, PhD
Cheon & Woo's Institute for Hand and Reconstructive Microsurgery, President, W Hospital, Dalseo Gu, Daegu, Korea

Contents

joints of the hand. Arthrodesis and arthroplasty come with a risk of postoperative infection. Superficial soft tissue infections can often be managed with oral antibiotics alone. Deep infections and osteomyelitis frequently require removal of hardware in addition to antibiotics and may require surgical revision once the infection is cleared. Selection of the most appropriate revision technique depends on the underlying cause of the initial failure, patients' functional and outcome needs, and surgeon preference.

Management of Complications of Ligament Injuries of the Wrist **267**

Sreenadh Gella, Jennifer L. Giuffre, and Tod A. Clark

Despite advances in understanding the anatomy and biomechanics of wrist motion, intrinsic carpal ligament injuries are difficult to diagnose and treat. Even when an accurate diagnosis is made, there is no consensus on the most appropriate and reliable treatment. Injury predisposes to a progressive decline in wrist function and a predictable pattern of degenerative arthritis. To prevent inadequate outcomes, many treatment options exist, all having inherent benefits and complications. This article reviews the complications of intrinsic carpal ligament injuries and complications of their treatment. Methods to prevent and principles to manage the complications are discussed.

Management of Complications of Wrist Arthroplasty and Wrist Fusion **277**

Michael P. Gaspar, Patrick M. Kane, and Eon K. Shin

The human wrist joint is unique from functional and anatomic standpoints. Numerous articulations exist within the wrist that allow for many options for partial wrist fusion and arthroplasty. In cases of pancarpal disease, fusion or arthroplasty of the entire wrist joint can be performed. Because of the high functional demand of the wrist, many of these surgical options can fail, leading to devastating complications. This article addresses the types of fusions and arthroplasties available for the wrist and discusses the potential complications associated with each. Methods to prevent these complications are presented and those to treat them once they have occurred are discussed.

Management of Complications of Flexor Tendon Injuries **293**

Nicholas Pulos and David J. Bozentka

Innovations in operative techniques, biomaterials, and rehabilitation protocols have improved outcomes after treatment of flexor tendon injuries. However, despite these advances, treatment of flexor tendon injuries remains challenging. This article highlights the complications of flexor tendon injuries and reviews the management of these complications.

Management of Complications of Extensor Tendon Injuries **301**

Kristina Lutz, Joey Pipicelli, and Ruby Grewal

Treatment goals for the management of extensor tendon injuries include restoration of function, minimizing disability, and decreasing the risk of complications. These goals can be achieved with an accurate understanding of the zone-specific concerns for extensor tendon injuries, early referral to hand therapy, and active communication between hand surgeons and therapists. This article reviews extensor tendon injuries by zone, outlines optimal management strategies that help prevent complications, and describes the treatment of these complications.

risk of infection after hand surgery include hand washing, skin preparation, sterile technique, and prophylactic antibiotics. The role of prophylactic antibiotics for small, clean, elective hand surgery procedures lasting less than 2 hours is debated.

Management of Complications of Congenital Hand Disorders **361**

Garet C. Comer and Amy L. Ladd

This article reviews treatment and presents complications seen in the treatment of 7 common congenital hand differences, including syndactyly, camptodactyly, ulnar and radial polydactyly, thumb hypoplasia, radial longitudinal deficiency, and epidermolysis bullosa. The management of these conditions is challenging but has evolved over the last several decades with refined understanding of the disease processes and treatments. The goal of this article is to synthesize prior knowledge and provide further insights into these conditions that will help the surgeon avoid treatment complications.

Index **377**

HAND CLINICS

FORTHCOMING ISSUES

August 2015
Management of Elbow Trauma
George S. Athwal, *Editor*

November 2015
Innovations in Intercarpal Ligament Repair and Reconstruction
Marco Rizzo, *Editor*

February 2016
Pain Management and Hand Surgery
Catherine Curtin, *Editor*

RECENT ISSUES

February 2015
New Developments in Management of Vascular Pathology of the Upper Extremity
Steven Moran, Karim Bakri and James Higgins, *Editors*

November 2014
Options for Surgical Exposure and Soft Tissue Coverage in Upper Extremity Trauma
Amitava Gupta, *Editor*

August 2014
Health Services Research and Evidence-Based Medicine in Hand Surgery
Jennifer F. Waljee and Kate Nellans, *Editors*

May 2014
Flap Reconstruction of the Traumatized Upper Extremity
Kevin C. Chung, *Editor*

RELATED INTEREST

Orthopedic Clinics of North America, January 2015 (Volume 46, Issue 1)

Preface

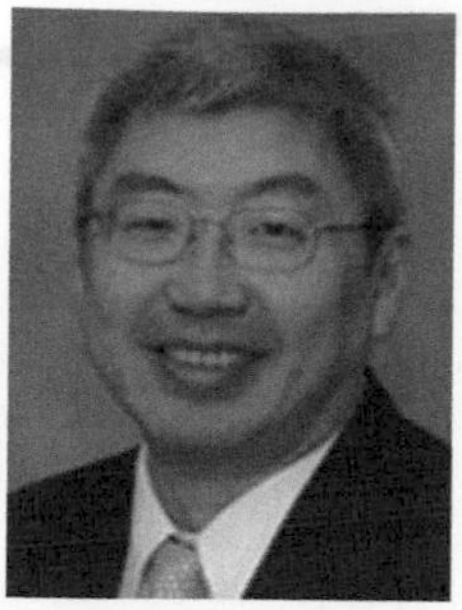

Kevin C. Chung, MD, MS
Editor

The word complication strikes fear in all of us. Not only does a complication delay the patient's recovery, but it also incurs great anguish to the surgeon and taxes the health care system with additional costs and efforts. Fortunately, complications are infrequent. The judge of a surgeon's character is to treat complications effectively when they do occur. Of course, careful preoperative planning and meticulous surgical techniques can avert many complications. This Issue of *Hand Clinics* is dedicated to preventing and solving surgical complications. The authors are all seasoned surgeons who have previously faced complications and who now unabashedly share their experiences to help us through these untoward events.

The practice of medicine needs to be transparent when adverse events and complications occur. The only way that we can improve outcomes as well as ourselves is to be introspective of our results and to discuss them openly without the fear of reprisal. Presenting complications in mortality and morbidity conferences, sharing them at national meetings for group consideration, and outlining the preventative measures and solutions in a volume such as this are the essential steps to instill confidence in our patients. Patients do accept that surgeons are not perfect, but each of us should arm ourselves with the necessary knowledge to face an unforeseen event and strive to be open with others if one should occur.

I appreciate the candor of my colleagues in offering their experiences. This issue is a collection of authoritative treaties on this topic that in the past were rarely discussed. I hope the readers will derive collective insight from my colleagues so that we can serve our patients even better.

Kevin C. Chung, MD, MS
University of Michigan Health System
Section of Plastic Surgery
Department of Surgery
1500 East Medical Center Drive
2130 Taubman Center, SPC 5340
Ann Arbor, MI 48109-5340, USA

E-mail address:
kecchung@med.umich.edu

Hand Clin 31 (2015) xiii
http://dx.doi.org/10.1016/j.hcl.2015.02.001
0749-0712/15/$ – see front matter

Erratum

In the February 2014 issue (Volume 31, Number 1), the article by Victor W. Wong, Ryan D. Katz and James P. Higgins was incorrectly titled as, "New Developments in Management of Vascular Pathology of the Upper Extremity". The correct title for this article is, "Interpretation of Upper Extremity Arteriography: Vascular Anatomy and Pathology".

Hand Clin 31 (2015) xv
http://dx.doi.org/10.1016/j.hcl.2015.01.013
0749-0712/15/$ – see front matter

Erratum

In the February 2014 issue (Volume 31, Number 1), the article by Victor W. Wong, Ryan D. Katz and James P. Higgins was incorrectly titled as: "New Developments in Management of Vascular Pathology of the Upper Extremity". The correct title for this article is, "Interpretation of Upper Extremity Arteriography: Vascular Anatomy and Pathology".

Hand Clin 31 (2015) xv
http://dx.doi.org/10.1016/j.hcl.2015.01.015

Complications of Compressive Neuropathy

Prevention and Management Strategies

Katherine B. Santosa, MD, Kevin C. Chung, MD, MS,
Jennifer F. Waljee, MD, MPH, MS*

KEYWORDS

- Median nerve • Ulnar nerve • Carpal tunnel syndrome • Carpal tunnel release
- Ulnar tunnel syndrome • Cubital tunnel syndrome • Complications

KEY POINTS

- Prevention of complications begins with a solid understanding of the normal anatomy and anatomic variations that may exist.
- Carpal tunnel release is among the most common hand surgical procedures performed, but complications occur in up to 25% of cases. Revision carpal tunnel surgery may be indicated in patients who present with recurrent, persistent, or new symptoms due to inadequate release, iatrogenic injury, recurrent symptoms, or perineural fibrosis.
- Cubital tunnel syndrome is the second most common compressive neuropathy, but recurrence or failed decompression occurs in 25% to 35% of patients. Frequently reported complications include injury to the medial antebrachial cutaneous (MABC) nerve, ulnar nerve subluxation, and recurrent symptoms because of inadequate release or perineural fibrosis.

Compressive neuropathies of the upper extremity are common and can result in profound disability if left untreated.[1–3] Nerve releases are frequently performed, but can be complicated by both iatrogenic events and progression of neuropathy. In this review, we examine the management of postoperative complications after 2 common nerve compression release procedures: carpal tunnel release and cubital tunnel release.

CARPAL TUNNEL SYNDROME

Carpal tunnel syndrome (CTS) is the most common compressive neuropathy, affecting 1.6% to 7.8% individuals.[4–6] Carpal tunnel release (CTR) is one of the most frequently performed outpatient procedures in the United States, and is typically considered to be a minor elective and routine procedure.[7] Complications are rare, but can result in devastating loss of hand function.

Intraoperative Complications

Normal anatomy of the carpal tunnel guides incision placement for open release; however, several anatomic variants exist, and can increase the risk of iatrogenic injury.[8–10] A solid understanding of the anatomic relationships of the proximal palm, carpal canal, and distal forearm can direct correct incision placement and prevent iatrogenic injury

Disclosures: None.
Supported in part by a Midcareer Investigator Award in Patient-Oriented Research (K24 AR053120) to Dr K.C. Chung.
Section of Plastic Surgery, Department of Surgery, University of Michigan Health System, 1500 East Medical Center Drive, Ann Arbor, MI 48109-5340, USA
* Corresponding author. Section of Plastic Surgery, University of Michigan Health System, 2130 Taubman Center, SPC 5340, 1500 East Medical Center Drive, Ann Arbor, MI 48109-5340.
E-mail address: filip@med.umich.edu

Hand Clin 31 (2015) 139–149
http://dx.doi.org/10.1016/j.hcl.2015.01.012
0749-0712/15/$ – see front matter

(**Fig. 1**).[11–17] Fortunately, injury to major neurovascular structures during CTR is exceedingly low. Permanent nerve injury more commonly occurs to the branches of the median nerve, including the palmar cutaneous branch (0.03%), the deep motor branch of the median nerve (0.01%), or the common digital nerves (0.12%), compared with injury to the median nerve proper (0.06%).[18]

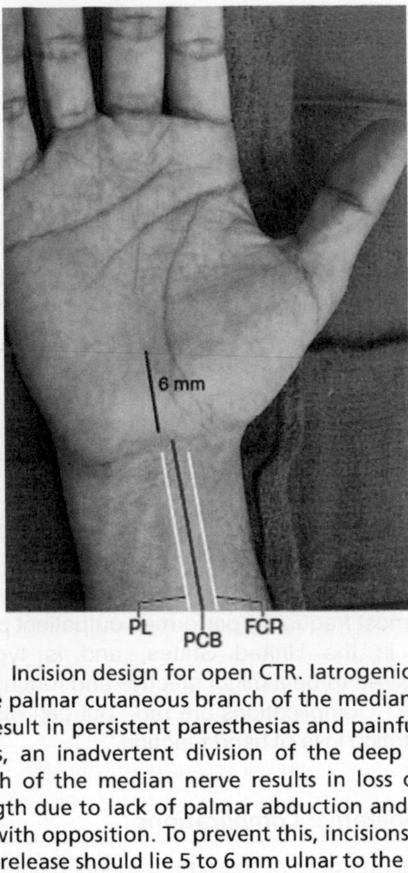

Fig. 1. Incision design for open CTR. Iatrogenic injury to the palmar cutaneous branch of the median nerve can result in persistent paresthesias and painful neuromas, an inadvertent division of the deep motor branch of the median nerve results in loss of grip strength due to lack of palmar abduction and weakness with opposition. To prevent this, incisions for an open release should lie 5 to 6 mm ulnar to the thenar crease, in line with the ulnar border of the middle finger. However, overcorrecting in the ulnar direction can result in entry into the more superficial Guyon canal, with potential injury to the ulnar neurovascular bundle. Inadvertent entry into the Guyon canal can be recognized if the dissection is carried down through the skin to reveal hypothenar fat, with diminutive palmar fascia, and no visualization of the transverse fibers of the transverse carpal ligament. Because the hand naturally is slightly pronated when placed on the hand table, entry into the Guyon canal can occur when the knife dissection is not perpendicular to the plane of the hand, but rather parallel to the transverse carpal ligament. FCR, flexor carpi radialis; PCB, palmar cutaneous branch; PL, palmaris longus. (*From* Sammer D. Open carpal tunnel release. In: Chung KC, editor. Operative techniques: hand and wrist surgery. vol. 2. Philadelphia: Elsevier Saunders; 2012; with permission.)

Injuries to adjacent structures, including the superficial palmar arch (0.1%), flexor tendons (0.1%), and the ulnar nerve (0.03%) also have been described.[18,19] Endoscopic techniques may result in a slightly higher rate of major nerve injury (0.13%–0.3%) versus open techniques (0.10%–0.2%).[18,20] However, other studies have not demonstrated a difference in major complications by technique. It is likely that overall complication rates are more dependent on surgeon experience with the specific technique.[21–23]

Postoperative Complications

A description of potential postoperative complications and etiologies of treatment failures are outlined in **Table 1**. Superficial and/or deep space infections are uncommon, and occur in only 0.4% of cases. Currently, perioperative antibiotic prophylaxis and operating room sterility is not indicated for CTR procedures, given the low rates of perioperative infection.[24,25] Symptomatic hypertrophic scarring and hypothenar "pillar" pain are more frequent, and have been correlated with perioperative mood disturbance. However, symptoms typically subside within 3 months, and can be managed by nonoperative techniques.[26] The incidence of pathologic pain syndromes, including complex regional pain syndrome (CRPS), has been described in up to 8% of patients after CTR.[27,28] Early recognition and referral to specialists experienced in the management of pathologic pain syndromes and CRPS is critical to prevent the propagation of symptoms and permanent disability. Less commonly, flexor tendon complications have been described after division of the transverse carpal ligament, including bowstringing, adhesions, and triggering.[29,30] Finally, wrist instability and pisotriquetral arthrosis has been reported in approximately 2% of patients, which often can be managed successfully with splinting, anti-inflammatory agents, and steroid injections. For those patients who have failed nonoperative measures, pisiform excision can be considered.[31]

Treatment Failure After Carpal Tunnel Release

After CTR, treatment failure can occur in up to 25% of patients, with approximately 12% of patients requiring secondary surgery.[1,32,33] Treatment failure refers to the presence of neuropathic symptoms, and can be considered in the following way: (1) persistent symptoms, (2) recurrent symptoms, or (3) the presence of an alternate diagnosis.[33] Persistent CTS refers to the presence of ongoing symptoms after CTR without improvement following release, and is more commonly

Table 1
Complications of carpal tunnel release

Complication	Description
Injury to anatomic structures	• Recurrent motor branch of the median nerve • Palmar cutaneous branch of the median nerve • Ulnar nerve injury due to inadvertent entry into the Guyon canal • Ulnar artery injury due to inadvertent entry into the Guyon canal • Superficial palmar arch injury • Flexor tendon injury
Soft tissue complications	• Hematoma • Infection • Skin necrosis • Scar hypertrophy
Pain	• Chronic regional pain syndrome • Hypothenar "pillar" pain
Other	• Flexor tendon bowstringing • Wrist instability: pisotriquetral subluxation
Persistent symptoms	• Persistent compression • Recurrent compression • Alternate diagnosis

encountered compared with recurrent symptoms. Persistent CTS following release is typically caused by an incomplete release of the flexor retinaculum distally or the antebrachial fascia proximally, and may be more common after endoscopic or limited incision techniques.[33–36] However, other prospective, randomized controlled studies have failed to demonstrate a difference in the incidence of persistent symptoms after CTR by release technique.[37,38]

Patients with recurrent CTS typically experience complete relief following primary release, but symptoms consistent with CTS recur after a period of at least 6 months or longer. The pathophysiology leading to recurrent CTS remains unclear, but is thought to be caused by scarring, fibrous proliferation, healing and reformation of the flexor retinaculum, or recurrent tenosynovitis.[39] Extraneural scarring impairs epineural blood flow, impedes nerve gliding, and can result in recurrent compression on the nerve. Recurrent symptoms account for nearly 20% of all revision surgeries, and are more common among patients with hypertension and diabetes.[39,40] It has been postulated that diabetes results in the glycosylation of connective tissues, increases collagen cross-linking, and causes stiffness and thickening of the transverse carpal ligament. Furthermore, microvascular disease associated with diabetes may render the median nerve more susceptible to injury by compression.[41] Similarly, hypertension has been shown to be a risk factor for CTS. Although the physiologic mechanism by which hypertension leads to CTS remains unclear, it is thought to be related to the use of β-blockers and comorbid conditions associated with hypertension, such as diabetes and vascular disease.[40,42]

Evaluation

Although adjunct diagnostic tests may be useful in the evaluation of patients with complications or treatment failure following CTR, a focused history and physical examination are the most important tools to guide the surgeon toward a treatment strategy. Patients who present with symptoms that are not congruent with prior symptoms of CTS should be evaluated for nerve injury or the presence of an alternative diagnosis. For example, patients with injury to the palmar cutaneous branch of the median nerve may present with localized numbness, and hyperalgesia across the scar with a positive Tinel sign along the course of the palmar cutaneous branch. Local anesthetic injection may help identify the lesion by temporary resolution of the discomfort.[43] Conservative therapies, such as desensitization, topical agents, and Botulinum A injections, may be initially helpful in suppressing symptoms.[43,44] However, patients with persistent symptoms despite conservative measures should undergo neuroma resection of the affected palmar cutaneous branch and nerve transposition. Similarly, injury to the digital nerves may present with anesthesia of the affected digit, or neuroma formation in the palm. Treatment includes exploration and identification of the injury, with repair of the nerve or neuroma resection and nerve grafting as indicated. Progressive weakness with thenar atrophy may suggest injury to the recurrent motor branch of the median nerve. Hyperalgesia, trophic changes, edema, and vasomotor asymmetries (ie, temperature and skin changes) may suggest development of CRPS.[28]

In addition to iatrogenic injury, the clinical examination can reveal alternate causes of symptoms. For example, the median nerve may be compressed more proximally in the forearm, such as at the ligament of Struthers (fibrous band between the medial epicondyle and supracondylar process), between the superficial and deep heads of the pronator teres, the arch of flexor digitorum superficialis (FDS), or the bicipital aponeurosis. Furthermore, vascular anomalies, tumors, Gantzer muscle (an accessory head of the flexor pollicis longus), palmaris profundus, or the presence of flexor carpi radialis brevis may all manifest with compressive symptoms.[45] Additionally, spinal pathology, such as cervical radiculopathy, spinal cord lesions, and thoracic outlet syndrome may all mimic symptoms of CTS. Systemic diseases, such as diabetic neuropathy, thyroid conditions, and hemodialysis-dependent renal failure due to microglobulin amyloid deposits, related neurologic sequelae, may manifest with symptoms similar to that of CTS.[46] Lesions resulting in a local mass effect at the carpal tunnel, such as ganglion cysts, arterial aneurysms, gouty tophi, amyloidosis, sarcoidosis, or fracture callus, may also result in diminished volume in the carpal canal and median nerve compression.

Among patients with no other competing diagnosis, it is critical to determine if the etiology of the treatment failure is due to the persistence or recurrence of symptoms after primary CTR. An interval of relief, followed by the recurrence of symptoms, is suggestive of perineural fibrosis and scarring. Patients with persistent symptoms are more likely to have symptoms that mirror their symptoms before primary CTR, whereas patients with recurrence may be more likely to present with scar hypersensitivity and pain.[47,48] Standard provocative maneuvers, including carpal compression and wrist flexion testing, may confirm the diagnosis of CTS, and provide information regarding the etiology of symptoms (**Table 2**).[35,49,50] Although response to steroid injection has been shown to be well correlated with relief among patients with primary CTS, its utility among patients with recurrent or persistent symptoms is less clear.[51] Recent evidence suggests that relief from steroid injection combined with positive provocative physical examination findings are predictive of relief for patients undergoing revision CTR for recurrent symptoms.[50]

Electrodiagnostic studies are useful to document the severity of compression, the presence of denervation of median nerve–innervated thenar musculature, and the presence of alternative locations of compression.[1] Additionally, electrodiagnostic testing can provide an objective parameter for long-term follow-up.[35,52,53] However, electrodiagnostic testing should not be taken in isolation, but rather in conjunction with the patient's clinical picture. For example, normal electrodiagnostic studies do not exclude the diagnosis of CTS, and electrodiagnostic studies can remain abnormal for a prolonged period after a successful surgical release.[53,54] In this context, electrodiagnostic studies may not be helpful in diagnosing recurrent CTS given the persistence of electrical changes in nerve conduction and motor response even after successful release, but can provide information regarding prognosis, recovery, and the presence of additional areas of nerve compression or injury.[50,55]

Table 2
Diagnostic testing for carpal tunnel syndrome

	Sensitivity, %	Specificity, %
Hand diagram	76	98
Night pain	96	100
Phalen	75	95
Tinel	64	99
Durkan	89	91
Semmes-Weinstein	65	88

Data from Szabo RM, Slater RR, Farver TB, et al. The value of diagnostic testing in carpal tunnel syndrome. J Hand Surg Am 1999;24(4):704–14.

Patients who have undergone prior CTR who present with persistent or recurrent symptoms should undergo plain radiographs to evaluate for the presence of fracture or dislocation contributing to compression on the median nerve. High-resolution ultrasonography may highlight the presence of space-occupying lesions contributing to median nerve compression, and can be further characterized with advanced imaging, such as MRI or computed tomography, as indicated.[56–58]

Treatment options In general, the decision to reoperate is based on signs and symptoms from the history and physical examination. For patients who present with clear signs of iatrogenic nerve injury (eg, dense anesthesia, motor function loss), immediate nerve exploration is indicated.[43,59] A short course of conservative measures is a helpful adjunct for patients with persistent or recurrent symptoms following CTR, and include splinting, steroid injections, desensitization, and range of motion exercises to promote nerve and tendon gliding.[35] However, most patients with recalcitrant symptoms will need surgical intervention.

Revision CTR is challenging, and robust evidence regarding the appropriate indications and timing is sparse.[50,60] The indications for reoperation include (1) persistent symptoms due to inadequate release of the flexor retinaculum or antebrachial fascia, (2) persistent symptoms due to more proximal nerve compression, (3) recurrent symptoms due to perineural scarring or reformation of the flexor retinaculum, and (4) suspected nerve injury. For patients who develop recurrent symptoms at 1 year or longer following primary release, repeat CTR is indicated.[35,59,61]

Revision surgery begins with an extension of the previous incision both proximally and distally for adequate exposure and to identify the nerve in normal tissue planes away from the scar tissue.[33] The incision should be extended proximally across the wrist crease, and created medially to the previous incision to enter the carpal canal along its ulnar aspect.[62] The median nerve is identified proximally and distally. The dissection proceeds into the carpal canal, noting that the median nerve may be adherent to the underside of the flexor retinaculum.[39,63] The transverse carpal ligament is explored, and released in its entirety.[61] External neurolysis is performed to free the median nerve from surrounding scar, and internal neurolysis also may be required to visualize normal fascicular anatomy.[33,35,39,59]

Following nerve release and neurolysis, the surgeon should assess the favorability of the wound bed surrounding the median nerve. Substantial scarring and poor vascularity may impede nerve gliding and predispose patients toward recurrent symptoms. To augment soft tissue coverage, several local flaps have been described, including the hypothenar fat pad, synovial flap, abductor digiti minimi, or the palmaris brevis, and regional or free flaps, including radial forearm, omentum, and lateral arm flaps, which may promote neovascularization, decreasing scar reformation, and enhance nerve regeneration.[65] Of these, the hypothenar fat pad is most commonly favored given its proximity to the wound bed, ease of dissection, and the robustness of the available tissue.[66] Following neurolysis, dissection proceeds between the dermis of the hypothenar skin and underlying fat. After the ulnar neurovascular structures are identified, the fat pad is elevated and mobilized to a region between the median nerve and transverse carpal ligament. In 62 patients with recalcitrant CTS, 58 reported excellent results after undergoing CTR, neurolysis, and hypothenar fat pad flap.[65] In another study, 41 of 45 patients with recurrent CTS experienced resolution of pain following neurolysis and hypothenar fat pad flap.[48] Recently, there has been growing enthusiasm for the use of vein grafts and synthetic substitutes to prevent scar formation following revision CTR and neurolysis.[67] Although these options may reduce operating room time and donor site morbidity, there is no evidence comparing the effectiveness of nerve wrapping with flap coverage, and synthetic options are substantially more expensive compared with autologous tissue coverage.[64]

Outcomes Reported outcomes among patients with complications following CTR vary widely. Some studies suggest that patients who are found to have an incomplete release of the transverse carpal ligament at reexploration have the most favorable prognosis, whereas patients with significant scarring and fibrosis fare much more poorly.[34,61] Similarly, patients who have undergone multiple revision procedures are less likely to experience relief, likely due to scarring and fibrosis in the wound bed.[39] Furthermore, patient factors likely mediate outcomes. For example, Hulsizer and colleagues[34] reported that only 18% of patients receiving worker's compensation who underwent revision experienced improvement postoperatively, compared with 84% of patients with conventional insurance. Therefore, it is essential to counsel patients regarding the probability of achieving relief so as to appropriately set expectations following any revision surgery.

CUBITAL TUNNEL SYNDROME

Cubital tunnel syndrome (CuTS), or compression of the ulnar nerve at the elbow, is the second most common compression neuropathy, and up to 75,000 decompression releases are performed in the United States yearly (**Fig. 2**).[68,69] Although multiple strategies are described, no single technique has emerged as superior, and in situ decompression and anterior transposition are most commonly performed.[69,70] Nerve transpositions may be performed subcutaneously, intramuscularly (within the flexor-pronator mass) and submuscularly (beneath the flexor-pronator mass). Recently, endoscopic in situ releases have been described, with the possibility of similar effectiveness, and earlier return to work.[71–74]

Postoperative Complications

Outcomes after primary cubital tunnel release (CuTR) are generally favorable, with good relief of symptoms in 80% to 90% of patients.[2,3] Patient-related risk factors, such as preoperative level of neuropathy, chronic neuropathy, older age (>50 years), and

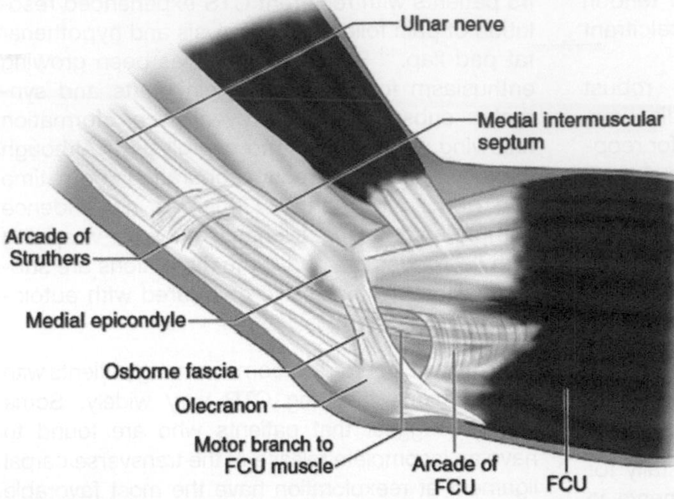

Fig. 2. Topography of ulnar nerve and sites of ulnar nerve compression. The ulnar nerve is derived from the ventral rami of cervical roots of C8 and T1 and becomes the terminal branch of the medial cord of the brachial plexus. The ulnar nerve then courses between the medial head of the triceps and the brachialis muscles. It travels posterior or medial to the brachial artery and posterior to the intramuscular septum. Approximately 8 cm from the medial epicondyle, the nerve is surrounded by the arcade of Struthers, which is a fascial band that connects the medial head of the triceps and the intramuscular septum. Here, it becomes superficial and pierces the medial intramuscular septum and enters the ulnar sulcus. It courses posterior to the medial condyle and medial to the olecranon and enters the cubital tunnel. The roof of the cubital tunnel is formed by the Osborne ligament. This is a thickened band between the humeral and ulnar head of the FCU. The medial collateral ligament of the elbow, elbow joint capsule, and olecranon make up the floor of the tunnel. Once through the cubital tunnel, the ulnar nerve travels deep to the humeral and ulnar heads of the FCU in the forearm. It goes through the FCU to the deep flexor-pronator aponeurosis distally. (*From* Lin PY, Sandeep SJ, Chung KC. In situ cubital tunnel decompression. In: Chung KC, editor. Operative techniques: hand and wrist surgery. vol. 2. Philadelphia: Elsevier Saunders; 2012; with permission.)

diabetes, are associated with a poor prognosis following surgery.[3,52] For patients with severe, chronic ulnar nerve compression, persistent dysesthesias and weakness are not uncommon, and complete recovery is unlikely, which should be discussed among surgeons and patients to ensure realistic patient expectations following release.[75] Therefore, discerning the best management for failed CuTR relies on appropriate diagnostic evaluation, patient counseling, careful operative approach, and discussion of the prognosis to address patient expectations. **Table 3** provides an overview of complications described following CuTR.

Nerve subluxation

Nerve subluxation is the most common cause of failed CuTR, reported in 2.4% to 20.0% of cases.[76–78] To prevent subluxation during an in situ release, the ulnar nerve should remain within its groove, and circumferential dissection should be avoided to prevent disruption of the surrounding areolar tissue and feeding blood vessels. Only the compressive fascial bands are released without neurolysis to avoid destabilizing the ulnar nerve. Following release, the elbow should be manipulated to check for subluxation, and anterior transposition should be performed if subluxation is noted.[13,69,76,78]

Treatment failure

Neuropathic symptoms in the distribution of the ulnar nerve occur in up to 30% of patients following CuTR, primarily due to inadequate release, most commonly at the medial intermuscular septum, or perineural fibrosis.[2,79,80] Pain radiating from the elbow scar to the small and ring fingers with numbness suggests recurrent compression, whereas patients who have persistent symptoms due to inadequate release do not experience any resolution in their symptoms.[81] In contrast, patients who may have recurrent symptoms due to perineural fibrosis may experience resolution of their symptoms initially, with symptom reappearance over time.

Iatrogenic injury

Iatrogenic injury to the medial antebrachial cutaneous (MABC) nerve has been reported as the leading cause of pain following CuTR (**Fig. 3**).[81] In a study examining intraoperative findings in revision CuTRs, nearly 73 of 100 cases had injury to the MABC nerve.[82] Pain in the scar associated with numbness in the posterior and medial elbow region is indicative of a neuroma of the MABC. Patients with a painful neuroma also experience radiating pain along the MABC territory with light tapping on the painful spot and experience pain relief and improvement in elbow function after a small injection of local anesthetic.[83] Initial management involves a 6-month trial of conservative measures with local massage, physiotherapy, and desensitization. If there is no significant

Table 3
Complications of cubital tunnel release (CuTR)

	Prevention Strategies	Treatment Options
Iatrogenic injury to medial antecubital cutaneous nerve	1. Knowledge of anatomy: 1.8 cm proximal to medial epicondyle and 3.1 cm distal to medial epicondyle (see **Fig. 2**) 2. Short 3–5-cm skin incisions	• Conservative management (massage, physiotherapy, desensitization) • Resection of neuroma • Nerve repair
Nerve subluxation	1. Secure ulnar nerve in its groove with subcutaneous tissue and feeding vessels 2. Check thoroughly intraoperatively by moving arm in various ways	• Revision CuTR (subcutaneous, intramuscular or submuscular transposition, or medial epicondylectomy)
Recurrent symptoms	1. Check for all possible sites of compression	• Revision CuTR (subcutaneous, intramuscular or submuscular transposition, or medial epicondylectomy) • Interposition grafts (vein wrapping)

improvement, the neuroma should be resected, and "cap" the ends of the nerve via electrocautery to prevent reformation of neuroma.[81–83] Microsurgical repair of the nerve also has been described,[78] although no studies have compared the effectiveness of repair versus resection.

Approach to revision cubital tunnel release

Failed release of the cubital tunnel is more frequent than carpal tunnel, and is also fraught with more challenges during revision surgery. Surgical options for failed CuTR include subcutaneous transposition, intramuscular transposition, submuscular transposition, and medial epicondylectomy. Secondary procedures largely depend on the technique that was used during the primary release (in situ release vs transposition). Similar to the approach for revision carpal tunnel, the elbow incision should be extended proximally and distally to maximize visualization of the nerve, while protecting the posterior branches of the MABC nerve. Exploration should include examination of MABC branches to rule out neuroma, and evaluation for any evidence of nerve subluxation. If the primary procedure was an in situ decompression, the ulnar nerve may be scarred, entrapped proximally (intermuscular septum) or distally (flexor carpi ulnaris), or subluxing over the medial epicondyle. The nerve should be released in an extended fashion, and external neurolysis is performed. Following external neurolysis, a transposition procedure should be performed. Currently,

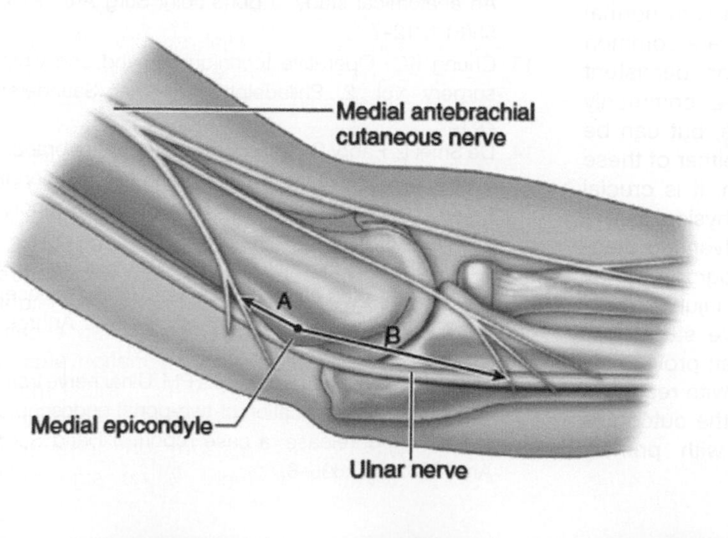

Fig. 3. Topography of the MABC nerve. The proximal crossing branch is found approximately 1.8 cm proximal to the medial epicondyle, and the distal crossing branch lies approximately 3.1 cm distal to the medial epicondyle. (*From* Lin PY, Sandeep SJ, Chung KC. In situ cubital tunnel decompression. In: Chung KC, editor. Operative techniques: hand and wrist surgery. vol. 2. Philadelphia: Elsevier Saunders; 2012; with permission.)

there are no comparative studies examining the effectiveness of transposition techniques (subcutaneous, intramuscular, submuscular) among patients with recurrent CuTS.[84] If the index procedure was a subcutaneous transposition, the nerve is usually found scarred along the medial epicondyle. After releasing the compression points, an intramuscular or submuscular transposition can be performed. Likewise, if a subcutaneous transposition was performed, the nerve should be dissected free before an intramuscular or submuscular transposition. Recently, there has been enthusiasm for creating a new soft tissue bed for the nerve by wrapping the ulnar nerve with vein or bioengineered synthetic devices to improve nerve gliding and minimize perineural fibrosis.[69] Although these adjuncts have shown encouraging results, comparative studies are not yet available.[85,86]

Outcomes

Compared with revision procedures for CTS, the outcomes following revision CuTR are much less predictable. The reasons for this are likely multifactorial. For example, ulnar nerve compression at the elbow often presents much later compared with other nerve compression conditions, and patients are more likely to have advanced, irreversible neuropathic changes. Furthermore, previous submuscular transposition, older age, and severe pain are poor prognostic indicators.[87] Although few patients experience complete relief, most patients report some improvement in symptoms following revision procedures.[88]

SUMMARY

Surgery for upper extremity compressive neuropathies is relatively common. To prevent iatrogenic injury, it is imperative for the surgeon to be aware of the structures associated with normal surgical anatomy and of those that are common variants. In addition, recurrent or persistent symptoms following a release are commonly associated with inadequate release, but can be associated with misdiagnosis. For either of these etiologies for failed decompression, it is crucial to perform a thorough history and physical examination with provocative testing. Advanced diagnostic testing, such as electromyography, may be helpful for comparison if nerve injury is suspected, especially if a preoperative study was conducted. Revision procedures can provide relief for many patients who present with recurrent or persistent symptoms, although the outcomes are less predictable compared with primary release.

REFERENCES

1. Neuhaus V, Christoforou D, Cheriyan T, et al. Evaluation and treatment of failed carpal tunnel release. Orthop Clin North Am 2012;43(4):439–47.
2. Dellon AL. Review of treatment results for ulnar nerve entrapment at the elbow. J Hand Surg Am 1989;14(4):688–700.
3. Mowlavi A, Andrews K, Lille S, et al. The management of cubital tunnel syndrome: a meta-analysis of clinical studies. Plast Reconstr Surg 2000;106(2):327–34.
4. Shiri R. The prevalence and incidence of carpal tunnel syndrome in US working populations. Scand J Work Environ Health 2014;40(1):101–2.
5. Tanaka S, Wild DK, Seligman PJ, et al. The US prevalence of self-reported carpal tunnel syndrome: 1988 National Health Interview Survey data. Am J Public Health 1994;84(11):1846–8.
6. Atroshi I, Gummesson C, Johnsson R, et al. Prevalence of carpal tunnel syndrome in a general population. JAMA 1999;282(2):153–8.
7. Leinberry CF, Rivlin M, Maltenfort M, et al. Treatment of carpal tunnel syndrome by members of the American Society for Surgery of the Hand: a 25-year perspective. J Hand Surg Am 2012;37(10):1997–2003.e3.
8. Lanz U. Anatomical variations of the median nerve in the carpal tunnel. J Hand Surg Am 1977;2(1):44–53.
9. Mitchell R, Chesney A, Seal S, et al. Anatomical variations of the carpal tunnel structures. Can J Plast Surg 2009;17(3):e3–7.
10. Hurwitz PJ. Variations in the course of the thenar motor branch of the median nerve. J Hand Surg Br 1996;21(3):344–6.
11. DaSilva MF, Moore DC, Weiss AP, et al. Anatomy of the palmar cutaneous branch of the median nerve: clinical significance. J Hand Surg Am 1996;21(4):639–43.
12. Taleisnik J. The palmar cutaneous branch of the median nerve and the approach to the carpal tunnel. An anatomical study. J Bone Joint Surg Am 1973;55(6):1212–7.
13. Chung KC. Operative techniques: hand and wrist surgery, vol. 2. Philadelphia: Elsevier Saunders; 2012.
14. De Smet L, Fabry G. Transection of the motor branch of the ulnar nerve as a complication of two-portal endoscopic carpal tunnel release: a case report. J Hand Surg Am 1995;20(1):18–9.
15. Luallin SR, Toby EB. Incidental Guyon's canal release during attempted endoscopic carpal tunnel release: an anatomical study and report of two cases. Arthroscopy 1993;9(4):382–6 [discussion: 381].
16. Nath RK, Mackinnon SE, Weeks PM. Ulnar nerve transection as a complication of two-portal endoscopic carpal tunnel release: a case report. J Hand Surg Am 1993;18(5):896–8.

17. Terrono AL, Belsky MR, Feldon PG, et al. Injury to the deep motor branch of the ulnar nerve during carpal tunnel release. J Hand Surg Am 1993;18(6):1038–40.
18. Boeckstyns ME, Sorensen AI. Does endoscopic carpal tunnel release have a higher rate of complications than open carpal tunnel release? An analysis of published series. J Hand Surg Br 1999;24(1):9–15.
19. Shinya K, Lanzetta M, Conolly WB. Risk and complications in endoscopic carpal tunnel release. J Hand Surg Br 1995;20(2):222–7.
20. Benson LS, Bare AA, Nagle DJ, et al. Complications of endoscopic and open carpal tunnel release. Arthroscopy 2006;22(9):919–24, 924.e1–2.
21. Michelotti B, Romanowsky D, Hauck RM. Prospective, randomized evaluation of endoscopic versus open carpal tunnel release in bilateral carpal tunnel syndrome: an interim analysis. Ann Plast Surg 2014; 73:S157–60.
22. Larsen MB, Sorensen AI, Crone KL, et al. Carpal tunnel release: a randomized comparison of three surgical methods. J Hand Surg Eur Vol 2013;38(6): 646–50.
23. Vasiliadis HS, Georgoulas P, Shrier I, et al. Endoscopic release for carpal tunnel syndrome. Cochrane Database Syst Rev 2014;(1):CD008265.
24. Leblanc MR, Lalonde DH, Thoma A, et al. Is main operating room sterility really necessary in carpal tunnel surgery? A multicenter prospective study of minor procedure room field sterility surgery. Hand (N Y) 2011;6(1):60–3.
25. Harness NG, Inacio MC, Pfeil FF, et al. Rate of infection after carpal tunnel release surgery and effect of antibiotic prophylaxis. J Hand Surg Am 2010;35(2):189–96.
26. Kim JK, Kim YK. Predictors of scar pain after open carpal tunnel release. J Hand Surg Am 2011;36(6): 1042–6.
27. da Costa VV, de Oliveira SB, Fernandes Mdo C, et al. Incidence of regional pain syndrome after carpal tunnel release. Is there a correlation with the anesthetic technique? Rev Bras Anestesiol 2011; 61(4):425–33.
28. Carroll I, Curtin CM. Management of chronic pain following nerve injuries/CRPS type II. Hand Clin 2013;29(3):401–8.
29. Netscher D, Dinh T, Cohen V, et al. Division of the transverse carpal ligament and flexor tendon excursion: open and endoscopic carpal tunnel release. Plast Reconstr Surg 1998;102(3):773–8.
30. Lee SK, Bae KW, Choy WS. The relationship of trigger finger and flexor tendon volar migration after carpal tunnel release. J Hand Surg Eur Vol 2014; 39(7):694–8.
31. Stahl S, Stahl S, Calif E. Latent pisotriquetral arthrosis unmasked following carpal tunnel release. Orthopedics 2010;33(9):673.
32. Cobb TK, Amadio PC. Reoperation for carpal tunnel syndrome. Hand Clin 1996;12(2):313–23.
33. Tung TH, Mackinnon SE. Secondary carpal tunnel surgery. Plast Reconstr Surg 2001;107(7):1830–43 [quiz: 1844, 1933].
34. Hulsizer DL, Staebler MP, Weiss AP, et al. The results of revision carpal tunnel release following previous open versus endoscopic surgery. J Hand Surg Am 1998;23(5):865–9.
35. Jones NF, Ahn HC, Eo S. Revision surgery for persistent and recurrent carpal tunnel syndrome and for failed carpal tunnel release. Plast Reconstr Surg 2012; 129(3):683–92.
36. Forman DL, Watson HK, Caulfield KA, et al. Persistent or recurrent carpal tunnel syndrome following prior endoscopic carpal tunnel release. J Hand Surg Am 1998;23(6):1010–4.
37. Atroshi I, Hofer M, Larsson GU, et al. Open compared with 2-portal endoscopic carpal tunnel release: a 5-year follow-up of a randomized controlled trial. J Hand Surg Am 2009;34(2):266–72.
38. Chen L, Duan X, Huang X, et al. Effectiveness and safety of endoscopic versus open carpal tunnel decompression. Arch Orthop Trauma Surg 2014; 134(4):585–93.
39. Zieske L, Ebersole GC, Davidge K, et al. Revision carpal tunnel surgery: a 10-year review of intraoperative findings and outcomes. J Hand Surg Am 2013; 38(8):1530–9.
40. Schreiber JE, Foran MP, Schreiber DJ, et al. Common risk factors seen in secondary carpal tunnel surgery. Ann Plast Surg 2005;55(3):262–5.
41. Fitzgibbons PG, Weiss AP. Hand manifestations of diabetes mellitus. J Hand Surg Am 2008;33(5): 771–5.
42. Emara MK, Saadah AM. The carpal tunnel syndrome in hypertensive patients treated with beta-blockers. Postgrad Med J 1988;64(749):191–2.
43. Braun RM, Rechnic M, Fowler E. Complications related to carpal tunnel release. Hand Clin 2002; 18(2):347–57.
44. Ranoux D, Attal N, Morain F, et al. Botulinum toxin type A induces direct analgesic effects in chronic neuropathic pain. Ann Neurol 2008;64(3):274–83.
45. Mazurek MT, Shin AY. Upper extremity peripheral nerve anatomy: current concepts and applications. Clin Orthop Relat Res 2001;(383):7–20.
46. Kwon HK, Pyun SB, Cho WY, et al. Carpal tunnel syndrome and peripheral polyneuropathy in patients with end stage kidney disease. J Korean Med Sci 2011;26(9):1227–30.
47. Stutz N, Gohritz A, van Schoonhoven J, et al. Revision surgery after carpal tunnel release–analysis of the pathology in 200 cases during a 2 year period. J Hand Surg Br 2006;31(1):68–71.
48. Mathoulin C, Bahm J, Roukoz S. Pedicled hypothenar fat flap for median nerve coverage in recalcitrant carpal tunnel syndrome. Hand Surg 2000; 5(1):33–40.

49. De Smet L. Recurrent carpal tunnel syndrome. Clinical testing indicating incomplete section of the flexor retinaculum. J Hand Surg Br 1993;18(2):189.
50. Beck JD, Brothers JG, Maloney PJ, et al. Predicting the outcome of revision carpal tunnel release. J Hand Surg Am 2012;37(2):282–7.
51. Edgell SE, McCabe SJ, Breidenbach WC, et al. Predicting the outcome of carpal tunnel release. J Hand Surg Am 2003;28(2):255–61.
52. Gellman H, Gelberman RH, Tan AM, et al. Carpal tunnel syndrome. An evaluation of the provocative diagnostic tests. J Bone Joint Surg Am 1986;68(5): 735–7.
53. Szabo RM, Slater RR Jr, Farver TB, et al. The value of diagnostic testing in carpal tunnel syndrome. J Hand Surg Am 1999;24(4):704–14.
54. Stutz NM, Gohritz A, Novotny A, et al. Clinical and electrophysiological comparison of different methods of soft tissue coverage of the median nerve in recurrent carpal tunnel syndrome. Neurosurgery 2008;62(3 Suppl 1):194–9 [discussion: 199–200].
55. Melvin JL, Johnson EW, Duran R. Electrodiagnosis after surgery for the carpal tunnel syndrome. Arch Phys Med Rehabil 1968;49(9):502–7.
56. Campagna R, Pessis E, Feydy A, et al. MRI assessment of recurrent carpal tunnel syndrome after open surgical release of the median nerve. AJR Am J Roentgenol 2009;193(3):644–50.
57. Wu HT, Schweitzer ME, Culp RW. Potential MR signs of recurrent carpal tunnel syndrome: initial experience. J Comput Assist Tomogr 2004;28(6):860–4.
58. Pastare D, Therimadasamy AK, Lee E, et al. Sonography versus nerve conduction studies in patients referred with a clinical diagnosis of carpal tunnel syndrome. J Clin Ultrasound 2009;37(7):389–93.
59. Mosier BA, Hughes TB. Recurrent carpal tunnel syndrome. Hand Clin 2013;29(3):427–34.
60. Amadio PC. Interventions for recurrent/persistent carpal tunnel syndrome after carpal tunnel release. J Hand Surg Am 2009;34(7):1320–2.
61. O'Malley MJ, Evanoff M, Terrono AL, et al. Factors that determine reexploration treatment of carpal tunnel syndrome. J Hand Surg Am 1992;17(4):638–41.
62. Dellon AL, Chang BW. An alternative incision for approaching recurrent median nerve compression at the wrist. Plast Reconstr Surg 1992; 89(3):576–8.
63. Green DP, Wolfe SW. Green's operative hand surgery. 6th edition. Philadelphia: Elsevier/Churchill Livingstone; 2011. Available at: http://proxy.lib.umich.edu/login?url=https://www.clinicalkey.com/dura/browse/bookChapter/3-s2.0-C20091589800.
64. Abzug JM, Jacoby SM, Osterman AL. Surgical options for recalcitrant carpal tunnel syndrome with perineural fibrosis. Hand (N Y) 2012;7(1):23–9.
65. Strickland JW, Idler RS, Lourie GM, et al. The hypothenar fat pad flap for management of recalcitrant carpal tunnel syndrome. J Hand Surg Am 1996; 21(5):840–8.
66. Soltani AM, Allan BJ, Best MJ, et al. A systematic review of the literature on the outcomes of treatment for recurrent and persistent carpal tunnel syndrome. Plast Reconstr Surg 2013;132(1):114–21.
67. Chou KH, Papadimitriou NG, Sarris I, et al. Neovascularization and other histopathologic findings in an autogenous saphenous vein wrap used for recalcitrant carpal tunnel syndrome: a case report. J Hand Surg Am 2003;28(2):262–6.
68. Fowler JR. Endoscopic cubital tunnel release. J Hand Surg Am 2014;39(10):2064–6.
69. Palmer BA, Hughes TB. Cubital tunnel syndrome. J Hand Surg Am 2010;35(1):153–63.
70. Zlowodzki M, Chan S, Bhandari M, et al. Anterior transposition compared with simple decompression for treatment of cubital tunnel syndrome. A meta-analysis of randomized, controlled trials. J Bone Joint Surg Am 2007;89(12):2591–8.
71. Tsai TM, Bonczar M, Tsuruta T, et al. A new operative technique: cubital tunnel decompression with endoscopic assistance. Hand Clin 1995; 11(1):71–80.
72. Cobb TK, Walden AL, Merrell PT, et al. Setting expectations following endoscopic cubital tunnel release. Hand (N Y) 2014;9(3):356–63.
73. Cobb TK, Sterbank PT, Lemke JH. Endoscopic cubital tunnel recurrence rates. Hand (N Y) 2010; 5(2):179–83.
74. Hoffmann R, Siemionow M. The endoscopic management of cubital tunnel syndrome. J Hand Surg Br 2006;31(1):23–9.
75. Ruchelsman DE, Lee SK, Posner MA. Failed surgery for ulnar nerve compression at the elbow. Hand Clin 2007;23(3):359–71, vi–vii.
76. Bartels RH, Menovsky T, Van Overbeeke JJ, et al. Surgical management of ulnar nerve compression at the elbow: an analysis of the literature. J Neurosurg 1998;89(5):722–7.
77. LeRoux PD, Ensign TD, Burchiel KJ. Surgical decompression without transposition for ulnar neuropathy: factors determining outcome. Neurosurgery 1990;27(5):709–14 [discussion: 714].
78. Nellans K, Tang P. Evaluation and treatment of failed ulnar nerve release at the elbow. Orthop Clin North Am 2012;43(4):487–94.
79. Holzner B, Kemmler G, Kopp M, et al. Preoperative expectations and postoperative quality of life in liver transplant survivors. Arch Phys Med Rehabil 2001; 82(1):73–9.
80. Hambleton RK, Swaminathan H, Rogers HJ. Fundamentals of item response theory. Newbury Park (CA): SAGE Publications, Inc; 1991.
81. Dellon AL, MacKinnon SE. Injury to the medial antebrachial cutaneous nerve during cubital tunnel surgery. J Hand Surg Br 1985;10(1):33–6.

82. Mackinnon SE, Novak CB. Operative findings in reoperation of patients with cubital tunnel syndrome. Hand (N Y) 2007;2(3):137–43.
83. Stahl S, Rosenberg N. Surgical treatment of painful neuroma in medial antebrachial cutaneous nerve. Ann Plast Surg 2002;48(2):154–8 [discussion: 158–60].
84. Ehsan A, Hanel DP. Recurrent or persistent cubital tunnel syndrome. J Hand Surg Am 2012;37(9): 1910–2.
85. Varitimidis SE, Vardakas DG, Goebel F, et al. Treatment of recurrent compressive neuropathy of peripheral nerves in the upper extremity with an autologous vein insulator. J Hand Surg Am 2001; 26(2):296–302.
86. Puckett BN, Gaston RG, Lourie GM. A novel technique for the treatment of recurrent cubital tunnel syndrome: ulnar nerve wrapping with a tissue engineered bioscaffold. J Hand Surg Eur Vol 2011; 36(2):130–4.
87. Gabel GT, Amadio PC. Reoperation for failed decompression of the ulnar nerve in the region of the elbow. J Bone Joint Surg Am 1990;72(2):213–9.
88. Aleem AW, Krogue JD, Calfee RP. Outcomes of revision surgery for cubital tunnel syndrome. J Hand Surg Am 2014;39(11):2141–9.

Management and Complications of Traumatic Peripheral Nerve Injuries

Matthew T. Houdek, MD, Alexander Y. Shin, MD*

KEYWORDS

• Nerve transection • Nerve repair • Traumatic nerve injury • Nerve and tendon transfers

KEY POINTS

- Peripheral nerve injuries can dramatically affect a patient's life.
- A detailed physical examination and ultrasound of nerve is recommended to assess for continuity of nerve in the early setting.
- If transection is found, early surgical repair is recommended. If nerve is in continuity, electromyography and clinical examination at 6 weeks after the injury is recommended.
- Autograft remains the standard for treatment of nerve defects.
- Tendon and transfers can improve patient function in the setting of irreparable nerve injuries and as an adjuvant to nerve repair.

INTRODUCTION

Occurring in up to 3% of all patients admitted to Level I trauma centers, traumatic injuries to peripheral nerves are devastating life-altering injuries that can lead to significant patient morbidity.[1,2] Typically seen in young adult men, these injuries occur after a variety of traumatic events, including penetrating trauma, crush injuries, traction events, and ischemia.[3] A great majority of injuries to peripheral nerves occur in the upper extremity, most commonly the radial, ulnar, and median nerves.[1,2,4,5] Although not as common as upper extremity injuries, lower extremity nerve injuries are typically associated with certain injuries, such as acetabular fractures and dislocations of the hip and knee that frequently affect the sciatic, femoral, and peroneal nerves.[1,5]

The management of traumatic peripheral nerve injuries is influenced by several factors, including type and severity of the injury, location of the injury, and timing from injury to presentation, as well as patient pain and function. This article reviews the types of peripheral nerve injuries, with a focus on the evaluation of a patient with a traumatic nerve injury, and the various treatment options and outcomes.

NERVE ANATOMY AND RESPONSE TO INJURY

Peripheral nerves are encased in a layer called the epineurium, which protects and nourishes the individual nerve fascicles. The epineurium surrounds the fascicles and runs between the fascicular groups. The major blood supply to the nerves lies on the outer surface of the epineurium and also in the inner epineurial layer. Within the inner epineurium, the individual fascicles are surrounded by a layer of connective tissue called the perineurium, which provides tensile strength

Conflicts of Interest: No conflicts of interest are declared by any author on this study.
Source of Funding: No funding was received for this work from the NIH, Wellcome Trust, or HHMI.
Division of Hand and Microvascular Surgery, Department of Orthopedic Surgery, Mayo Clinic, 200 First Street Southwest, Rochester, MN 55905, USA
* Corresponding author.
E-mail address: shin.alexander@mayo.edu

Hand Clin 31 (2015) 151–163
http://dx.doi.org/10.1016/j.hcl.2015.01.007
0749-0712/15/$ – see front matter

to the nerves. Inside the fascicles is a loose connective tissue matrix known as the endoneurium that protects and nourishes the individual axons (**Fig. 1**). In the endoneurium, there is a capillary network from the epineurial vasculature that acts an extension of the blood-brain barrier.

Following transection of the nerve, the cell body swells, releases Nissl granules, and the nucleus is dispersed to the periphery of the cell, switching the metabolic activity to regeneration. Forty-eight hours following nerve transection, Wallerian degeneration occurs, with breakdown of the axon distal to the level of transection (**Fig. 2**). Schwann cells proliferate and break down myelin and debris from the axons. Schwann cells also begin the reparative process by aligning longitudinally. This forms Büngner bands, providing a scaffold for the axon to regenerate. At the distal end of these bands is the growth cone, which is the regenerative fascicle. The regenerative fascicle attempts to join with the distal transected segment to complete regeneration. When the perineurium is damaged, the regenerative nerve fascicles can escape their normal regenerative process.[6] This leads to a proliferation of fibroblasts and Schwann cells in a disorganized fashion, leading to a neuroma formation.[6] Similarly, pressure to the nerve can lead to epineurial damage, fascicular escape, and neuroma formation.[7]

CLASSIFICATION OF PERIPHERAL NERVE INJURY

The Seddon and Sunderland classifications (**Table 1**) are typically used to define these injuries

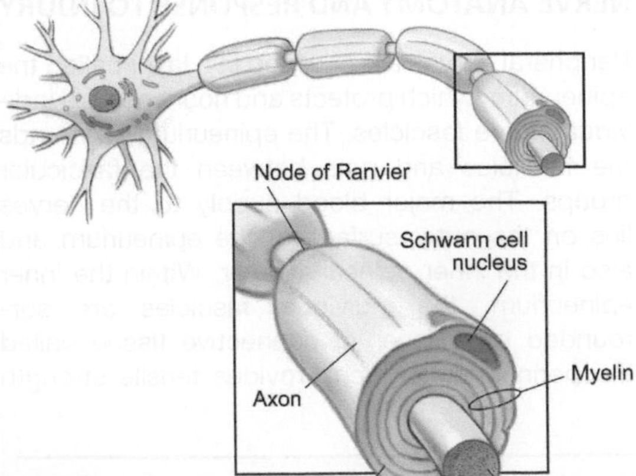

Fig. 1. Myelinated axons are surrounded by Schwann cells to form a protective layer of myelin. Individual nerve fibers are encased in the individual axons. (*Copyright* Mayo Foundation for Medical Education and Research; with permission.)

and are based on the response of injury.[8,9] The Seddon[8] classification is based on the ability of the nerve to transmit nerve signal and the architecture of the nerve. Sunderland[9] expanded on this classification to further divide axonotmesis based on the continuity of the endoneurium, perineurium, and epineurium. This is an important consideration because when the endoneurium is disrupted the scaffold of peripheral nerve created by Schwann cells becomes deformed, inhibiting successful nerve regeneration.[9] In a second-degree injury, the endoneurium is maintained and axons are able to regenerate along the course of the nerve. In an injury of the third, fourth, or fifth degree, damage to the endoneurium leads to destruction of the neurons and neuroma formation. Because traumatic injuries are typically combined injuries, Boyd and colleagues[10] added a sixth-degree to the Sunderland classification for mixed injuries.

CLINICAL EXAMINATION OF PATIENTS WITH SUSPECTED PERIPHERAL NERVE INJURY

The cornerstone for evaluating patients with a peripheral nerve injury is the history and physical examination, with grading of individual muscle groups based on levels of innervations undertaken and graded based on British Medical Research Council (**Table 2**).[11] A detailed, recorded, serial, and systematic examination by the same examiner is required to determine if there are any subtle changes in function. Localization of a Tinel sign over the site of nerve injury is an important feature. In a first-degree injury there is no Tinel sign. Second-degree injuries are associated with muscle atrophy and a Tinel sign will move distally at a rate of an inch per month, indicating the advancement of axonal growth. Third-degree injuries will atrophy and have a Tinel sign that migrates distally; however, it is slower than an inch per month. In fourth-degree and fifth-degree injuries, there is rapid and severe atrophy and a Tinel sign that does not move distally.

Radiographic imaging of peripheral nerve injuries is performed with MRI or ultrasound.[12–14] MRI can be used to examine peripheral nerves that are not accessible by ultrasound and provides valuable information concerning muscle atrophy, presence of tumors, and it characterizes surrounding soft-tissue structures.[12] Owing to its low cost, speed of examination, and ability to image the nerve in continuity, ultrasound is considered the imaging modality of choice for peripheral nerve injuries.[12–14] Ultrasound is valuable in the care of traumatic nerve injuries, especially acute injuries, when diagnosing nerve continuity. The use of ultrasound has changed the course of management

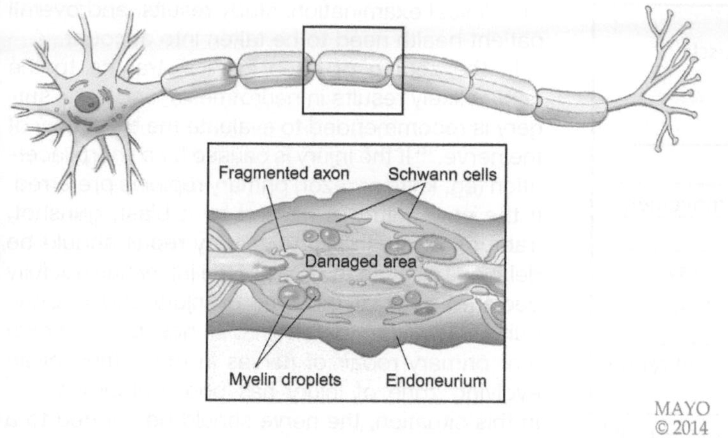

Fig. 2. Following nerve injury, the reparative process is signaled by the Schwann cells in response to fragmentation of the axon and wallerian degeneration. (*Copyright* Mayo Foundation for Medical Education and Research; with permission.)

in more than 50% of patients by showing a nerve in either continuity or discontinuity (**Fig. 3**).[13,14]

Electrodiagnostic tests such as electromyography (EMG) and nerve conduction study (NCS) are helpful in diagnosing the location, estimating the severity, and predicting the recovery of the nerve injury. NCS can be used immediately to localize an injury; however, an EMG is typically withheld until 3 to 6 weeks following injury because no degenerative change will occur during this period. Following the 3-week to 6-week mark, a baseline EMG should be obtained, followed by sequential EMGs (6–12-week intervals) to document any recovery of the involved nerve. EMG can detect evidence of reinnervation weeks to months before the physical examination. Motor unit potentials (MUPs) are action potentials recorded from the motor units innervated by a single anterior horn cell and are identified on EMG. When the nerve is damaged they are disrupted. At the early signs of reinnervation, unstable MUPs are frequently observed with various patterns and amplitudes and increased MUP duration. When the nerve has healed, the MUP will return to a preinjury appearance with a prolonged duration. The EMG can be helpful in planning time for surgery based on the rate of nerve growth and the distance from the injury to the most critical site of reinnervation. Because a nerve grows approximately 1 mm per day or an inch per month, the surgeon can use this information to estimate the time it will take for the nerve to regenerate.[15]

TYPES AND TIMING OF REPAIR OF TRAUMATIC NERVE INJURIES

The type of nerve injury is critical in determining the need for urgent surgical exploration versus observation. The simplest classification is whether the injury is open or closed, and whether the overlying soft tissue is intact. Closed injuries are typically characterized by nerves in continuity and associated with neurapraxia or axonotmesis.[15] With these injuries, a spontaneous recovery is

Table 1
Classification of peripheral nerve injuries

Sunderland Classification	Seddon Classification	Process	Recovery
First-degree	Neurapraxia	Segmental demyelination	Full
Second-degree	Axonotmesis	Axon severed, intact endoneurium	Full
Third-degree	—	Axon severed, endoneurium not intact, perineurium-fascial arrangement preserved	Variable
Fourth-degree	—	Axon, endoneurium, perineurium-fascicle discontinuity, epineurium intact	None
Fifth-degree	Neurotmesis	Discontinuity of entire nerve	None
Sixth-degree	—	Mixed	Unpredictable

Adapted from Seddon H. Three types of nerve injuries. Brain 1943;66:237–88; and Sunderland S, editor. Nerve injuries and their repair: a critical appraisal. New York: Churchill Livingstone; 1991.

Table 2
British Medical Research Council muscle grading

Grade	Muscle Function
0	No motor function
1	Muscle fasciculation but no movement
2	Gravity-eliminated motion
3	Full range of motion against gravity
4	Motion against resistance through a range of motion
5	Normal muscle power with a full range of motion

From O'Brien M. Aids to the examination of the peripheral nervous system. Philadelphia: W.B. Saunders; 2000; with permission.

possible and observation for 6 weeks is recommended. If there is no recovery by 6 weeks, an EMG and ultrasound should be obtained for a baseline evaluation. If the nerve is transected, surgical exploration should be undertaken. If the nerve is in continuity and at 12 weeks after injury there is no recovery, the patient should have a repeat EMG. If there are electrical signs of reinnervation by the presence of MUPs, spontaneous reinnervation of the muscle should be expected. If there is no evidence of reinnervation 3-6 months from the injury, the nerve should be explored surgically. In the setting of a stretch injury, there is the potential for a lengthy injury, resulting in patients typically followed for up to 5 to 6 months before surgical exploration. Unfortunately, the decision to operate is not as straight forward as surgeons would like. All factors related to the injury, the clinical examination, study results, and overall patient health need to be taken into account.

In the setting of open injuries, trauma to the nerves likely results in neurotmesis, and early surgery is recommended to evaluate the continuity of the nerve.[15] If the injury is caused by a sharp laceration (eg, knife or razor) primary repair is preferred. If the open injury is caused by a blast, gunshot, fracture, or crush injury, primary repair should be delayed because the zone of the injury has not fully declared itself at the time of injury and is often quite difficult to determine. It has been shown that primary repair of nerves in the setting of an evolving zone of injury has poor outcomes.[16,17] In this situation, the nerve should be sutured to a local structure, such as a tendon or fascia, to prevent retraction and facilitate repair at a later time. It is important to delay treatment of these injuries because of the inflammatory nature of the surrounding tissue and nerve, as well as to allow neuroma formation so the scarred nerve can be resected back to healthy nerve tissue at the time of repair. Evolving nerve deficits are another indication for early surgical exploration. Typically, these are caused by blunt injury and associated with entrapment of a nerve from swelling, such as the median nerve at the wrist.

PRINCIPLES AND INTRAOPERATIVE CONSIDERATIONS OF NERVE REPAIR

Nerve repair has improved significantly with microsurgical techniques and an operating microscope should be used for nerve repair whenever possible. With the use of an operative microscope, it is possible to perform group fascicular repair

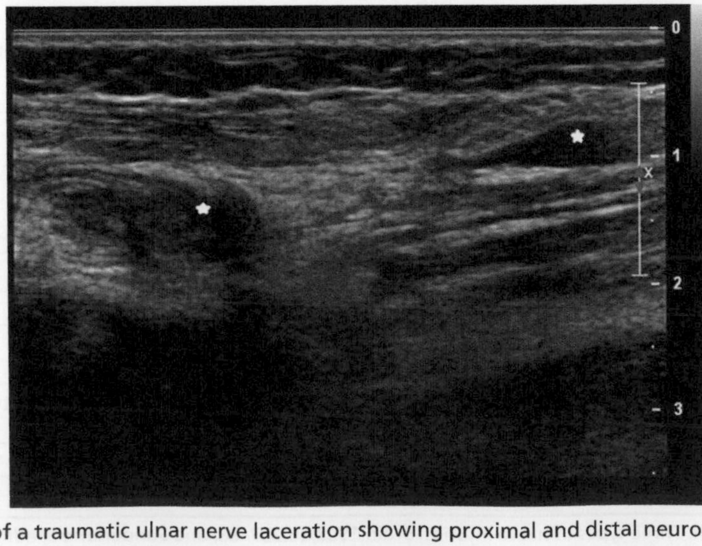

Fig. 3. Ultrasound of a traumatic ulnar nerve laceration showing proximal and distal neuromas (*stars*) along with a 14 mm nerve gap.

over an epineurial repair. In the setting of a traumatic injury this can be difficult and prospective studies have shown no difference in outcomes of epineurial versus fascicular repair for most peripheral nerves.[18–20] Similarly, it is often difficult to distinguish between motor and sensory nerve fascicles. However, in the distal forearm, repair of an ulnar nerve injury is based on the fascicular motor and sensory grouping.[21] The internal topography of the distal ulnar nerve has been extensively studied, with the sensory group of fascicles found on the radial side of ulnar nerve. Just ulnar to the sensory nerve lies the smaller deep motor branch of the ulnar nerve. When performing a repair of the ulnar nerve, the authors recommend finding the cleavage plane between the fascicles at the level of the wrist. At this level the motor group is located at a dorsoulnar position. This can be traced proximally to allow appropriate fascicular repair.

Repairs should be performed under a microscope or high-power loupe magnification using an 8-0 or 9-0 monofilament suture. Cadaveric studies have shown 9-0 nylon sutures prevented the most gapping, versus a 10-0 monofilament suture, and did not typically fail under tension or pull out of the repaired nerve ending.[22] Fibrin glue can be used to enhance the strength of the repair site. Fibrin glue (**Fig. 4**) has been shown to improve the resistance to gapping at the repair site and theoretically provides a barrier to scar formation.[23–26] The nerve ends should be transected sharply to create a clean end (see **Fig. 4**), after which a tension-free nerve repair is done. Tension at the repair site has been shown to be detrimental to the repair by causing gapping of the repair site, connective tissue proliferation, scar formation, and ischemia.[27] The involved extremity should be put through a range of motions to make sure there is not significant tension at the repair site at different functional positions.

Important Considerations of Primary Repair

When performing a primary repair of a transection or following removal of a neuroma-in-continuity (NIC) it is important that the repair site has very little to no tension. To ensure a tension-free repair, the authors recommend transposition and proximal or distal dissection of the nerve. This will provide additional nerve length. Under no circumstances should a repair be performed under tension. If there is not enough nerve excursion to perform a primary repair, the authors would manage the gap with an autograft (see later discussion).

MANAGEMENT OF NERVE GAPS

Nerve gaps occur following transection of a nerve or following the removal of an NIC.[28] If there is no significant tension at the repair site, a nerve gap can be overcome through primary repair of the nerve. For repairs without significant tension, an end-to-end repair is desired, allowing the regenerating to only cross 1 site of repair as opposed to 2, as would be the case with a graft. If there is tension at the repair site, or for an NIC that does not transmit nerve action potentials (NAPs), nerve grafting is indicated. Nerve grafting is undertaken using a

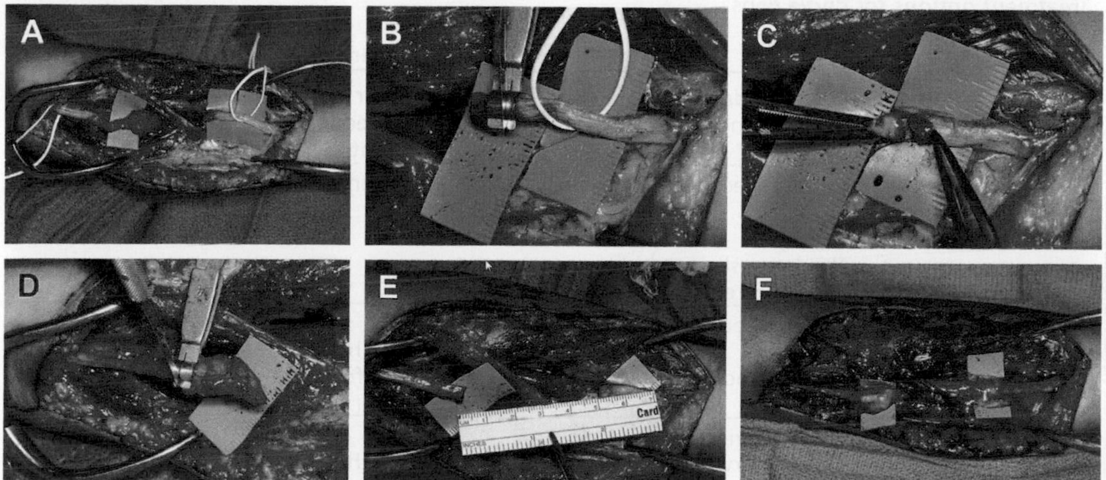

Fig. 4. Intraoperative proximal and distal neuroma, along with a substantial nerve gap in the ulnar nerve following a traumatic transection (*A*). To prepare the nerve ends for grafting, a nerve cutting device was used to resect the neuromas (*B, D*) back to the level of individual fascicle bundles (*C*). Following neuroma transection, a 6 cm nerve graft was left (*E*). This was repaired using an autologous sural nerve graft and the repair site was supplemented with fibrin glue (*F*).

variety of graft material, including autograft, allograft, and conduits (**Table 3**).

Autograft

Autograft remains the standard for grafting of peripheral nerve injuries (see **Fig. 4**). Autograft is preferred because it contains host Schwann cells, provides neurotrophic growth factors, and lacks immunogenicity.[29] For a graft to survive, it must be revascularized. Therefore, cutaneous nerves that are thin are the donors of choice for autograft material. The autograft should be placed in a well-vascularized tissue bed and should be created 10% to 20% longer than the defect site to avoid tension at the repair site and to account for any scarring that will occur at the repair site. The sural nerve is considered the workhorse autograft material, providing up to 40 cm of graft material. Other graft options include the lateral and anterior medial antebrachial cutaneous nerves, and the superficial radial nerve. Autograft harvest does have some drawbacks, including a second scar, sensory loss, neuroma formation, and inferior results compared with a tension-free repair. To accommodate for diameter differences, the sural nerve can be cut into appropriate length segments and used as cables to fit the recipient nerve (see **Fig. 4**).

Although sensory nerves make up most of the available nerve autografts, there is consideration for modality-specific regeneration (MSR).[30–32] This is based on the idea that, when given the choice, motor axons prefer to regenerate down motor grafts as opposed to sensory grafts, and vice versa.[31–33] However, in a large animal study, there was no difference in nerve regeneration when performing MSR versus mixing motor and sensory grafts.[34] At this time, the authors do not think there is enough clinical information for performing MSR instead of the traditional sensory autograft.

Allograft

Allografts are of particular interest to treat a traumatic nerve gap or following resection of an NIC. There is the potential for an abundant supply of nerve graft material, they can be banked for future use, and there is no need to sacrifice a donor nerve. The major drawback of allografts is the need for immunosuppression.[35] Immunosuppression is needed because nerve regeneration in allografts requires viable Schwann cells to support remyelination. The donor Schwann cells are immunogenic to the host, so immunosuppression is needed for 24 months after transplant. Tacrolimus is a commonly used agent for immunosuppression and has been shown to modulate nerve regeneration.[36–39] Mackinnon and colleagues[36] have shown pretreatment of nerve allografts with tacrolimus or cold preserving (4–5° C for 7 days) the allografts, will lead to reliable clinical outcomes similar to autograft when used for the treatment of nerve gaps.

Table 3
Treatment options for nerve gaps

Material	Advantages	Disadvantages
Nerve Autograft	• Gold standard • Nonimmunogenic	• Donor site morbidity • Limited length • Potential neuroma
Tissue Allograft	• Potential equivalent recovery to autograft • Supply • No donor site morbidity • Schwann cells	• Immunosuppression
Acellular Allograft	• Potential equivalent recovery to autograft • No immunosuppression	• Cost • No Schwann cells • Only for small diameter nerves • Motor reconstruction results unknown
Conduits	• Nonimmunogenic • Guides nerve growth • Can prevent fibrosis at site of repair	• Cost • No Schwann cells or nerve matrix • Only used for small sensory nerves
Nerve Transfers	• Early motor and sensation	• Donor site morbidity • Need for motor reeducation
Tendon Transfers	• Restores motor function	• Donor site morbidity • No sensation

To circumvent the need for immunosuppression, processed acellular allografts can be used to bridge these gaps.[40,41] The use of detergents removes the donor Schwann cells, while leaving the extracellular matrix for nerve regeneration. Decellularized allografts have shown promise in the setting of traumatic injury and following resection of an NIC in digital sensory nerves by providing adequate sensation to the digit, with a reported 2-point discrimination of 4 to 6 mm.[42,43] However, use of decellularized allografts in motor nerve reconstruction should be used guardedly because animal studies have not demonstrated favorable results in motor nerve reconstruction[44] and current clinical studies are flawed owing to their retrospective natures.[45,46]

Nerve Conduits

Various types of autologous and synthetic nerve conduits have been used to provide a framework for nerve regeneration to occur in nerve gaps less than 3 cm.[29,41,47–50] Although they have minimal donor morbidity, conduits are currently limited in their use for nerve gaps.[51] Weber and colleagues,[49] as well as Agnew and Dumanian,[50] have shown promising results with the use of conduits for sensory nerve gaps. Animal models have also shown that wrapping sites of nerve repairs with conduits reduces scar formation.[52,53] The limitations to conduits are related to their cost, lack of Schwann cells, and neurotrophic factors that are critical to nerve regeneration. Animal models examining the use of conduits in motor nerves have not shown promising results with 3-cm defects.[51,54]

Nerve Transfers

When there is a long segment of injured nerve, the distance to the target muscle may be too long for regeneration after nerve repair before permanent muscle damage occurs. In this situation, nerve transfer can be performed (**Table 4**). The principle for nerve transfers for peripheral nerve injuries is to convert a proximal injury into a distal injury by transferring a nerve close to the site of denervation.[55,56] Transfers provide the advantages of potentially restoring both sensory and motor function, reinnervation of multiple muscle groups, operating outside the zone of traumatic injury, and decreasing the time to reinnervation.[56] The use of nerve transfers for restoration of distal function in the upper and lower extremity has shown promising results, with patients typically reaching Grade III muscle strength.[55,57–65] In addition to motor function, sensory nerve transfers are also possible to restore sensation to the fingers.[56,59]

Important Considerations of Nerve Gap Management

When performing a repair of a nerve gap, it is possible to encounter a situation in which there is not enough graft material. In this situation, the authors recommend transposition and dissection of the proximal and distal nerve stumps to obtain the maximal excursion of the nerve endings. Care should be taken to avoid stretching the graft because this would cause undue tension at the repair sites. If possible, the authors harvest additional autograft and recommend replacing the initial autograft altogether. It is important to avoid

Table 4
Nerve transfers for traumatic peripheral nerve injuries

Injured Nerve	Functional Deficit	Donor Nerve	Recipient Nerve
Ulnar	Hand intrinsic	Terminal AIN to PQ PIN to ECU/EDM	Deep ulnar motor branch
Median	Thumb opposition Finger flexion	Terminal AIN to PQ Ulnar to FCU MC to brachialis	Recurrent median AIN
	Pronation	PIN to ECRB Ulnar to FCU Median to FDS	Pronator quadratus branch of median
Radial	Wrist extension Finger extension	Median to FCR Median to FDS	ECRB branch of PIN PIN
Femoral	Knee extension	Anterior obturator Superior gluteal to TFL	Rectus femoris branch of femoral Vastus medialis branch of femoral
Peroneal	Ankle dorsiflexion	Tibial	Deep motor branch of peroneal

Abbreviations: AIN, anterior interosseous nerve; ECRB, extensor carpi radialis brevis; ECU, extensor carpi ulnaris; EDM, extensor digiti minimi; FCR, flexor carpi radialis; FCU, flexor carpi ulnaris; FDS, flexor digitorum superficialis; MC, musculocutaneous; PIN, posterior interosseous nerve; PQ, pronator quadratus; TFL, tensor fasciae latae.

using an interposition graft (autograft, allograft, or conduit) between the initial graft and the proximal and/or distal nerve endings. Other sites of potential autograft include sural nerve, intercostal nerve, lateral and anterior medial antebrachial cutaneous nerves, and the superficial radial nerve. Currently, the authors recommend against using a nerve conduit for large (>3 cm) nerve gaps and against the use of allograft, even in this setting.

OUTCOMES OF TRAUMATIC NERVE REPAIR

The outcomes of nerve repair following a traumatic injury are commonly affected by factors outside of the control of surgeon. The age of the patient, location of the injury, and the timing of presentation after injury all have a significant effect on the outcome.[9,66,67] Sunderland[9] reported on the results of his 40 years of nerve repair and showed younger patients, early repair, single functional repair, distal repairs, and short nerve grafts were all associated with improved patient outcomes. For primary repair of nerves in the upper extremity, the results are typically favorable, with most patients recovering at least Grade III muscle strength and sensory recovery, with ulnar nerve injuries typically fairing worse than radial or median nerve injuries.[68–77]

In the lower extremity, factors affecting the results for nerve repair and grafting are similar to those in the upper extremity, with a shorter time after injury to repair and distal repair sites associated with favorable outcomes.[78–82] It has been shown that traumatic peroneal nerve injuries treated with either repair or grafting fare worse than tibial nerve injuries.[78–83] It is thought that the worse outcomes observed in the peroneal nerve are related to its lateral location, making the nerve more prone to severe injury. Similarly, the tibial nerve is more elastic, has a better vascular supply and regenerative potential, and innervates fewer muscle groups than the peroneal nerve.[84]

MANAGEMENT OF COMPLICATIONS OF PERIPHERAL NERVE INJURY

Neuroma-in-Continuity

Occurring after Sunderland third-degree and fourth-degree injuries, an NIC represents the body's attempt at repair. Typically, an NIC follows a blunt injury and can be followed clinically and electrically for 8 to 12 weeks. An EMG is extremely useful in this setting and, if at the EMG, action potential is able to transverse an NIC at 12 weeks, the potential for spontaneous recovery is high. On the other hand, if there is no signal across the NIC, there is a need for exploration of the neuroma, followed by repair or grafting.

Once the decision to explore the NIC is made, it is surgically important to gain exposure of the neuroma well proximal and distal. This allows for 360° visualization of the nerve and helps with dissection of the lesion off adherent structures. Beginning at either the proximal or distal end of the nerve, dissection of the nerve from any adherent is performed sharply through the mesoneurium, taking care to minimize handling of the nerve. Once the NIC is exposed, we perform an external neurolysis in a circumferential manner both proximal and distal to the level of injury, releasing any sites of entrapment. Following the neurolysis, it is important to document intraoperative NAPs.

NAPs provide valuable information about nerve function and determine if a nerve can be treated with neurolysis alone or if nerve grafting will be needed. NAPs beyond the site of injury indicate preserved function or regeneration of the axons, indicating the potential for clinical recovery. The absence of NAPs beyond the site of injury is a poor indicator for nerve recovery and regeneration.[85,86] The presence or absence of NAPs around an NIC are important to determine if there are any functional axons in the neuroma to provide motor function distal to the site of injury.[87] If NAPs are present, an internal neurolysis can be used to identify the intact motor fibers proximal and distal, which allows removal of the damaged segment of nerves and repair of the injured segments with split fascicular grafting.

If the NAPs do not transverse the neuroma, the authors recommend excising the neuroma. It is important to trim the nerve endings to a level at which the fascicular detail is clearly apparent. We would then free the proximal and distal stumps from surrounding soft tissues and transpose the stumps, if needed, to obtain maximal excursion of the ends. If possible, we attempt a primary nerve repair. However, if there is undue tension at the site, use of sural nerve autograft is recommended to repair the gap. In our practice, we supplement the repair sites with a conduit sleeve and fibrin glue. We believe this reduces scar formation and strengthens the repair site.

Pain Associated with Traumatic Nerve Injury

Pain following traumatic nerve injuries can be debilitating. Following a traumatic event there are 2 types of pain syndromes: complex regional pain syndrome (CRPS) and neuritic pain.[15,88] There are 2 types of CRPS. Type I is more common and usually due to soft-tissue injury and not associated with a nerve injury. Type II occurs where there is a discernable nerve lesion. CRPS is characterized by pain and limited range of motion, along with autonomic manifestations, including swelling, vasomotor changes, skin changes, and bone demineralization. Neuritic pain, on the other hand, is associated with nerve injury and is a deep, constant, pulsating pain.

The treatment of nerve pain is multimodal. Typically, sympathetic and stellate ganglion blocks are used to treat CRPS. However, if these do not relieve the pain, sympathetectomy may be the only way to treat the pain. Studies have shown that vitamin C given after a distal radius fracture or ankle fracture can help prevent the development of CRPS.[89–93] For neuritic pain, early mobilization of the limb and transcutaneous electrical neurostimulation has been shown to help. Unlike CPRS, neuritic pain can be eased with surgical neurolysis; however, the risk of further loss of function is a complication following neurolysis.

At the authors' institution, CRPS is treated by a multimodal team to manage patients' symptoms as early as possible. When a diagnosis of CRPS is suspected, we have patients evaluated by physical therapy and pain management to assist with range of motion, mobilization, and pharmacologic intervention. If, however, patients are debilitated by CRPS, we will perform a nerve block or epidural to allow the patient to begin aggressive physical therapy.

OPTIONS IF NERVE REPAIR OR GRAFTING FAIL

Revising the Nerve Transfer or Nerve Graft

Revising the nerve transfer or nerve graft is often a very difficult decision. It should be made after sufficient time has lapsed to call the index nerve surgery a failure, yet before there is an irreversible denervation of muscle. If the nerve graft or transfer is for sensory nerves, revision can be considered years after index procedure. However, if it is a motor reconstruction, 9 to 12 months after injury is about the latest a revision nerve procedure should be considered.

Tendon Transfers

Tendon transfers are indicated if a patient presents with signs of severe distal muscle atrophy, when functional recovery does not occur after nerve repair or grafting, or to supplement function after nerve repair. Early tendon transfer can assist a nerve repair by providing an internal "splint" by substituting for the paralyzed muscle groups.[94,95] In the traumatic setting, tendon transfers in the upper extremity are typically used to restore thumb, finger flexion or extension, and wrist extension (**Table 5**). In the lower extremity, tendon transfers are used to prevent knee buckling, prevent patellar subluxation, and restore ankle extension and flexion.[96–99] A typical patient will improve following tendon transfer. A thorough discussion with the patient on the timing of tendon transfers is necessary. Early tendon transfers can restore function earlier than waiting for a nerve to regenerate but may not result in normal function. Late tendon transfers can restore some function but time lost in waiting for the nerve to recover may be unacceptable for some patients.

Table 5
Tendon transfers for traumatic nerve injuries

Nerve	Function	Tendon Transfer
Radial	Wrist extension	PT to ECRB
	Finger extension	FCU or FCR to EDC
		FDS of ring or middle finger to EDC of index, long, ring and small finger
	Thumb extension	PL to EPL
		FDS long or middle finger to EPL
Median or Ulnar	Finger flexion	ECRL to FDP (2-5)
	Thumb flexion	Brachioradialis to FPL
Femoral	Knee extension	Biceps femoris/semitendinosus to patella
Peroneal	Ankle dorsiflexion	PTT to lateral cuneiform
		PT to TA
		FDL to EDL/EHL
Tibial	Ankle plantarflexion	TA to calcaneus

Abbreviations: ECRB, extensor carpi radialis brevis; ECRL, extensor carpi radialis longus; EDC, extensor digitorum communis; EDL, extensor digitorum longus; EHL, extensor hallucis longus; EIP, extensor indicis proprius; EPL, extensor pollicis longus; FCR, flexor carpi radialis; FCU, flexor carpi ulnaris; FDL, flexor digitorum longus; FDP, flexor digitorum profundus; FDS, flexor digitorum superficialis; FPL, flexor pollicis longus; PL, palmaris longus; PT, pronator teres; PTT, posterior tibial tendon; TA, tibialis anterior.

SUMMARY

Overall, the management of traumatic peripheral nerve injuries varies depending on the type of injury, location of injury, and mechanism of injury. The authors recommend early surgical exploration and repair for clean, open injuries. However, in the setting of closed injuries, with a significant zone of injury, we recommend observation. When primary repair is not possible, autograft is the standard for nerve grafting. However, advances in allografts (tissue or decellularized) hold promise for future treatment options for these devastating injuries. At this time, we recommend against the use of conduits for nerve gaps greater than 3 cm. In patients with proximal injuries or who present late, we would consider nerve or tendon transfers, alone or in combination, to restore function.

REFERENCES

1. Noble J, Munro CA, Prasad VS, et al. Analysis of upper and lower extremity peripheral nerve injuries in a population of patients with multiple injuries. J Trauma 1998;45(1):116–22.
2. Taylor CA, Braza D, Rice JB, et al. The incidence of peripheral nerve injury in extremity trauma. Am J Phys Med Rehabil 2008;87(5):381–5.
3. Robinson LR. Traumatic injury to peripheral nerves. Suppl Clin Neurophysiol 2004;57:173–86.
4. Fassler PR, Swiontkowski MF, Kilroy AW, et al. Injury of the sciatic nerve associated with acetabular fracture. J Bone Joint Surg Am 1993;75(8):1157–66.
5. Kouyoumdjian JA. Peripheral nerve injuries: a retrospective survey of 456 cases. Muscle Nerve 2006;34(6):785–8.
6. Yuksel F, Kişlaoğlu E, Durak N, et al. Prevention of painful neuromas by epineural ligatures, flaps and grafts. Br J Plast Surg 1997;50(3):182–5.
7. Sunderland S. The anatomy and physiology of nerve injury. Muscle Nerve 1990;13(9):771–84.
8. Seddon H. Three types of nerve injuries. Brain 1943;66:237–88.
9. Sunderland S, editor. Nerve injuries and their repair: a critical appraisal. New York: Churchill Livingstone; 1991.
10. Boyd KU, Nimigan AS, Mackinnon SE. Nerve reconstruction in the hand and upper extremity. Clin Plast Surg 2011;38(4):643–60.
11. O'Brien M. Aids to the examination of the peripheral nervous system. Philadelphia: W.B. Saunders; 2000.
12. Zaidman CM, Seelig MJ, Baker JC, et al. Detection of peripheral nerve pathology: comparison of ultrasound and MRI. Neurology 2013;80(18):1634–40.
13. Padua L, Di Pasquale A, Liotta G, et al. Ultrasound as a useful tool in the diagnosis and management of traumatic nerve lesions. Clin Neurophysiol 2013;124(6):1237–43.
14. Hollister AM, Simoncini A, Sciuk A, et al. High frequency ultrasound evaluation of traumatic peripheral nerve injuries. Neurol Res 2012;34(1):98–103.
15. Dubuisson A, Kline DG. Indications for peripheral nerve and brachial plexus surgery. Neurol Clin 1992;10(4):935–51.
16. Ring D, Chin K, Jupiter JB. Radial nerve palsy associated with high-energy humeral shaft fractures. J Hand Surg 2004;29(1):144–7.
17. Zachary LS, Dellon AL. Progression of the zone of injury in experimental nerve injuries. Microsurgery 1987;8(4):182–5.
18. Young L, Wray RC, Weeks PM. A randomized prospective comparison of fascicular and epineural digital nerve repairs. Plast Reconstr Surg 1981;68(1):89–93.
19. Lundborg G, Rosén B, Dahlin L, et al. Tubular versus conventional repair of median and ulnar nerves in the human forearm: early results from a prospective, randomized, clinical study. J Hand Surg 1997;22(1):99–106.
20. Lundborg G, Rosén B, Dahlin L, et al. Tubular repair of the median or ulnar nerve in the human forearm: a 5-year follow-up. J Hand Surg 2004;29(2):100–7.
21. Chow JA, Van Beek AL, Bilos ZJ, et al. Anatomical basis for repair of ulnar and median nerves in the distal part of the forearm by group fascicular suture and nerve-grafting. J Bone Joint Surg Am 1986;68(2):273–80.
22. Giddins GE, Wade PJ, Amis AA. Primary nerve repair: strength of repair with different gauges of nylon suture material. J Hand Surg 1989;14(3):301–2.
23. Isaacs JE, McDaniel CO, Owen JR, et al. Comparative analysis of biomechanical performance of available "nerve glues". J Hand Surg 2008;33(6):893–9.
24. Ornelas L, Padilla L, Di Silvio M, et al. Fibrin glue: an alternative technique for nerve coaptation—Part II. Nerve regeneration and histomorphometric assessment. J Reconstr Microsurgery 2006;22(2):123–8.
25. Martins RS, Siqueira MG, Da Silva CF, et al. Overall assessment of regeneration in peripheral nerve lesion repair using fibrin glue, suture, or a combination of the 2 techniques in a rat model. Which is the ideal choice? Surg Neurol 2005;64(Suppl 1). S1:10–S1:16. [discussion: S1:16].
26. Narakas A. The use of fibrin glue in repair of peripheral nerves. Orthop Clin North Am 1988;19(1):187–99.
27. Millesi H. Healing of nerves. Clin Plast Surg 1977;4(3):459–73.
28. Millesi H. The nerve gap. Theory and clinical practice. Hand Clin 1986;2(4):651–63.
29. Ray WZ, Mackinnon SE. Management of nerve gaps: autografts, allografts, nerve transfers, and

end-to-side neurorrhaphy. Exp Neurol 2010;223(1): 77–85.
30. Brenner MJ, Hess JR, Myckatyn TM, et al. Repair of motor nerve gaps with sensory nerve inhibits regeneration in rats. Laryngoscope 2006;116(9):1685–92.
31. Hoke A, Redett R, Hameed H, et al. Schwann cells express motor and sensory phenotypes that regulate axon regeneration. J Neurosci 2006;26(38): 9646–55.
32. Chu TH, Du Y, Wu W. Motor nerve graft is better than sensory nerve graft for survival and regeneration of motoneurons after spinal root avulsion in adult rats. Exp Neurol 2008;212(2):562–5.
33. Brushart TM. Preferential reinnervation of motor nerves by regenerating motor axons. J Neurosci 1988;8(3):1026–31.
34. Kawamura DH, Johnson PJ, Moore AM, et al. Matching of motor-sensory modality in the rodent femoral nerve model shows no enhanced effect on peripheral nerve regeneration. Exp Neurol 2010;223(2): 496–504.
35. Ansselin AD, Pollard JD. Immunopathological factors in peripheral nerve allograft rejection: quantification of lymphocyte invasion and major histocompatibility complex expression. J Neurol Sci 1990;96(1):75–88.
36. Mackinnon SE, Doolabh VB, Novak CB, et al. Clinical outcome following nerve allograft transplantation. Plast Reconstr Surg 2001;107(6):1419–29.
37. Gold BG, Katoh K, Storm Dickerson T. The immunosuppressant FK506 increases the rate of axonal regeneration in rat sciatic nerve. J Neurosci 1995; 15(11):7509–16.
38. Feng FY, Ogden MA, Myckatyn TM, et al. FK506 rescues peripheral nerve allografts in acute rejection. J Neurotrauma 2001;18(2):217–29.
39. Moore AM, Ray WZ, Chenard KE, et al. Nerve allotransplantation as it pertains to composite tissue transplantation. Hand (N Y) 2009;4(3):239–44.
40. Dumont CE, Hentz VR. Enhancement of axon growth by detergent-extracted nerve grafts. Transplantation 1997;63(9):1210–5.
41. Whitlock EL, Tuffaha SH, Luciano JP, et al. Processed allografts and type I collagen conduits for repair of peripheral nerve gaps. Muscle Nerve 2009;39(6):787–99.
42. Karabekmez FE, Duymaz A, Moran SL. Early clinical outcomes with the use of decellularized nerve allograft for repair of sensory defects within the hand. Hand (N Y) 2009;4(3):245–9.
43. Guo Y, Chen G, Tian G, et al. Sensory recovery following decellularized nerve allograft transplantation for digital nerve repair. J Plast Surg Hand Surg 2013;47(6):451–3.
44. Giusti G, Willems WF, Kremer T, et al. Return of motor function after segmental nerve loss in a rat model: comparison of autogenous nerve graft, collagen conduit, and processed allograft (AxoGen). J Bone Joint Surg Am 2012;94(5):410–7.
45. Cho MS, Rinker BD, Weber RV, et al. Functional outcome following nerve repair in the upper extremity using processed nerve allograft. J Hand Surg 2012;37(11):2340–9.
46. Brooks DN, Weber RV, Chao JD, et al. Processed nerve allografts for peripheral nerve reconstruction: a multicenter study of utilization and outcomes in sensory, mixed, and motor nerve reconstructions. Microsurgery 2012;32(1):1–14.
47. Chiu DT, Janecka I, Krizek TJ, et al. Autogenous vein graft as a conduit for nerve regeneration. Surgery 1982;91(2):226–33.
48. Chiu DT, Strauch B. A prospective clinical evaluation of autogenous vein grafts used as a nerve conduit for distal sensory nerve defects of 3 cm or less. Plast Reconstr Surg 1990;86(5):928–34.
49. Weber RA, Breidenbach WC, Brown RE, et al. A randomized prospective study of polyglycolic acid conduits for digital nerve reconstruction in humans. Plast Reconstr Surg 2000;106(5):1036–45 [discussion: 1046–8].
50. Agnew SP, Dumanian GA. Technical use of synthetic conduits for nerve repair. J Hand Surg 2010;35(5): 838–41.
51. Moore AM, Kasukurthi R, Magill CK, et al. Limitations of conduits in peripheral nerve repairs. Hand (N Y) 2009;4(2):180–6.
52. Kim PD, Hayes A, Amin F, et al. Collagen nerve protector in rat sciatic nerve repair: a morphometric and histological analysis. Microsurgery 2010;30(5):392–6.
53. Lee JY, Parisi TJ, Friedrich PF, et al. Does the addition of a nerve wrap to a motor nerve repair affect motor outcomes? Microsurgery 2014;34:562–7.
54. Sahakyants T, Lee JY, Friedrich PF, et al. Return of motor function after repair of a 3-cm gap in a rabbit peroneal nerve: a comparison of autograft, collagen conduit, and conduit filled with collagen-GAG matrix. J Bone Joint Surg Am 2013;95(21):1952–8.
55. Brown JM, Tung TH, Mackinnon SE. Median to radial nerve transfer to restore wrist and finger extension: technical nuances. Neurosurgery 2010;66(3 Suppl Operative):75–83 [discussion: 83].
56. Tung TH, Mackinnon SE. Nerve transfers: indications, techniques, and outcomes. J Hand Surg 2010;35(2):332–41.
57. Lee JY, Kircher MF, Spinner RJ, et al. Factors affecting outcome of triceps motor branch transfer for isolated axillary nerve injury. J Hand Surg 2012; 37(11):2350–6.
58. Giuffre JL, Bishop AT, Spinner RJ, et al. Partial tibial nerve transfer to the tibialis anterior motor branch to treat peroneal nerve injury after knee trauma. Clin Orthop Relat Res 2012;470(3):779–90.
59. Brown JM, Yee A, Mackinnon SE. Distal median to ulnar nerve transfers to restore ulnar motor and

sensory function within the hand: technical nuances. Neurosurgery 2009;65(5):966–77 [discussion: 977–8].
60. Ustun ME, Oğün TC, Büyükmumcu M, et al. Selective restoration of motor function in the ulnar nerve by transfer of the anterior interosseous nerve. An anatomical feasibility study. J Bone Joint Surg Am 2001;83-A(4):549–52.
61. Ray WZ, Mackinnon SE. Clinical outcomes following median to radial nerve transfers. J Hand Surg 2011; 36(2):201–8.
62. Novak CB, Mackinnon SE. Distal anterior interosseous nerve transfer to the deep motor branch of the ulnar nerve for reconstruction of high ulnar nerve injuries. J Reconstr Microsurgery 2002; 18(6):459–64.
63. Wang Y, Zhu S. Transfer of a branch of the anterior interosseus nerve to the motor branch of the median nerve and ulnar nerve. Chin Med J 1997;110(3): 216–9.
64. Tung TH, Chao A, Moore AM. Obturator nerve transfer for femoral nerve reconstruction: anatomic study and clinical application. Plast Reconstr Surg 2012; 130(5):1066–74.
65. Tung TH, Barbour JR, Gontre G, et al. Transfer of the extensor digiti minimi and extensor carpi ulnaris branches of the posterior interosseous nerve to restore intrinsic hand function: case report and anatomic study. J Hand Surg 2013;38(1):98–103.
66. Lundborg G, Rosen B. Sensory relearning after nerve repair. Lancet 2001;358(9284):809–10.
67. Lundborg G, Rosen B. Hand function after nerve repair. Acta Physiol (Oxf) 2007;189(2):207–17.
68. Kline DG. Surgical repair of peripheral nerve injury. Muscle Nerve 1990;13(9):843–52.
69. Mailander P, Berger A, Schaller E, et al. Results of primary nerve repair in the upper extremity. Microsurgery 1989;10(2):147–50.
70. Kallio PK, Vastamaki M. An analysis of the results of late reconstruction of 132 median nerves. J Hand Surg 1993;18(1):97–105.
71. Roganovic Z, Pavlicevic G. Difference in recovery potential of peripheral nerves after graft repairs. Neurosurgery 2006;59(3):621–33 [discussion: 621–33].
72. Roganovic Z. Missile-caused median nerve injuries: results of 81 repairs. Surg Neurol 2005;63(5):410–8 [discussion: 418–9].
73. Roganovic Z. Missile-caused ulnar nerve injuries: outcomes of 128 repairs. Neurosurgery 2004;55(5): 1120–9.
74. Roganovic Z, Petkovic S. Missile severances of the radial nerve. Results of 131 repairs. Acta Neurochir (Wien) 2004;146(11):1185–92.
75. Taha A, Taha J. Results of suture of the radial, median, and ulnar nerves after missile injury below the axilla. J Trauma 1998;45(2):335–9.
76. Kim DH, Kam AC, Chandika P, et al. Surgical management and outcomes in patients with median nerve lesions. J Neurosurg 2001;95(4):584–94.
77. Young C, Hudson A, Richards R. Operative treatment of palsy of the posterior interosseous nerve of the forearm. J Bone Joint Surg Am 1990;72(8): 1215–9.
78. Roganovic Z. Missile-caused complete lesions of the peroneal nerve and peroneal division of the sciatic nerve: results of 157 repairs. Neurosurgery 2005;57(6):1201–12 [discussion: 1201–12].
79. Roganovic Z, Pavlicevic G, Petkovic S. Missile-induced complete lesions of the tibial nerve and tibial division of the sciatic nerve: results of 119 repairs. J Neurosurg 2005;103(4):622–9.
80. Taha A, Taha J. Results of suture of the sciatic nerve after missile injury. J Trauma 1998;45(2):340–4.
81. Wood MB. Peroneal nerve repair. Surgical results. Clin Orthop Relat Res 1991;(267):206–10.
82. Kline DG, Kim D, Midha R, et al. Management and results of sciatic nerve injuries: a 24-year experience. J Neurosurg 1998;89(1):13–23.
83. Kim DH, Ryu S, Tiel RL, et al. Surgical management and results of 135 tibial nerve lesions at the Louisiana State University Health Sciences Center. Neurosurgery 2003;53(5):1114–24 [discussion: 1124–5].
84. Murovic JA. Lower-extremity peripheral nerve injuries: a Louisiana State University Health Sciences Center literature review with comparison of the operative outcomes of 806 Louisiana State University Health Sciences Center sciatic, common peroneal, and tibial nerve lesions. Neurosurgery 2009;65(4 Suppl):A18–23.
85. Tiel RL, Happel LT Jr, Kline DG. Nerve action potential recording method and equipment. Neurosurgery 1996;39(1):103–8 [discussion: 108–9].
86. Oberle JW, Antoniadis G, Rath SA, et al. Value of nerve action potentials in the surgical management of traumatic nerve lesions. Neurosurgery 1997; 41(6):1337–42 [discussion: 1342–4].
87. Kline DG. Timing for exploration of nerve lesions and evaluation of the neuroma-in-continuity. Clin Orthop Relat Res 1982;(163):42–9.
88. Stanton-Hicks M, Jänig W, Hassenbusch S, et al. Reflex sympathetic dystrophy: changing concepts and taxonomy. Pain 1995;63(1):127–33.
89. Jaiman A, Lokesh M, Neogi DS. Effect of vitamin C on prevention of complex regional pain syndrome type I in foot and ankle surgery. Foot Ankle Surg 2011;17(3):207.
90. Besse JL, Gadeyne S, Galand-Desmé S, et al. Effect of vitamin C on prevention of complex regional pain syndrome type I in foot and ankle surgery. Foot Ankle Surg 2009;15(4):179–82.
91. Shah AS, Verma MK, Jebson PJ. Use of oral vitamin C after fractures of the distal radius. J Hand Surg 2009;34(9):1736–8.

92. Zollinger PE, Tuinebreijer WE, Kreis RW, et al. Effect of vitamin C on frequency of reflex sympathetic dystrophy in wrist fractures: a randomised trial. Lancet 1999;354(9195):2025–8.
93. Zollinger PE, Tuinebreijer WE, Breederveld RS, et al. Can vitamin C prevent complex regional pain syndrome in patients with wrist fractures? A randomized, controlled, multicenter dose-response study. J Bone Joint Surg Am 2007;89(7):1424–31.
94. Burkhalter WE. Early tendon transfer in upper extremity peripheral nerve injury. Clin Orthop Relat Res 1974;(104):68–79.
95. Omer GE Jr. Tendon transfers in combined nerve lesions. Orthop Clin North Am 1974;5(2):377–87.
96. Fansa H, Meric C. Reconstruction of quadriceps femoris muscle function with muscle transfer. Handchir Mikrochir Plast Chir 2010;42(4):233–8 [in German].
97. Cush G, Irgit K. Drop foot after knee dislocation: evaluation and treatment. Sports medicine and arthroscopy review 2011;19(2):139–46.
98. Wiesseman GJ. Tendon transfers for peripheral nerve injuries of the lower extremity. Orthop Clin North Am 1981;12(2):459–67.
99. Vigasio A, Marcoccio I, Patelli A, et al. New tendon transfer for correction of drop-foot in common peroneal nerve palsy. Clin Orthop Relat Res 2008;466(6):1454–66.

Management of Complications with Hand Fractures

Varun K. Gajendran, MD[a,*], Vishal K. Gajendran, BS[b], Kevin J. Malone, MD[a]

KEYWORDS

• Hand fractures • Phalanx fractures • Metacarpal fractures • Complications • Stiffness • Malunion • Nonunion • Infection

KEY POINTS

- The most relevant complications of metacarpal and phalangeal fractures include stiffness, malunion, nonunion, arthritis, infection, and complex regional pain syndrome.
- These complications can occur with both operative and nonoperative treatments.
- Surgical treatment can often be challenging because of the complex anatomy and the need to simultaneously address the bone, joint, and soft tissues to achieve good outcomes.
- With careful attention to detail, surgery can produce good to excellent outcomes, although salvage operations may be necessary in some cases.

INTRODUCTION

Fractures of the metacarpals and phalanges account for more than 40% of all upper extremity fractures and are associated with tremendous financial burden and societal costs.[1] A recent epidemiologic study from the Netherlands revealed that hand fractures were the most expensive subgroup of all fractures, resulting in an excess of $278 million in annual costs and loss of productivity.[2] Because of the intricate anatomy within a confined area, surgical treatment can be challenging and complications are not uncommon with both operative and nonoperative treatments.[3–12] Therefore, the treating hand surgeon must be able to promptly recognize complications and treat them effectively to optimize functional outcomes. Stiffness is by far the most common complication, followed by malunion, posttraumatic arthritis, nonunion, infection, and chronic pain syndromes.[3,6,7,11]

Nonoperative management of these fractures, while appropriate in many instances, can lead to complications and severely compromise hand function.[3] Operative treatment has the potential to mitigate these complications and optimize mechanics and function, but it also has the potential to cause those very same complications, as well as others such as infection, hardware-related issues, and nonunion.[3,6,7,11,12] Therefore, all of these risks must be carefully considered in the context of the injury, along with specific patient characteristics such as age, activity level, occupation, and vocational interests to optimize outcomes and minimize complications.

STIFFNESS

Stiffness is not only the most common complication encountered, but it is also unfortunately the most difficult to treat.[13] High-energy and open

Disclosures: No disclosures (V.K. Gajendran, V.K. Gajendran); Paid consultant for Synthes and instructor/lecturer for AO (K.J. Malone).

[a] Department of Orthopedic Surgery, MetroHealth Medical Center, 2500 MetroHealth Drive, Cleveland, OH 44109, USA; [b] University of Toledo College of Medicine, 2801 West Bancroft Street, Toledo, OH 43606, USA
* Corresponding author.
E-mail address: varun182@gmail.com

Hand Clin 31 (2015) 165–177
http://dx.doi.org/10.1016/j.hcl.2014.12.001
0749-0712/15/$ – see front matter

fractures are at greater risk for developing stiffness, as are crush injuries and those with extensive injury to the surrounding soft tissue envelope, as illustrated in **Fig. 1**.[4,7,12] Phalanx fractures, particularly those around the proximal interphalangeal (PIP) joint, are more predisposed to developing stiffness than metacarpal fractures.[12,14] Immobilization for 4 weeks or greater is also likely to result in stiffness, so early active motion must be instituted under the care of a skilled hand therapist. Therefore, stable fracture fixation with careful handling of the soft tissue envelope is desirable to allow early motion.[7,11]

There is considerable debate about the use of specific types of implants and their implications for early motion and prevention of stiffness. Ring[15] and Page and Stern[4] advocated the use of larger implants, particularly in the phalanges, to provide added stability and allow early active motion to avoid stiffness. This concept has been supported by other studies showing good results and relatively low complication rates with plate fixation in the metacarpals and phalanges.[16] However, a few studies have raised concerns about the possibly higher rates of complications including stiffness, malunion, nonunion, tendon rupture, and infection that have been observed in nearly 50% of cases of plate fixation, requiring secondary procedures.[8,10,12,14] K-wire fixation, while more biologically friendly, can have problems with infection and loss of fixation that may lead to malunion, nonunion, stiffness, and compromised function.[17–19] Ultimately, there are advantages and drawbacks to each technique and implant that must be matched with the patient and fracture type. K-wire fixation is preferable in acute fractures when it achieves adequate stability to allow early

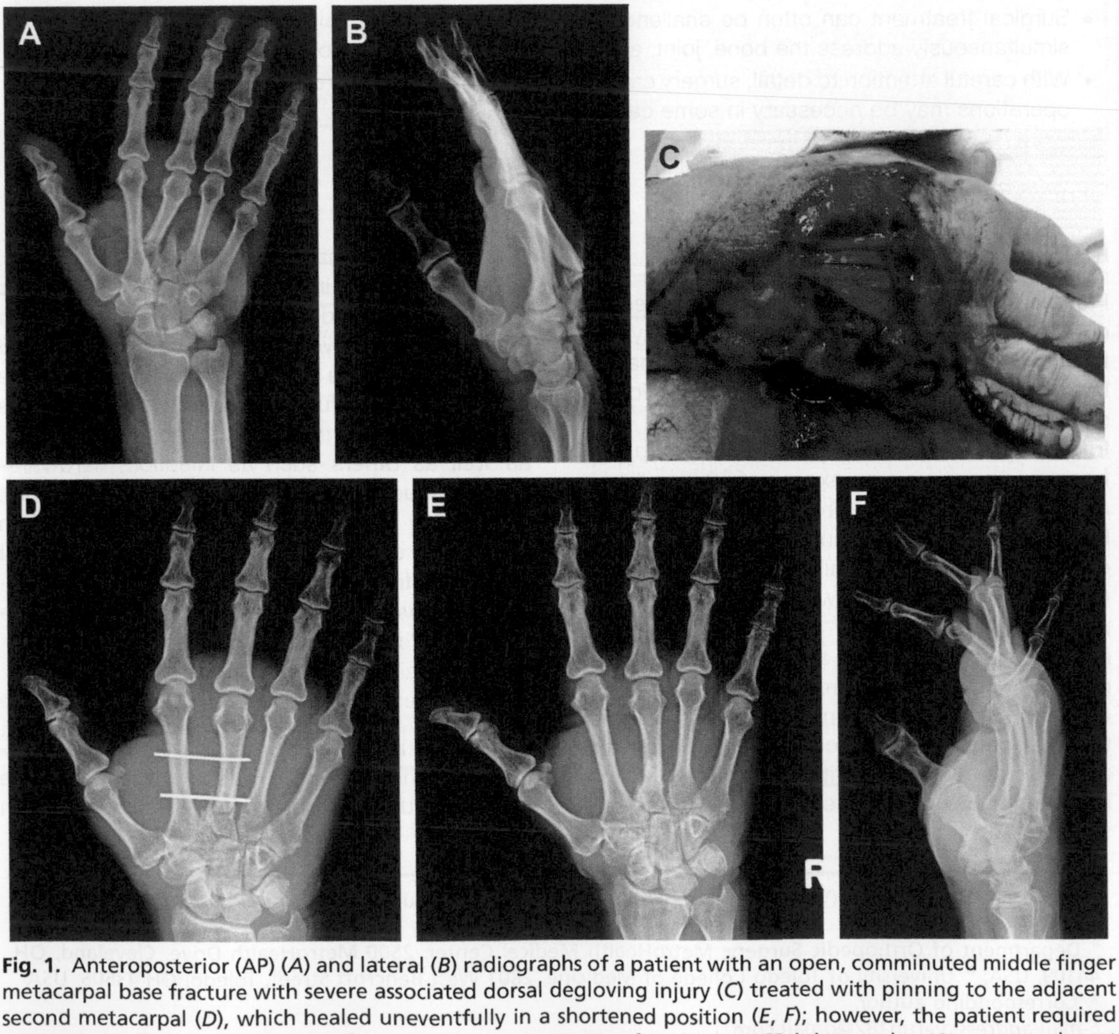

Fig. 1. Anteroposterior (AP) (*A*) and lateral (*B*) radiographs of a patient with an open, comminuted middle finger metacarpal base fracture with severe associated dorsal degloving injury (*C*) treated with pinning to the adjacent second metacarpal (*D*), which healed uneventfully in a shortened position (*E, F*); however, the patient required extensor tenolysis 6 months later for extension contractures of multiple MCP joints and a 10° extensor lag at the middle finger MCP joint, which allowed her to regain full motion.

motion, but larger implants such as plates become more useful when treating complications of hand fractures, as will be discussed later.

Stiffness with both active and passive motion indicates a capsular contracture, whereas stiffness with active motion alone is caused by tendon adhesions to the surrounding soft tissues, capsule, bone, or implants. The initial treatment of stiffness is through intensive hand therapy with an experienced therapist to gain as much motion as possible. Often, sufficient motion can be regained to allow the patient to be functional.[20] However, in cases when motion has plateaued after at least 3 months following fracture fixation and hand therapy, surgical treatment is indicated. It is critical for the skin and soft tissue envelope to be mature and supple, and for the fracture to be consolidated before any surgical procedure. The patient must be informed of the intensive postoperative rehabilitation and be dedicated to participating in this process.

Flexor tendon adhesions most commonly occur within zone 2 in association with proximal and middle phalanx fractures wherein there is significant injury to the surrounding soft tissues.[21,22] After failed conservative management, tenolysis can be performed as described by Yamazaki and colleagues[23] through a volar approach using a zigzag incision from the distal palmar crease to the distal finger crease. A z-plasty can be performed when there is significant contracture and concern about skin closure. The adhesions between the skin and tendon sheath are released. The tendon sheath is opened using multiple transverse incisions, which are placed proximal to the A2 pulley, distal to the A2 pulley, and through the middle of the A2 pulley. Every effort should be made to preserve the A2 and A4 pulleys. The flexor tendons are freed from adhesions to each other and the underlying capsule and bone using curved blades (**Fig. 2**) or fine periosteal elevators. If there is a persistent flexion contracture, the checkrein ligaments, accessory collateral ligaments, and the volar aspect of the collateral ligaments are sequentially released in that order until the joint can be adequately extended. In most cases, all 3 structures will need to be released to regain full extension. If the patient is awake with local anesthesia, active motion can be demonstrated by having the patient make a fist; otherwise, the tendons can be pulled proximally at the wrist to check active motion. Using the algorithm described above, Yamazaki and colleagues[23] noted average improvement in total active motion (TAM) of 107° and mostly excellent and good clinical outcomes. In the series by Hahn and colleagues,[24] 84% of fingers that underwent flexor tenolysis in the setting of stiffness following fracture achieved a mean postoperative TAM of 189° at a mean follow-up of 10 months compared with a preoperative TAM of 79°.

Extensor tendon adhesions are more common than flexor tendon adhesions because the surgical approach and plating are usually performed dorsally or laterally in most cases. Freeland and Orbay[25] advocated the use of miniplates and screws to create a more stable construct and demonstrated that as little as 1.7 mm of tendon excursion may decrease adhesions and prevent stiffness. They described a technique of excising the lateral band and oblique fibers of the extensor apparatus on the side of the plate to expose the proximal phalanx and limit adhesions (**Fig. 3**). Various techniques have been described, but common to all of them is a curvilinear dorsal skin incision, sharp release of the skin from the underlying extensor mechanism, and separation of the central slip, lateral slip, and intrinsic apparatus from each other and the underlying bone and capsule with blades or elevators. A dorsal capsulotomy can be added if necessary after carefully dissecting out the radial and ulnar aspects of the extensor mechanism and freeing it from the underlying dorsal capsule.[6,26] After dorsal capsulotomy, the dorsal half of the collateral ligaments can be released for further correction if necessary.[7] Gould and Nicholson[27] performed capsulectomies for stiffness involving

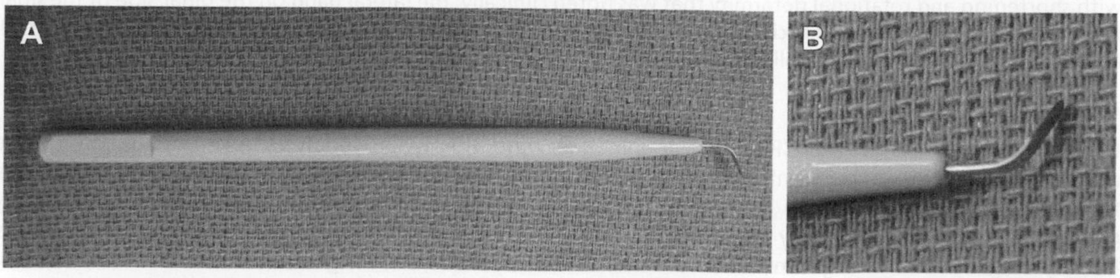

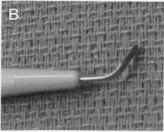

Fig. 2. Curved blades like the one pictured in (*A*) and (*B*) are useful for negotiating the tight spaces around a tendon to perform a complete release of the surrounding adhesions.

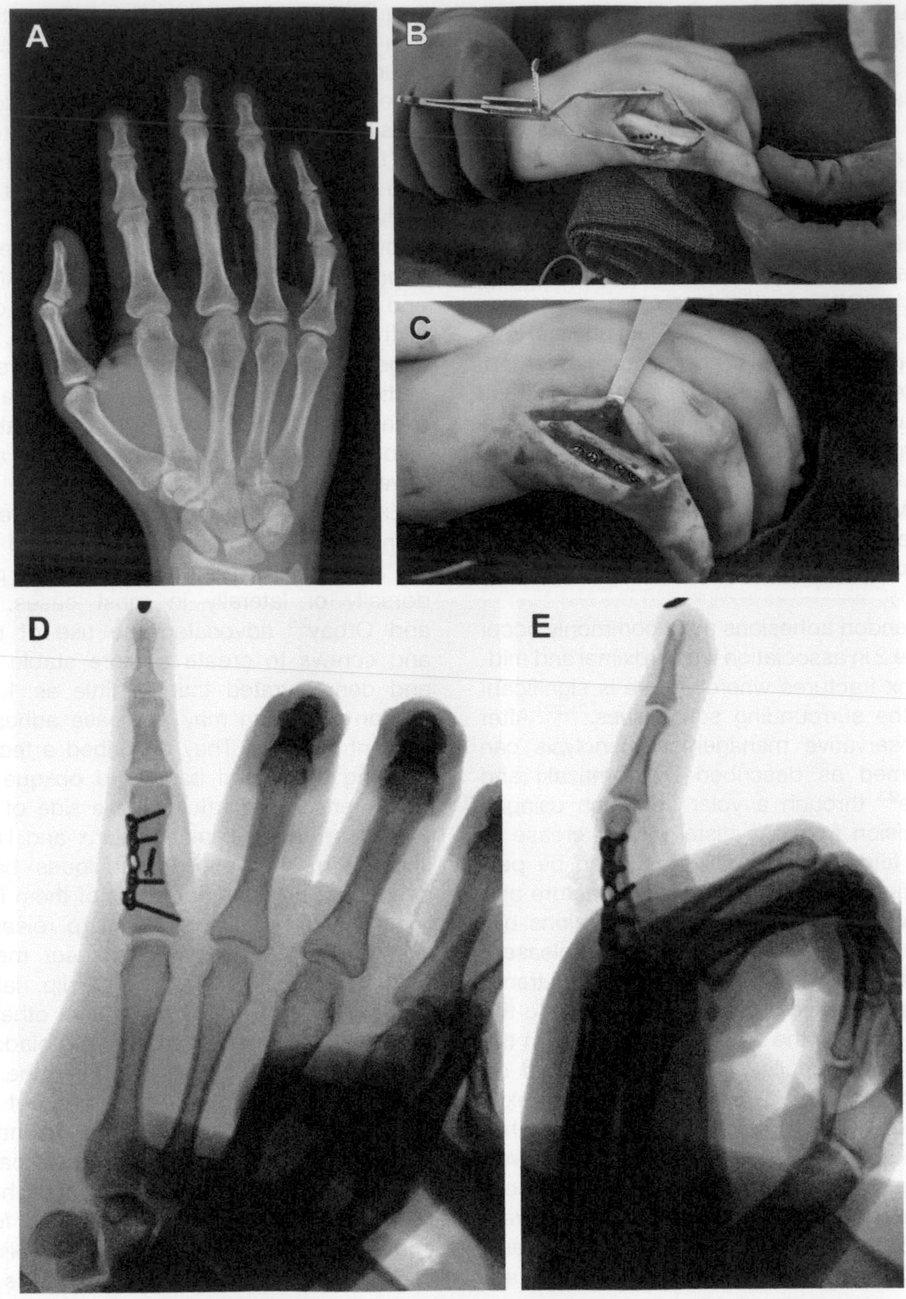

Fig. 3. AP of the hand (*A*) shows a displaced, oblique, and unstable proximal phalanx shaft fracture associated with shortening and rotational deformity that was noted clinically; the lateral band on the ulnar side of the small finger was marked out (*B*) and excised (*C*) to expose and plate the fracture as shown in the intraoperative AP (*D*) and lateral (*E*) images of the small finger.

the metacarpophalangeal (MCP) and PIP joints, and patients who underwent the procedure following fractures and crush injuries achieved gains in active motion that they found to be functionally significant. Creighton and Steichen[6] achieved good outcomes with increases in TAM of about 50° when tenolysis alone was performed and 30° when tenolysis and capsulotomy were performed, presumably because the latter cases had more longstanding contractures, which may have led to higher recurrence rates. Other authors have also shown good results with reliable restoration of active and passive motion using similar techniques.[26,28]

Postoperatively, pain management and edema control with early active motion are crucial for a successful outcome. The patient must also be fully engaged with hand therapy early and throughout the postoperative course until the soft tissues have stabilized and motion is maintained.[29] When there are both flexor and extensor tendon adhesions, it may be prudent to perform extensor tenolysis first, followed by a period of intensive therapy, and then perform flexor tenolysis after the soft tissues are again stable. When surgical treatment fails to restore adequate motion, fusion in a more functional position may be a salvage option.

MALUNION

Deformities caused by malunions can range from the mild, aesthetically displeasing to the severe and functionally disabling. They can be caused by a combination of shortening, malrotation, and angulation in the coronal and/or sagittal plane, but one deformity usually predominates. Surgical correction is indicated for functionally disabling deformities and should be tailored to the specific patient to fit his or her goals. Surgical planning should include the approach, the osteotomy site and type, choice of implant, and postoperative rehabilitation.[3,6,7,11,15,29-37]

Metacarpal Malunion

Metacarpal malunions are generally apex dorsal due to the deforming forces of the intrinsics muscles and extrinsic flexors. There can be a rotational component as well, which is assessed with the fingers flexed. Oblique and comminuted metacarpal fractures can also have shortening present.[7,11,15] Although up to 6 mm of shortening can be tolerated owing to the ability of the MCP joint to hyperextend and compensate, every subsequent 2 mm of shortening results in a 7° extensor lag.[38] Shortening also compromises power, with 2 mm of shortening causing a mild 8% loss of power and 10 mm of shortening leading to a more significant 45% loss of power.[39]

Although the exact guidelines are variable, index and middle finger angular deformities of up to 10°, and ring and small finger angular deformities of 20° and 30°, respectively, can generally be tolerated.[7] Coronal plane deformity can be tolerated as long as the digits do not impinge, and border digits are more tolerant of coronal plane angulation because of the increased spacing.[29] Osteotomies can be performed at the site of the original fracture or away from the fracture. The advantages of performing the osteotomy at the old fracture site are the ability to restore normal anatomy without creating a zigzag deformity, access to the soft tissues for concurrent tenolysis and capsulectomy, and the ability to correct multiple deformities. Therefore, osteotomies should generally be performed at the old fracture site whenever possible.[15] Both opening and closing wedge osteotomies may be performed for angular deformities. Closing wedge ostetotomies are easier and more reliable, but they shorten the metacarpal. Opening wedge osteotomies may be used when there is also shortening present that needs to be corrected, and cancellous grafts are adequate as long as the fixation is robust.[11,15,29,36,37,40-42] Although K-wires can be used for stabilization, plates and screws are preferred to allow early motion, particularly in opening wedge osteotomies where the added stability is crucial.[15]

Rotational malunions can lead to overlapping of the digits, and the adjacent joints cannot compensate for the deformity, so they are less well tolerated. As little as 5° of malrotation can produce 1.5 cm of digital overlap.[7] The rotational osteotomy can be performed either at the site of the old fracture or proximally at the base as described by Weckesser[43] to produce a correction of up to 18° for the index, long, and ring metacarpals, and 30° for the small metacarpal.[44] If there is a significant angular deformity, osteotomy at the fracture site may be preferable to address both deformities. Another excellent option for a primarily rotational deformity is a proximal step-cut osteotomy, as first described by Manktelow and Mahoney,[45] which allows for a greater surface area of bone apposition and fixation with lag screws without use of a bulky plate.[42,46] Fixation can be in the form of K-wires or plate and screws, with the latter potentially creating a more stable construct to allow early motion.[7,11,15,45] Many series have been published on the outcomes of osteotomies for correction of rotational malunions using the above techniques, and they report uniformly good outcomes with high rates of healing, deformity correction, and patient satisfaction, with a small percentage of patients undergoing secondary procedures for stiffness as expected.[37,41-43,45-48]

Phalangeal Malunion

Phalangeal malunions, similar to metacarpal malunions, can exhibit deformities in the coronal and sagittal planes, malrotation, and shortening.[7] Proximal phalangeal malunions characteristically have an apex volar deformity due to the lumbricals flexing up the proximal fragment and the central slip extending the distal fragment.[21] Biomechanically, the dorsal surface of the bone is shortened relative to the length of the extensor tendon when volar angulation exceeds 15°, and this creates an extensor lag of about 12° per 1 mm of shortening.[21,49] When angulation exceeds 25°, both flexion and extension are compromised.[22] Because of the extensor lag at the PIP joint and its proclivity for stiffness, fixed flexion contractures can rapidly develop. Middle phalangeal malunions are apex dorsal if the fracture is proximal to the flexor digitorum superficialis (FDS) insertion and apex volar if the fracture is distal to the FDS insertion. Apex volar angulation is more commonly seen and it can significantly affect flexor tendon biomechanics.[21,29]

In general, phalangeal malunions are best treated at the level of the fracture rather than elsewhere in the phalanx or at the metacarpal level because of the benefit of being able to concurrently perform tenocapsulolysis and address the source of the deformity. However, consideration may be given to performing osteotomies at the proximal phalanx base rather than close to the PIP joint to lower the risk of contracture.[30] For apex volar malunions, a closing wedge osteotomy hinged on the dorsal periosteum is a good option, because it maintains the length of the bone relative to the extensor tendon and allows for good opposition of the bone ends during healing.[3] A lateral plate can then be applied away from the tendons to reduce adhesions, and early motion can begin. For severely angulated malunions in which the bone is significantly shortened relative to the tendon, a dorsal opening wedge osteotomy should be performed and stabilized with a dorsal plate. Although this theoretically restores the original length of the bone, it has a higher risk of adhesion formation and stiffness. Coronal plane malunions are often due to bone loss on the concave side. Opening wedge osteotomies with interposed bone graft, sparing the cortex on the convex side, followed by fixation with a lateral plate, have demonstrated good results.[31] Rotational deformities may be present and should be addressed while addressing the angular deformities and shortening.

In their series of phalangeal malunions, Buchler and colleagues[31] reported a 100% union rate and deformity correction, but concurrent tenolysis and/or capsulectomy was performed in 50% of cases because of the high incidence of tendon adhesions and joint contractures. Good to excellent outcomes ranged from 64% to 96% depending on whether the bone alone was involved or additional structures had to be treated. Trumble and Gilbert[50] similarly recommended in situ osteotomy of the phalanx at the level of the old fracture rather than at the metacarpal because of the ability to perform simultaneous tenolysis and capsulotomy, which is needed in most cases. All of their patients healed and had full correction of their deformities, with PIP joint motion improving by 15° and distal interphalangeal (DIP) joint motion improving by 10°. Therefore, treatment of phalangeal malunions is more challenging than metacarpal malunions because of the surrounding intrinsic apparatus and extrinsic tendons, the tendency for tendon adhesions, and the development of PIP joint contractures. Surgical treatment can substantially improve function and lead to patient satisfaction.

ARTHRITIS

Posttraumatic arthritis can be the result of intra-articular malunion or chondral injury from the moment of impaction. Although chondral injury may be irreversible, articular incongruity can be surgically corrected, and it is much easier to do so in the acute setting.[30,31,51] Established intra-articular malunions can be very challenging to treat.[15,30] The treatment options depend on the patient, the deformity, the involved joint, and the presence of arthrosis, and they include osteotomies, various types of arthroplasties, and arthrodeses.[15,30,35]

There are 2 general approaches to the correction of intra-articular malunions. When the malunion is within 8 to 10 weeks old and the old fracture line can still be defined, an osteotomy can be performed through the fracture to reverse the deformity and make the articular surface more congruous.[30] This osteotomy may, however, require manipulating and fixing of small, unstable articular fragments, which may in theory result in the disruption of biology, as well as compromised fixation. On the other hand, chronic malunions where the fracture line is no longer apparent requires special techniques by incorporating creative osteotomies to reduce the articular surface.[15,30,31,51,52] Teoh and colleagues[52] have described one such technique that involves resecting a wedge of bone from the intercondylar area and creating a larger condylar piece that contains the diaphysis. This technique allows for easier correction of the articular malunion and fixation of a larger fragment after advancement, thereby reducing the theoretic risk of fixation failure, nonunion, and osteonecrosis (**Fig. 4**). Subcondylar closing wedge osteotomy just proximal to the collateral ligament insertion has also been described with good results.[29,30,33,53] Another approach advocated by Ring[15] and Harness and colleagues[53] is accepting the articular malunion and instead performing an extra-articular osteotomy to counteract the angular or rotational deformity produced by the articular malunion. This

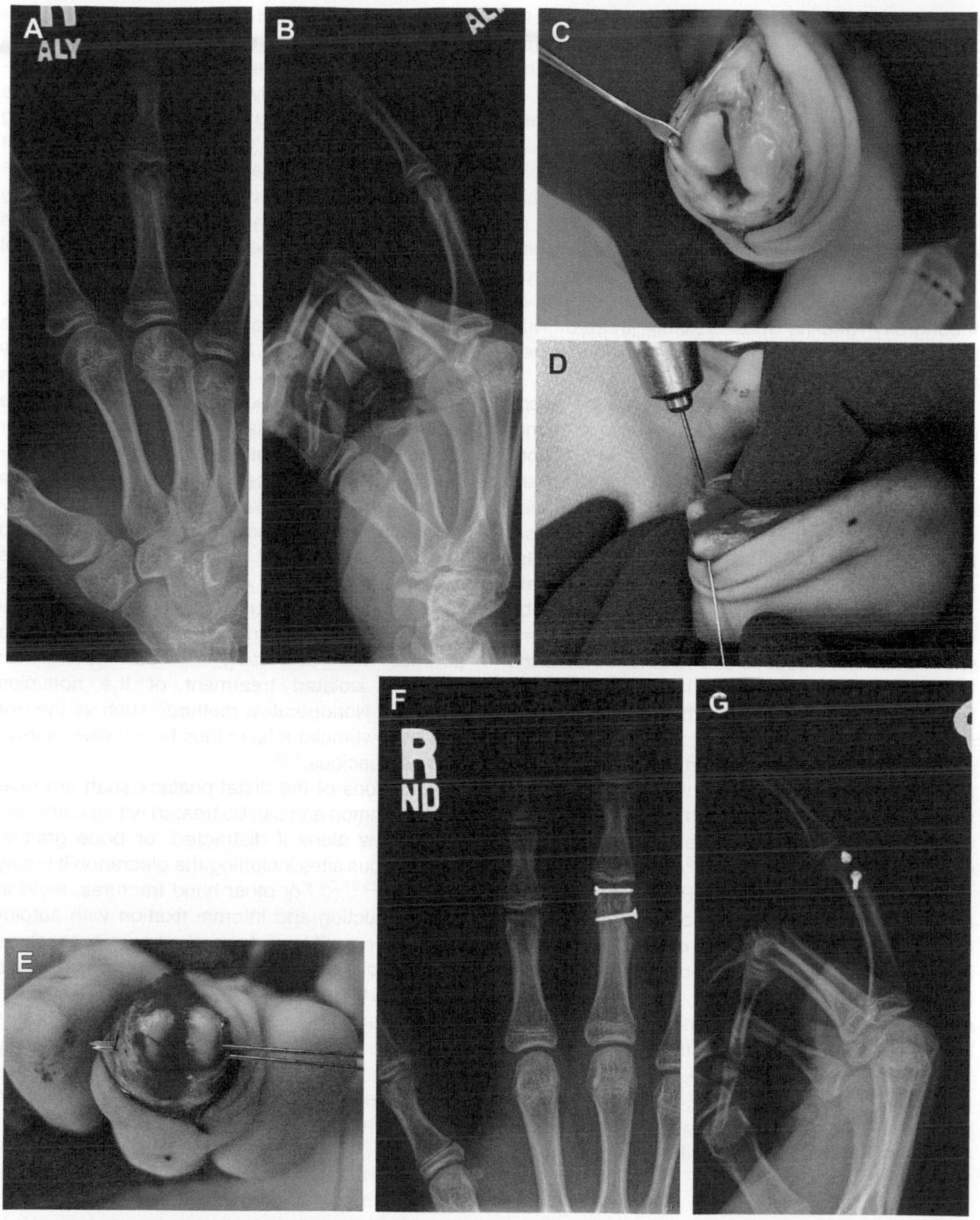

Fig. 4. AP (*A*) and lateral (*B*) radiographs of the long finger showing a displaced proximal phalanx unicondylar fracture that presented late with an intra-articular malunion, which was also evident intraoperatively (*C*); a wedge of bone was resected from the intercondylar area (*D*) and the malunited fragment was then reduced to the intact condyle and fixed with 2 screws, resulting in improved articular congruity intraoperatively (*E*), also seen on the AP (*F*) and lateral (*G*) radiographs. The fracture went on to heal with a good clinical and radiographic outcome.

extra-articular osteotomy could potentially approximate normal joint biomechanics and produce more favorable joint contact forces. For the most severe deformities or when arthrosis is already present, arthrodesis and arthroplasty are excellent options.[7,15,30]

Intra-articular malunions at the DIP joint are usually due to bony mallet injuries. The main concern with these injuries is the development of an extensor lag at the DIP joint and subsequent PIP joint hyperextension, resulting in a Swan-neck deformity. Arthrosis can also develop because of incongruity and is most reliably treated with arthrodesis in 5° to 10° of flexion when symptomatic.[35,54]

Malunions around the PIP joint can be associated with stiffness and angular and rotational deformities that can severely limit hand function. The treatment options, as outlined above, are extra-articular and intra-articular osteotomies depending on the deformity. In the case of dorsal PIP fracture, dislocations with loss of the volar articular surface of the middle phalanx, volar plate arthroplasty, or hemi-hamate arthroplasty can be used. Volar plate arthroplasty can have problems with flexion contractures and recurrent instability, but hemihamate arthroplasty has been shown to be effective for articular surface loss of up to 50%.[55] When the deformity cannot be reconstructed or there is already arthrosis present, the index finger is best treated with arthrodesis to provide a stable base for pinch, and the remaining fingers can be treated with arthroplasty to preserve motion, or arthrodesis.[35]

Malunions around the MCP joint occur more infrequently, but they can also be challenging to treat. Again, the treatment options consist of intra-articular and extra-articular osteotomies. Arthrodesis and arthroplasty are used for the severe, uncorrectable deformities or if there is pre-existing arthrosis. As with the PIP joint, it may be preferable to fuse the index MCP joint to provide stability during pinch, but the other MCP joints should be treated with arthroplasty because motion at the MCP joints is vital for normal hand function.[35]

NONUNION

Because of the rich vascular network supplying the hand, nonunion is fortunately a rare complication in the metacarpals and phalanges. When it occurs, it is usually seen in complex injuries such as open fractures and crush injuries where there are concomitant injuries to the nerves, blood vessels, and tendons. Stiffness from tendon adhesions and capsular contractures is usually present as well, leading to a hand that has severely compromised function. Most nonunions in the hand are atrophic and associated with bone loss or infection.[15] They are usually the sequelae of operative treatment and caused by vascular insult during exposure and fracture fixation, or malreduction of the fracture in a distracted position.[56] Hypertrophic nonunions are less common and can simply be treated with revision of the reduction to achieve bone contact followed by more stable internal fixation.[7,35]

The diagnosis of nonunion can be challenging, as radiolucent lines can be seen on radiographs for more than a year in fractures that ultimately unite radiographically. Moreover, most patients are clinically healed and return to work well before radiographic healing is noted.[3] Therefore, other factors such as pain, instability, deformity, and failure of fixation should be considered along with the radiographs when making the diagnosis. Regardless of the time required for union, the hand should never be immobilized for greater than 6 weeks because of the risk of developing contractures.[15] Many cases of nonunion will require salvage procedures such as arthrodesis or amputation to address the coexisting injuries rather than requiring isolated treatment of the nonunion alone.[7,15] Nonoperative methods such as the use of a bone stimulator have thus far not been shown to be efficacious.[7,35]

Nonunions of the distal phalanx shaft are relatively common and can be treated with a compression screw alone if distracted, or bone grafting from various sites including the olecranon if purely atrophic.[35,57,58] For other hand fractures, revision open reduction and internal fixation with autologous bone graft is performed along with tenolysis and arthrolysis for the coexisting stiffness in cases where the finger is expected to be nearly fully functional after surgery. Autologous bone graft is the standard, and cancellous autograft is generally sufficient to stimulate healing unless there is a large defect that requires load sharing, in which case a structural autograft may be used. A semi-structural bone peg can also be fashioned by compacting cancellous autograft using a syringe, and this may be adequate for most hand fractures.[15,59] Technically, all atrophic and nonviable bone must be resected until there is bleeding bone. Implants used for internal fixation in the setting of a nonunion should be slightly larger than those that are typically used for acute fractures in that location to provide added mechanical stability. Periarticular and fixed angle plates may be used around the joints.[3,7,15,56] Few studies have reported on the outcomes after surgical management of nonunions with internal fixation and bone grafting, but the results are not encouraging. In the series by Jupiter and colleagues[56] of 25 patients with nonunions, 15 patients had complex injuries. Although plate and screw fixation provided better stability than K-wire fixation, few digits ultimately achieved good function. The authors' experience has been similar, as illustrated by the case in **Fig. 5** of an open metacarpal fracture from a gunshot wound with significant soft tissue injury and bone loss that ultimately resulted in a persistent nonunion despite multiple procedures.

Given the limited success of nonunion repair with bone grafting and revision internal fixation, arthrodesis and amputation play important roles in the surgical treatment of nonunion. Arthrodesis is appropriate for intra-articular and periarticular nonunions with severe stiffness that would preclude a good functional result after bone grafting and revision internal fixation alone. Amputation is indicated for significant bone loss, chronic infection, permanent sensory loss, and poor soft tissue coverage. Stiff fingers are often bypassed during the use of the hand and adversely affect function. They also require protection and cause stiffness of the adjacent fingers. Therefore, amputation is a good solution for these patients and almost universally improves their function.[7,15,56]

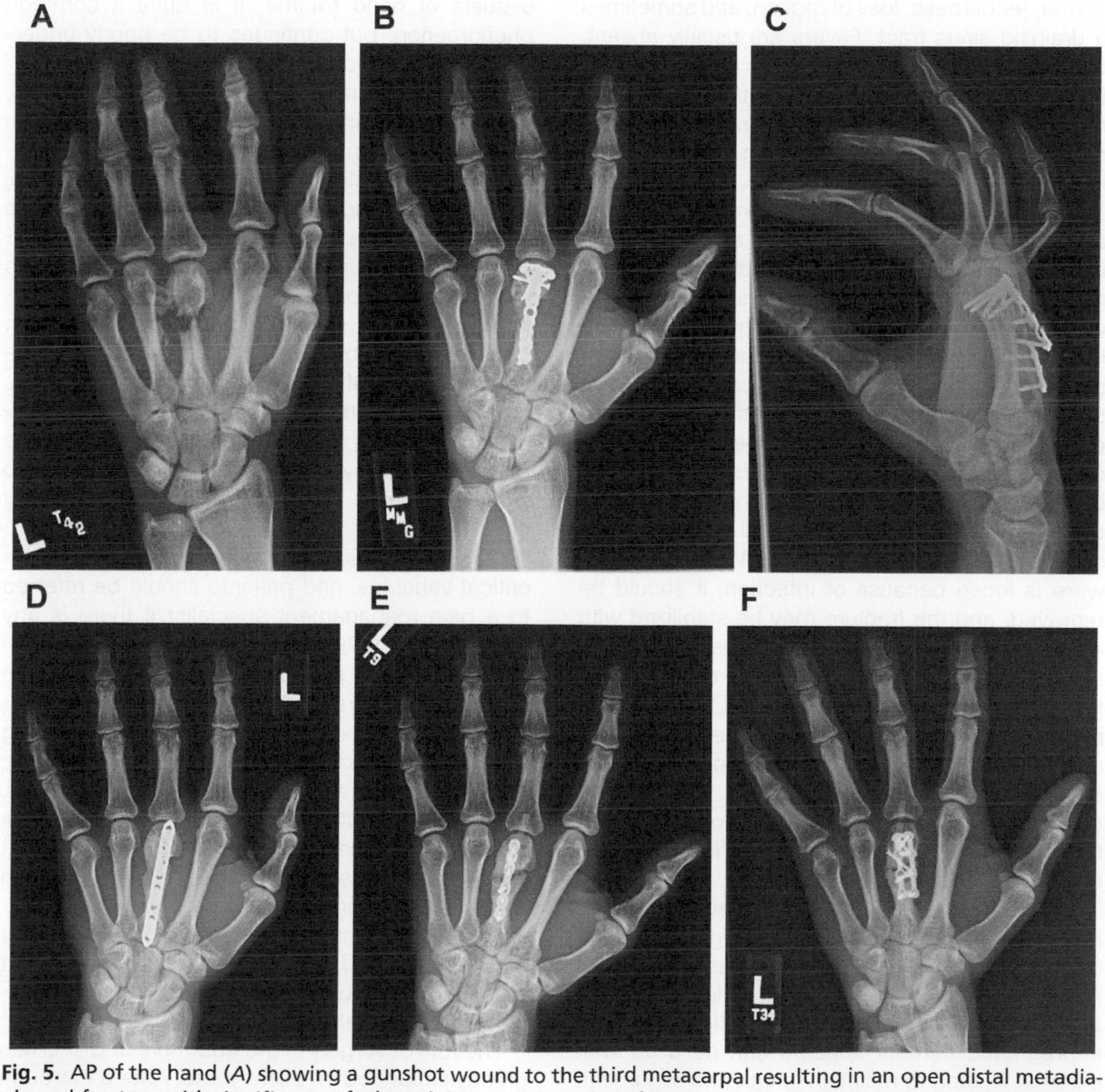

Fig. 5. AP of the hand (*A*) showing a gunshot wound to the third metacarpal resulting in an open distal metadiaphyseal fracture with significant soft tissue injury and bone loss that was treated initially with plate fixation and subsequently bone grafted for delayed union at 4 months, but continued to remain nonunited, resulting in hardware failure (*B, C*). The patient thereafter failed to heal after 3 more procedures: the first with a spanning plate and structural bone graft (*D*), followed by 2 more revisions of the plate fixation with bone grafting (*E, F*).

INFECTION

Infection rates after hand fractures correlate directly with the extent of the soft tissue injury and contamination of the wound. Open fractures are associated with deep infection rates as high as 11% after operative treatment.[60,61] Devitalization of the surrounding soft tissues and periosteal stripping create an environment that is vulnerable to infection after bacterial inoculation. Osteomyelitis can follow when the bone becomes involved, and treatment can be challenging with amputation rates reported by some to be around 40%.[62]

The definitive diagnosis of osteomyelitis is made with cultures obtained from a bone biopsy. Clinically, patients present with swelling, warmth, erythema, tenderness, loss of motion, and sometimes a draining sinus tract. Fevers are usually absent, but inflammatory markers such as C-reactive protein are elevated although the white blood count may be normal or elevated. Radiographs are initially normal, but may reveal sequestrum and involucrum in chronic cases.[9]

The treatment of acute osteomyelitis without abscess formation is parenteral antibiotics with close monitoring of the clinical status and inflammatory markers, followed by a short course of oral antibiotics once the inflammatory markers have normalized. Surgery is indicated when nonsurgical management fails, or in cases of chronic osteomyelitis or acute osteomyelitis with an associated abscess. The goals of surgery are to eradicate all infected and nonviable tissues including bone, effectively obliterate the dead space, sufficiently stabilize the skeleton, and provide stable soft tissue coverage for healing. When the hardware is loose because of infection, it should be removed, and the fracture may be stabilized with external fixation. If the fracture has healed, the hardware should be removed. If, on the other hand, the fracture has not yet united, the hardware may be retained until union while the patient is on chronic suppressive antibiotics. The dead space can be managed with antibiotic impregnated cement spacers with external fixation as needed for stability, and flaps can be used for soft tissue coverage as necessary.[7,9,11,61,62]

Infected nonunions that are being salvaged rather than amputated should undergo a thorough debridement and removal of all devitalized and necrotic tissue including bone, followed by the administration of parenteral antibiotics. Antibiotic impregnated cement spacers can be used with external fixation to maintain length and alignment. If the skin and soft tissues are compromised, flaps may be necessary for soft tissue coverage and to improve local vascularity for eradication of the infection. The definitive reconstructive procedure may be performed after the infection has been cleared and should follow the principles outlined above for treating nonunions.[15]

CHRONIC PAIN

Although the exact incidence is unknown, complex regional pain syndrome (CRPS) is a common entity in the upper extremity. It has been reported to occur after distal radius fractures and fasciectomy for Dupuytren disease.[63,64] Although it can occur after hand fractures, the current literature has little information about CRPS in this setting. Cold sensitivity, a known symptom of CRPS, has been extensively reported in the literature as a sequela of hand trauma. It is quite a common phenomenon, but continues to be poorly understood and is difficult to treat.[65,66]

CRPS is characterized by trophic changes, autonomic dysfunction, and impaired function. In the hand, it can manifest as persistent pain well after the injury, delayed bone healing or nonunion, stiffness, swelling, atrophy, cold sensitivity, and osteopenia on radiographs. CRPS can be attributed to nerve injury during surgery or sympathetic overactivity without a specific nerve injury. Therefore, diagnostic injections with local anesthetic may be useful for identifying neuromas or compressed nerves if the symptoms are in a specific nerve distribution. In other cases, several diagnostic modalities can be used, including a 3-phase bone scan and sympatholytic challenge testing to identify patients whose pain is sympathetically driven.[66]

Early recognition and treatment are the most critical variables, and patients should be referred to a pain management specialist if there is any suspicion for CRPS. Initial treatment consists of hand therapy to prevent stiffness, along with an oral medication regimen that can include antidepressants, anticonvulsants, membrane-stabilizing agents, calcium-channel blockers, and adrenergic agents. Parenteral agents have also been used, but there are limited data on their outcomes. The exact regimen that is appropriate for each patient is beyond the scope of this article. Although patients may seem uncooperative with hand therapy, their continued participation is critical for maintaining hand motion and function. Contrast baths and transcutaneous electrical nerve stimulation units may help with pain control.[11,66]

The role of surgery in the treatment of CRPS has greatly expanded in recent years. After a thorough workup and identification of a specific nerve as the trigger, neurolysis, nerve decompression, or neuroma excision can be performed.[67] For patients with generalized sympathetic overactivity confirmed on sympatholytic challenge testing, surgical sympathectomy may provide benefit. In the worst cases when all other treatments have failed and stiffness is adversely affecting adjacent fingers and overall hand function, an amputation may be necessary.[63,66]

SUMMARY

Both operative and nonoperative management of hand fractures can lead to complications that can be challenging to treat. Therefore, all hand surgeons should have a keen understanding of the nature of these complications, how to avoid them, and how to treat them when they do occur. This knowledge can ultimately give the patient an acceptable, and oftentimes even an excellent outcome, despite the initial complication.

REFERENCES

1. Chung KC, Spilson SV. The frequency and epidemiology of hand and forearm fractures in the United States. J Hand Surg Am 2001;26(5):908–15.
2. de Putter CE, Selles RW, Polinder S, et al. Economic impact of hand and wrist injuries: health-care costs and productivity costs in a population-based study. J Bone Joint Surg Am 2012;94(9):e56.
3. Green DP. Complications of phalangeal and metacarpal fractures. Hand Clin 1986;2(2):307–28.
4. Page SM, Stern PJ. Complications and range of motion following plate fixation of metacarpal and phalangeal fractures. J Hand Surg Am 1998;23(5):827–32.
5. Kozin SH, Thoder JJ, Lieberman G. Operative treatment of metacarpal and phalangeal shaft fractures. J Am Acad Orthop Surg 2000;8(2):111–21.
6. Creighton JJ Jr, Steichen JB. Complications in phalangeal and metacarpal fracture management. Results of extensor tenolysis. Hand Clin 1994;10(1):111–6.
7. Balaram AK, Bednar MS. Complications after the fractures of metacarpal and phalanges. Hand Clin 2010;26(2):169–77.
8. Fusetti C, Meyer H, Borisch N, et al. Complications of plate fixation in metacarpal fractures. J Trauma 2002;52(3):535–9.
9. Gaston RG, Kuremsky MA. Postoperative infections: prevention and management. Hand Clin 2010;26(2):265–80.
10. Kurzen P, Fusetti C, Bonaccio M, et al. Complications after plate fixation of phalangeal fractures. J Trauma 2006;60(4):841–3.
11. Markiewitz AD. Complications of hand fractures and their prevention. Hand Clin 2013;29(4):601–20.
12. Stern PJ, Wieser MJ, Reilly DG. Complications of plate fixation in the hand skeleton. Clin Orthop Relat Res 1987;(214):59–65.
13. Meals C, Meals R. Hand fractures: a review of current treatment strategies. J Hand Surg Am 2013;38(5):1021–31 [quiz: 1031].
14. Duncan RW, Freeland AE, Jabaley ME, et al. Open hand fractures: an analysis of the recovery of active motion and of complications. J Hand Surg Am 1993;18(3):387–94.
15. Ring D. Malunion and nonunion of the metacarpals and phalanges. Instr Course Lect 2006;55:121–8.
16. Bannasch H, Heermann AK, Iblher N, et al. Ten years stable internal fixation of metacarpal and phalangeal hand fractures-risk factor and outcome analysis show no increase of complications in the treatment of open compared with closed fractures. J Trauma 2010;68(3):624–8.
17. Botte MJ, Davis JL, Rose BA, et al. Complications of smooth pin fixation of fractures and dislocations in the hand and wrist. Clin Orthop Relat Res 1992;(276):194–201.
18. Hsu LP, Schwartz EG, Kalainov DM, et al. Complications of K-wire fixation in procedures involving the hand and wrist. J Hand Surg Am 2011;36(4):610–6.
19. Faruqui S, Stern PJ, Kiefhaber TR. Percutaneous pinning of fractures in the proximal third of the proximal phalanx: complications and outcomes. J Hand Surg Am 2012;37(7):1342–8.
20. Young VL, Wray RC Jr, Weeks PM. The surgical management of stiff joints in the hand. Plast Reconstr Surg 1978;62(6):835–41.
21. Agee J. Treatment principles for proximal and middle phalangeal fractures. Orthop Clin North Am 1992;23(1):35–40.
22. Coonrad RW, Pohlman MH. Impacted fractures in the proximal portion of the proximal phalanx of the finger. J Bone Joint Surg Am 1969;51(7):1291–6.
23. Yamazaki H, Kato H, Uchiyama S, et al. Results of tenolysis for flexor tendon adhesion after phalangeal fracture. J Hand Surg Eur Vol 2008;33(5):557–60.
24. Hahn P, Krimmer H, Muller L, et al. Outcome of flexor tenolysis after injury in zone 2. Handchir Mikrochir Plast Chir 1996;28(4):198–203.
25. Freeland AE, Orbay JL. Extraarticular hand fractures in adults: a review of new developments. Clin Orthop Relat Res 2006;445:133–45.
26. Schneider LH. Tenolysis and capsulectomy after hand fractures. Clin Orthop Relat Res 1996;(327):72–8.
27. Gould JS, Nicholson BG. Capsulectomy of the metacarpophalangeal and proximal interphalangeal joints. J Hand Surg Am 1979;4(5):482–6.
28. Uhl RL. Salvage of extensor tendon function with tenolysis and joint release. Hand Clin 1995;11(3):461–70.
29. Seitz WH Jr, Froimson AI. Management of malunited fractures of the metacarpal and phalangeal shafts. Hand Clin 1988;4(3):529–36.

30. Freeland AE, Lindley SG. Malunions of the finger metacarpals and phalanges. Hand Clin 2006;22(3):341–55.
31. Buchler U, Gupta A, Ruf S. Corrective osteotomy for post-traumatic malunion of the phalanges in the hand. J Hand Surg Br 1996;21(1):33–42.
32. Diaz-Garcia R, Waljee JF. Current management of metacarpal fractures. Hand Clin 2013;29(4):507–18.
33. Froimson AI. Osteotomy for digital deformity. J Hand Surg Am 1981;6(6):585–9.
34. Gollamudi S, Jones WA. Corrective osteotomy of malunited fractures of phalanges and metacarpals. J Hand Surg Br 2000;25(5):439–41.
35. Hammert WC. Treatment of nonunion and malunion following hand fractures. Clin Plast Surg 2011;38(4):683–95.
36. Kollitz KM, Hammert WC, Vedder NB, et al. Metacarpal fractures: treatment and complications. Hand (N Y) 2014;9(1):16–23.
37. van der Lei B, de Jonge J, Robinson PH, et al. Correction osteotomies of phalanges and metacarpals for rotational and angular malunion: a long-term follow-up and a review of the literature. J Trauma 1993;35(6):902–8.
38. Strauch RJ, Rosenwasser MP, Lunt JG. Metacarpal shaft fractures: the effect of shortening on the extensor tendon mechanism. J Hand Surg Am 1998;23(3):519–23.
39. Meunier MJ, Hentzen E, Ryan M, et al. Predicted effects of metacarpal shortening on interosseous muscle function. J Hand Surg Am 2004;29(4):689–93.
40. Sanders RA, Frederick HA. Metacarpal and phalangeal osteotomy with miniplate fixation. Orthop Rev 1991;20(5):449–56.
41. Menon J. Correction of rotary malunion of the fingers by metacarpal rotational osteotomy. Orthopedics 1990;13(2):197–200.
42. Jawa A, Zucchini M, Lauri G, et al. Modified step-cut osteotomy for metacarpal and phalangeal rotational deformity. J Hand Surg Am 2009;34(2):335–40.
43. Weckesser EC. Rotational osteotomy of the metacarpal for overlapping fingers. J Bone Joint Surg Am 1965;47:751–6.
44. Gross MS, Gelberman RH. Metacarpal rotational osteotomy. J Hand Surg Am 1985;10(1):105–8.
45. Manktelow RT, Mahoney JL. Step osteotomy: a precise rotation osteotomy to correct scissoring deformities of the fingers. Plast Reconstr Surg 1981;68(4):571–6.
46. Pichora DR, Meyer R, Masear VR. Rotational step-cut osteotomy for treatment of metacarpal and phalangeal malunion. J Hand Surg Am 1991;16(3):551–5.
47. Pieron AP. Correction of rotational malunion of a phalanx by metacarpal osteotomy. J Bone Joint Surg Br 1972;54(3):516–9.
48. Botelheiro JC. Overlapping of fingers due to malunion of a phalanx corrected by a metacarpal rotational osteotomy–report of two cases. J Hand Surg Br 1985;10(3):389–90.
49. Vahey JW, Wegner DA, Hastings H 3rd. Effect of proximal phalangeal fracture deformity on extensor tendon function. J Hand Surg Am 1998;23(4):673–81.
50. Trumble T, Gilbert M. In situ osteotomy for extra-articular malunion of the proximal phalanx. J Hand Surg Am 1998;23(5):821–6.
51. Lester B, Mallik A. Impending malunions of the hand. Treatment of subacute, malaligned fractures. Clin Orthop Relat Res 1996;(327):55–62.
52. Teoh LC, Yong FC, Chong KC. Condylar advancement osteotomy for correcting condylar malunion of the finger. J Hand Surg Br 2002;27(1):31–5.
53. Harness NG, Chen A, Jupiter JB. Extra-articular osteotomy for malunited unicondylar fractures of the proximal phalanx. J Hand Surg Am 2005;30(3):566–72.
54. Tomaino MM. Distal interphalangeal joint arthrodesis with screw fixation: why and how. Hand Clin 2006;22(2):207–10.
55. Oak N, Lawton JN. Intra-articular fractures of the hand. Hand Clin 2013;29(4):535–49.
56. Jupiter JB, Koniuch MP, Smith RJ. The management of delayed union and nonunion of the metacarpals and phalanges. J Hand Surg Am 1985;10(4):457–66.
57. Ozcelik IB, Kabakas F, Mersa B, et al. Treatment of nonunions of the distal phalanx with olecranon bone graft. J Hand Surg Eur Vol 2009;34(5):638–42.
58. Meijs CM, Verhofstad MH. Symptomatic nonunion of a distal phalanx fracture: treatment with a percutaneous compression screw. J Hand Surg Am 2009;34(6):1127–9.
59. Kim J, Ki SH, Cho Y. Correction of distal phalangeal nonunion using PEG bone graft. J Hand Surg Am 2014;39(2):249–55.
60. Chow SP, Pun WK, So YC, et al. A prospective study of 245 open digital fractures of the hand. J Hand Surg Br 1991;16(2):137–40.
61. McLain RF, Steyers C, Stoddard M. Infections in open fractures of the hand. J Hand Surg Am 1991;16(1):108–12.
62. Reilly KE, Linz JC, Stern PJ, et al. Osteomyelitis of the tubular bones of the hand. J Hand Surg Am 1997;22(4):644–9.
63. Li Z, Smith BP, Smith TL, et al. Diagnosis and management of complex regional pain syndrome

complicating upper extremity recovery. J Hand Ther 2005;18(2):270–6.
64. Reuben SS. Preventing the development of complex regional pain syndrome after surgery. Anesthesiology 2004;101(5):1215–24.
65. Nijhuis TH, Smits ES, Jaquet JB, et al. Prevalence and severity of cold intolerance in patients after hand fracture. J Hand Surg Eur Vol 2010;35(4):306–11.
66. Li Z, Smith BP, Tuohy C, et al. Complex regional pain syndrome after hand surgery. Hand Clin 2010;26(2):281–9.
67. Jupiter JB, Seiler JG 3rd, Zienowicz R. Sympathetic maintained pain (causalgia) associated with a demonstrable peripheral-nerve lesion. Operative treatment. J Bone Joint Surg Am 1994;76(9):1376–84.

Management of Complications of Periarticular Fractures of the Distal Interphalangeal, Proximal Interphalangeal, Metacarpophalangeal, and Carpometacarpal Joints

Alex G. Dukas, MD, MA, Jennifer Moriatis Wolf, MD*

KEYWORDS

• Periarticular fractures • Complication • Treatment • Management • CMC • DIP • PIP • MCP

KEY POINTS

- Stiffness is a common complication of treatment of periarticular fractures; early motion is critical to its prevention.
- Instability can be a feature of periarticular fractures that must be considered.
- Posttraumatic arthritis is a common complication of periarticular fractures.

INTRODUCTION

Fractures of the hand are among the most common injuries resulting in emergency room visits. These injuries comprise up to 10% to 25% of all fracture-related visits to the emergency room.[1] In order of occurrence, distal phalanx fractures occur most commonly out of all hand fractures, followed by metacarpal, proximal phalanx, and middle phalanx fractures.[1] The vast majority of hand fractures are periarticular. For the most part, fractures of the hand have relatively good outcomes whether treated operatively or nonoperatively. However, complications do arise, and the hand surgeon must be able to recognize and treat them.

Distal Phalangeal Periarticular Fractures

Periarticular fractures of the distal interphalangeal (DIP) joint most commonly involve the insertion site of extensor or flexor tendon. These injuries are common in athletes.

Mallet finger fractures

- Definition: Disruption of the terminal extensor insertion results in a DIP extension lag that is termed a mallet finger. A volarly directed force

Funding Sources: None (Dr A.G. Dukas); Grants from American Foundation for Surgery of the Hand and Dept. of Defense (DOD-CDMRP-OR130096) (Dr J.M. Wolf).
Conflict of Interest: None (Dr A.G. Dukas); Salary, J Hand Surgery Deputy Editor; Salary, Elsevier Updates Editor (Dr J.M. Wolf).
Department of Orthopedic Surgery, UConn Health Center, New England Musculoskeletal Institute, Medical Arts & Research Building, 263 Farmington Avenue, Farmington, CT 06030, USA
* Corresponding author.
E-mail address: jmwolf@uchc.edu

Hand Clin 31 (2015) 179–192
http://dx.doi.org/10.1016/j.hcl.2015.01.009
0749-0712/15/$ – see front matter

to the tip of the finger, typically as the finger is actively extending, causes an acute flexion moment that ruptures the terminal extensor tendon.

- Bony mallet injuries result when the extensor insertion site is avulsed from the distal phalanx with a bony articular fragment (**Fig. 1**). Treatment of bony mallet injuries is based on whether the fracture is stable or unstable.
- For closed fractures involving less than 30% of the joint surface and no subluxation on imaging, full-time extension splinting is recommended for 6 weeks, followed by 6 weeks of nighttime splinting, with protective splinting during demanding activities. Fracture fragments of more than 30% of the articular surface or volar subluxation have been associated with permanent deformity.[2] Instability has been attributed to fracture fragments involving 30% to 50% of the articular surface.[2]
- Operative treatment usually consists of closed reduction and pinning, with options including simple pin fixation in extension or extension block pinning techniques.[3,4]

Both nonoperative and operative treatments have described risks of complications. The most frequently encountered issues include:

- Dorsal skin complications (irritation, maceration, ulceration, superficial infection);
- Recurrence of flexion deformity; and
- Cosmetic "bump" at the dorsal DIP joint.

Stern and Kastrup[5] reported a 45% skin complication rate with splinting. These complications were usually transient and consisted mainly of ulcerations, maceration, and pain. In the majority of cases, splint complications can be managed by changing the splint type, providing a custom splint, or readjusting the splint.

Persistence of extensor lag after treatment of mallet finger is common and not necessarily considered a complication. Crawford defined a good outcome as 10° or less after treatment.[6] During surgical correction, tendon balance is critical, because as little as 1 mm of terminal tendon lengthening can result in proximately 25° of DIP joint extension lag. Some extensor lag can be expected after treatment, is usually tolerated well, and typically causes no functional deficit or patient dissatisfaction.[7]

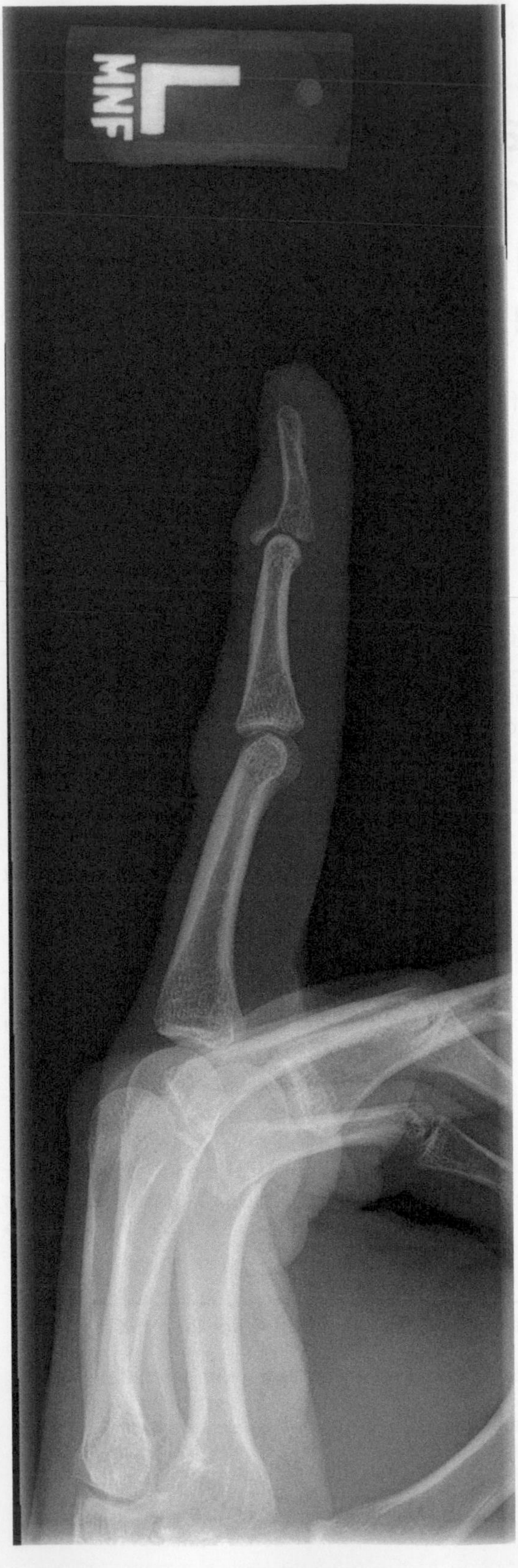

Fig. 1. Bony mallet injuries result when the extensor insertion site is avulsed from the distal phalanx with a bony articular fragment.

Operative intervention is indicated if the patient is dissatisfied with the appearance of the deformity or there is a functional deficit.[8] The senior author's preferred technique for correction of persistent lag is extensor repair or tenodermodesis with Kirschner wire fixation.[9] However, the patient is always warned that mild extensor lag is still a potential outcome, and with a salvage option of fusion of the DIP joint.

Other complications of bony mallet fractures include:

- Poor motion
- Pain.

These adverse outcomes may require DIP arthrodesis if symptomatic enough. The senior author's preferred technique is a "dorsal H"–type incision with cannulated screw fixation.

Finally, complications of pin fixation and arthrodesis include:

- Nailbed injury if the Kirschner wire or screw is placed too dorsally,[5] and
- Nonunion, requiring revision.[10] Nonunions are typically not symptomatic, owing to the fibrous tissue stabilization, but if painful, revision may be required.

Jersey finger fracture

- Definition: Disruption of the terminal flexor digitorum profundus (FDP) tendon insertion on the distal phalanx.
- Occurs less commonly than mallet finger.
- Most frequently seen in athletes, caused by an acute extension moment applied to the DIP while the FDP is firing.
- The ring finger is the most prone to this injury.[11] Diagnosis is often obscured by acute swelling and may be missed, as there is no pathognomonic deformity
- Physical examination reveals loss of active DIP flexion with the finger remaining in a position of relative extension compared with other digits and loss of passive tenodesis to the affected finger.

FDP ruptures with or without an associated bony avulsion were classified by Leddy and Packer into 3 types based on FDP location[12]:

- Type I: the tendon is retracted to the level of the distal palmar crease;
- Type II: the tendon end retracts to the proximal interphalangeal joint; and
- Type III: the tendon has an associated small bone fragment, which lies at the level of the DIP joint.
- Since their initial classification, a type IV injury was added, and is defined as a fracture with concomitant avulsion of the FDP tendon from the fracture fragment.[13]

All FDP avulsions require surgical repair of the tendon with either fixation or excision of the bony fragment based on size. In cases of Leddy IV injuries, the tendon repair can be combined with a grasping core suture stitch and Keith needle delivery through the sterile matrix with sutures tied over a button.

Complications of fixation that arise during treatment of Leddy III and IV injuries include:

- Loss of fixation;
- Nail ridging, which can be prevented by placement of the button distal to the germinal matrix area; and
- Flexor adhesions, which can be prevented potentially by early tendon rehabilitation, if possible.

Loss of fixation or nonunion is treated with open debridement, bone grafting, and fixation revision with Kirschner wires or compression screw.[14] Salvage of a failed FDP repair is achieved by DIP arthrodesis.

Periarticular Fractures About the Proximal Interphalangeal Joint

The proximal interphalangeal (PIP) joint is a hinge joint and is the most commonly injured joint of the hand.[15] Stability of the joint is provided:

- Dorsally by the extensor tendon central slip and lateral bands;
- Laterally by the collateral ligaments, accessory collateral ligaments, and the conjoined lateral bands; and
- Volarly by the volar plate, flexor tendons, and the fibro-osseous flexor tendon sheath.

Ligamentous disruption, volar plate avulsion, and any articular incongruity resulting from fractures disrupt this delicate balance. Fractures about the PIP joint pose a great challenge to the hand surgeon because of the predilection of this joint for stiffness, pain, arthritis, and residual deformities caused by soft tissue imbalance or adhesions. Fractures of the PIP joint often result from fracture dislocations. An axial and dorsally directed blow to the fully extended digit results in a dorsal fracture dislocation, where the middle phalanx volar plate insertion is avulsed, with associated metaphyseal comminution or impaction. Less common, but analogous to dorsal dislocations, volar fracture dislocations result from an axial shear loading of the extended digit resulting in an avulsion of the dorsal lip of the middle phalanx with possible impaction and comminution. Pilon fractures can result from a pure axial load on the extended PIP joint and are characterized by involvement of both the volar and dorsal cortical margins of the middle phalangeal base, with extensive comminution and depression of the central articular surface, making them highly unstable.

Volar plate injuries

Hyperextension of the PIP joint is prevented by the volar plate. The volar plate is a thick, ligamentous structure that forms the floor of the PIP joint. The volar plate originates proximally as laterally thickened cords anchored to the periosteum of the proximal phalanx and inserts distally on the volar aspect of the proximal middle phalanx.

Forced hyperextension with varying amounts of corresponding axial load to the joint may lead to various types of injury, ranging from a partial tear of the volar plate to an avulsion fracture of the phalanx (**Fig. 2**) and the possible corresponding dorsal dislocation. Dorsal PIP joint dislocations are the most common dislocations of the hand.

Hyperextension injuries are classified according to the Eaton classification for injuries of the volar plate and avulsion fractures:

- Type I: hyperextension injury to the volar plate and collateral ligaments, with no dislocation of the joint or presence of fracture;
- Type II: presence of dorsal dislocation of the PIP joint associated with volar plate and collateral ligament injury; and
- Type III: presence of fracture (typically at the base of the middle phalanx), associated with a hyperextension injury.

If the PIP joint is dislocated dorsally, a reduction maneuver using a combination of traction and hyperextension followed by flexion is typically effective. For dislocation to occur, the volar plate and at least one of the collateral ligaments must be disrupted. Most often the volar plate is avulsed from the distal insertion; however, a proximal avulsion is rare and, when it occurs, can become interposed in the joint blocking reduction. After reduction, stability of the joint must be assessed. The first step in avoiding complications is to determine the stability of the joint. This is obtained by clinical evaluation, and radiographic parameters.[16,17]

With Eaton type III fractures, the size of the articular fragment correlates with stability.[18] Generally, lateral x-rays of the PIP joint demonstrating:

- Thirty percent of the middle phalanx articular surface or less are stable.
- When 30% to 50% of the middle phalanx articular surface is involved, clinical evaluation is needed to determine stability.
- Fractures with greater than 50% involvement are unstable.
- Other radiographic signs of instability include loss of collinear alignment of the proximal and middle phalanx dorsal cortices as well as the dorsal "V" sign.[19]

If the PIP joint is stable, nonoperative treatment is indicated. This is treated routinely in an extension block splint and buddy taping to initiate early motion. For tenuous injuries that tend to subluxate in near full extension, extension block splinting can be used. In this scenario, an extension block splint is set at 10° less extension than the point at which instability occurs. Joint congruity is confirmed on x-rays. These injuries require close follow-up.

This method of treatment becomes less practical as the degree of necessary flexion to maintain joint stability becomes greater. Flexion beyond 60° impedes even minimal active arc of motion and can cause stiffness. Injuries of this type should be treated by operative means.[20]

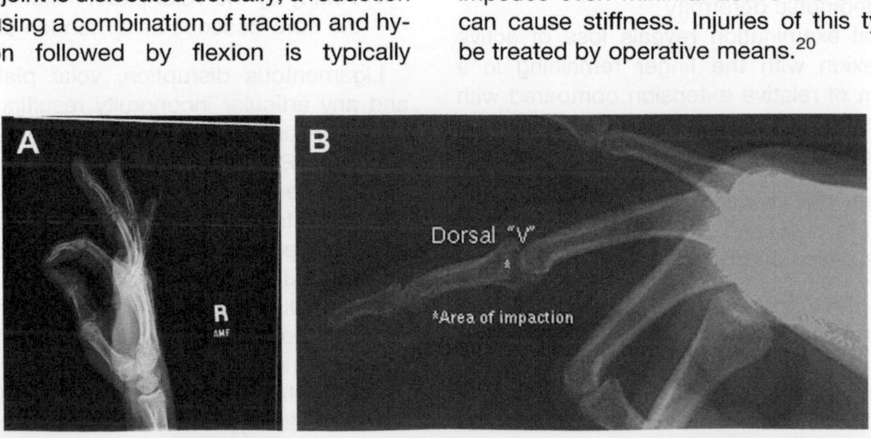

Fig. 2. (*A, B*) Forced hyperextension with varying amounts of corresponding axial load to the joint may lead to various types of injury, ranging from a partial tear of the volar plate to an avulsion fracture of the phalanx.

Surgical options include:

- Open reduction and internal fixation;
- Extension block pinning;
- Volar plate arthroplasty;
- Hemihamate arthroplasty; and
- External fixation.

There are a variety of ways to treat these fractures operatively. The ideal treatment strives to achieve a concentric reduction, allows for early motion, and minimizes edema and soft tissue disruption.

For larger fragments that can accommodate mini-screws, open reduction and internal fixation can provide anatomic reduction of the articular surface.[21] The rigid fragment fixation permits early mobilization (**Fig. 3**); however, the exposure required may increase the risk of stiffness, and precise bone reduction of the small bone fragments can be challenging.

External fixation and newer external fixators that provide dynamic traction allow for protected movement and supportive stability.[22] Complications include pin tract infections, loss of alignment or articular reduction, and pin site loosening, and require diligent follow-up.[22,23]

For extensively comminuted volar lip fractures or chronic dislocations owing to inadequate bony congruency, buttress support either by hemihamate arthroplasty or volar plate arthroplasty is a good option. Typically, volar plate arthroplasty is utilized in fractures involving less than 50% of the articular surface, whereas hemihamate arthroplasty can be used in fractures involving greater than 50% articular surface.[24–27] Volar plate arthroplasty requires removing comminuted fragments and advancing the volar plate to fill the defect to achieve stability. Reports of dislocation and coronal plane angulation have been reported in the

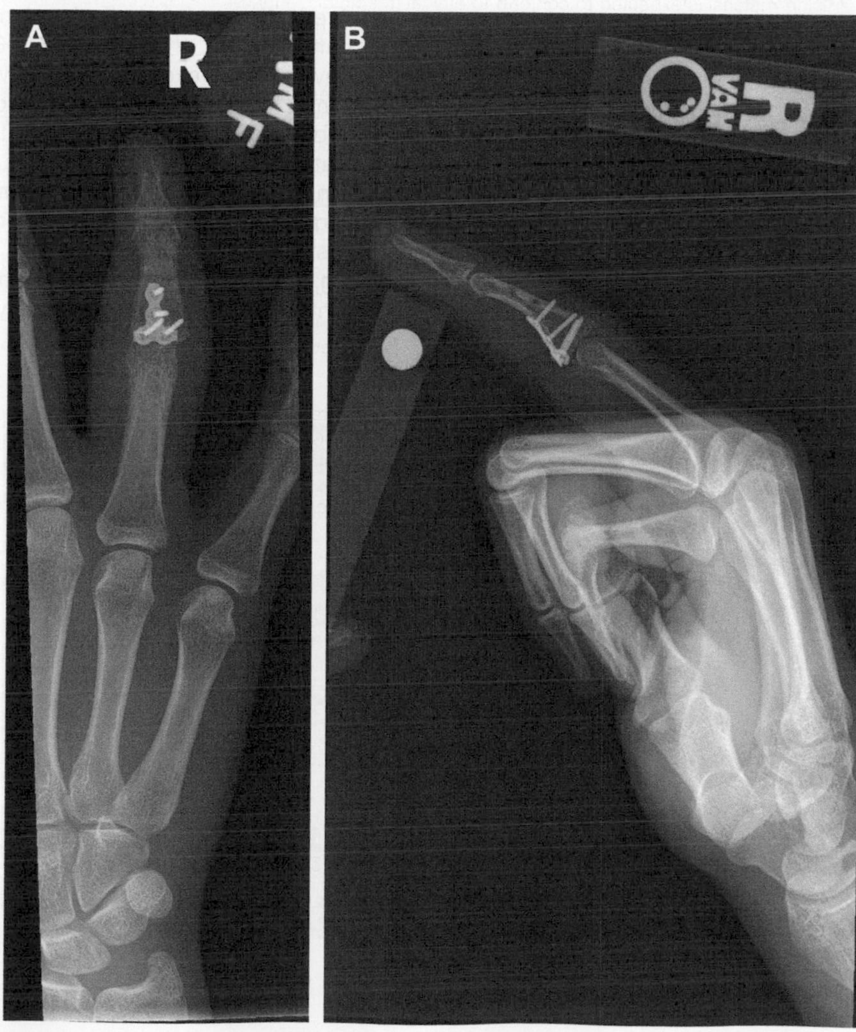

Fig. 3. (*A, B*) Rigid fragment fixation permits early mobilization.

literature.[18,25] Hemihamate arthroplasty has been used successfully to recreate the damaged portion of the volar articular surface and achieve stability. Redislocation has been reported.[17,26]

Extension block pinning limits motion at the PIP joint. When utilizing this technique, the surgeon can control the range of motion, but as with any percutaneous procedure, pin tract infections, loosening, and stiffness are possible complications.[20,28,29]

Bony central slip and boutonniere injuries

Dorsal lip fractures are not as common as volar lip fractures. If a dorsal base fracture involves the central slip insertion, this can present with acute boutonniere deformity (**Fig. 4**).[30] As with volar fractures, joint stability must be assessed and determined before treatment.[20] If the fracture is displaced, operative intervention is indicated.[30,31]

Fixation is typically accomplished through open reduction with mini-screw fixation or Kirschner wire fixation and immobilization. Usually open fixation is used for fractures involving larger fragments with less comminution, and Kirschner wire fixation reserved for smaller fragments. Zhang and colleagues[31] described their success with a technique in which a steel wire is looped under the central hood to provide fixation for the fragment. Complications include loss of reduction, joint extension lag, skin breakdown, pain, stiffness, and infections.[30–32]

PIP fracture–dislocations

Treatment of PIP fracture–dislocations includes:

- Initial closed reduction of the joint and assessment for stability through the arc of motion.
- Injuries requiring increased flexion to maintain stability are considered unstable and should be treated operatively.
- Presence of associated fracture of greater than 30% or continued subluxation on radiographic images indicates an unstable injury and necessitates operative intervention.
- Surgical options include:
    - Percutaneous pinning (avoiding the need for extensive soft tissue mobilization and dissection); and
    - Open reduction and internal fixation that provides interfragmentary compression and the option for earlier mobilization.

Eberlin and colleagues[33] reported outcomes for closed reduction and periarticular pinning of base and shaft fractures, showing that 63% were able to achieve good to excellent results with minimal loss of motion. The most common complication of closed pinning is stiffness. The best preventive and treatment for this complication is aggressive early range of motion and occupational therapy, including static progressive extension or flexion methods, serial casting, dynamic and static splinting, heat treatment, and edema control. The contribution of soft tissue injury increases

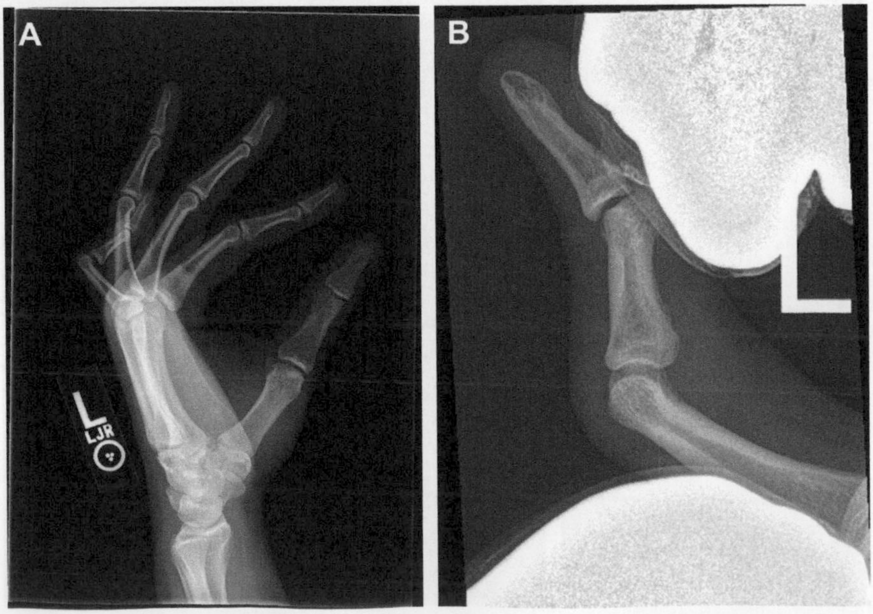

Fig. 4. (*A*, *B*) Soft tissue boutonniere deformity without dorsal base fracture.

the risk of complications in these injuries as well.[34,35]

Persistent PIP joint contracture can be treated operatively. Before operative intervention is pursued, it must be determined whether or not the contracture is caused by soft tissue imbalance or malunion resulting in a block to motion. Jupiter and colleagues[36] postulated that stiff digits are often caused by bony deformity and soft tissue injury. If this is the case, osseous abnormalities must be corrected before addressing soft tissue contracture.

Simple excision of bony spurs blocking joint motion can be performed with a small incision over the location of the spur and careful soft tissue handling. Light[37] noted that, in early osteotomy of intraarticular malunions, careful curettage of the maturing callus at the fracture site often allows excellent visualization of the articular incongruity. Reestablishment of the articular surface can be accomplished by early callus takedown. Mobilization of fracture fragments and packing of the bone void with cancellous autograft from the distal radius or olecranon can also be used.

The senior author's preferred treatment for bony contracture caused by phalangeal malunion is a volar approach when possible, which avoids violation of the extensor mechanism and allows excellent visualization of the articular surface. With intraarticular step-off, depressed pieces are elevated and then autograft obtained from Lister tubercle is placed. We use the lowest profile hardware that achieves fixation, such as countersunk screws with a small L- or T-shaped plate, which can be bent to fit the profile of the phalanx.

If loss of motion is caused by soft tissue contracture or imbalance of flexor or extensor tendon adhesions, tenolysis is performed. Many authors recommend limiting the contracture release to either the flexor or extensor side but not both, because this can potentially cause swelling and hinder the postoperative therapy program. As shown in **Table 1**, Jupiter and colleagues described 6 types of finger stiffness, with an additional 2 types contributed by Kaplan. Although described for the PIP joint, this classification can be expanded for evaluation of any hand joint. If both the flexor and extensor side of the joint must be addressed, staged release is recommended. The senior author's preference is to address the flexor side first, owing to the ability to safely expose the joint and to address more easily adhesions volarly as well as radially and ulnarly.

Chronic PIP joint fracture–dislocations represent a difficult problem, and treatment is fraught with complications. Operative options include hemihamate arthroplasty or volar plate arthroplasty if no osteoarthritis of the remnant joint is present. Volar plate arthroplasty is an option when 50% or less of the articular surface is preserved, with risk for recurrent subluxation and flexion contracture with greater involvement of the joint surface.[16] Calfee and colleagues[27] reported on a series of PIP fracture–dislocations treated with hemihamate arthroplasty in both the acute and chronic setting. The patients with chronic dislocations treated by hemihamate arthroplasty regained a similar arc of motion compared with those treated in the acute setting. The authors recommend hemihamate arthroplasty when more than 50% of the articular joint surface is involved.[27]

If the articular surface is arthritic or otherwise not reconstructable, salvage procedures are recommended. Joint fusion or arthroplasty are good options to eliminate pain and restore motion.

For PIP joint fusion, the position chosen depends on the finger affected. Conventionally, the recommended angle of fusion is[38]:

- 20° to 25° of flexion for the index finger;
- 30° of flexion in the middle finger;
- 40° of flexion and the ring finger; and
- 40° to 50° of flexion in the small finger.

For PIP arthroplasty, options include:

- Silicone;
- Metal-polyethylene implants; and
- Pyrocarbon.

Silicone has stood the test of time as an arthroplasty material, although complications include fracture, dislocation, and loss of motion.[39] Metal and polyethylene implants are used less commonly. Finally, the use of pyrocarbon implants at the PIP joint has had reported complications of loosening, squeaking, and failure.[40]

Metacarpophalangeal Dislocations and Periarticular Metacarpal Fractures

Simple dislocations or fracture–dislocations of the metacarpophalangeal (MCP) joint (**Fig. 5**) generally require operative intervention. In a simple dislocation, the proximal phalanx becomes dorsally dislocated over the metacarpal head and the volar plate ruptures proximally with resultant interposition between the articular surfaces.[16] Attempts at closed reduction by longitudinal traction often further incarcerate the metacarpal head between the lumbrical radially and the flexor tendons ulnarly.[16]

Irreducible fracture–dislocations are best approached through a dorsal incision. Care must

Table 1
Classification of digital stiffness

Stiffness	Motion on Examination	Dorsal Abnormality	Volar Abnormality	Treatment
Type 1	Limited passive flexion Passive extension	Extensor tendon adhesions Dorsal capsular or collateral ligament contracture	Volar plate tightness Contracture of checkrein or accessory collateral ligaments Skin deficiency A2 pulley insufficiency	Stage 1: release extensor adhesions and dorsal capsulectomy Stage 2: flexor tenolysis/tendon reconstructive procedures; release of volar plate and checkrein ligaments
Type 2	Limited passive flexion Limited active extension	Dorsal capsular or collateral ligament contracture Extensor tendon adhesions	Dorsal abnormality precludes reliable assessment of flexor mechanism	Stage 1: release extensor adhesions and dorsal capsulectomy. Evaluate for flexor insufficiency Stage 2: flexor tenolysis or reconstruction
Type 3	Limited active flexion, full passive flexion Limited passive extension		Flexor adhesions or partial rupture Volar plate or accessory collateral contracture; skin deficiency/contracture A2 pulley insufficiency	Tenolysis or reconstruction of flexor mechanism Volar plate/accessory collateral/checkrein release pulley reconstruction Skin release, lengthening, graft
Type 4	Limited active flexion or extension	Incompetent or overlengthened extensor mechanism	Intrasynovial flexor adhesions or flexor insufficiency	Stage 1: extensor tendon reconstruction Stage 2: flexor tendon lysis of adhesions or reconstruction
Type 5	Limited passive extension		Volar plate contracture Volar scarring Dupuytren contracture	Splinting Surgical release of contractile tissue
Type 6	Limited active flexion		Flexor adhesions or flexor insufficiency	Flexor tenolysis or flexor reconstruction
Type 7	Limited passive flexion	Burn or scar contracture	Bone block	Skin and contracture release
Type 8	Limited active extension	Extensor injury (central slip or distal extensor rupture)		Splinting (early) Extensor repair or reconstruction

Courtesy of American Society for Surgery of the Hand, Chicago, Illinois; with permission.

be taken to protect the radial digital neurovascular bundle because it is often tented superficially over the metacarpal head.[41] Flexor tendons are generally found ulnar to the metacarpal head. A freer is then used to remove the interposed volar plate with subsequent joint reduction. There are minimal data on outcomes after these injuries,[16] although most patients are reported to regain full motion within 4 to 6 weeks after injury.

Metacarpal fractures make up about approximately one-third of all hand fractures.[1] The small finger ray is most commonly affected. The bony anatomy of the metacarpals forms the transverse and longitudinal arches of the hand. Metacarpals

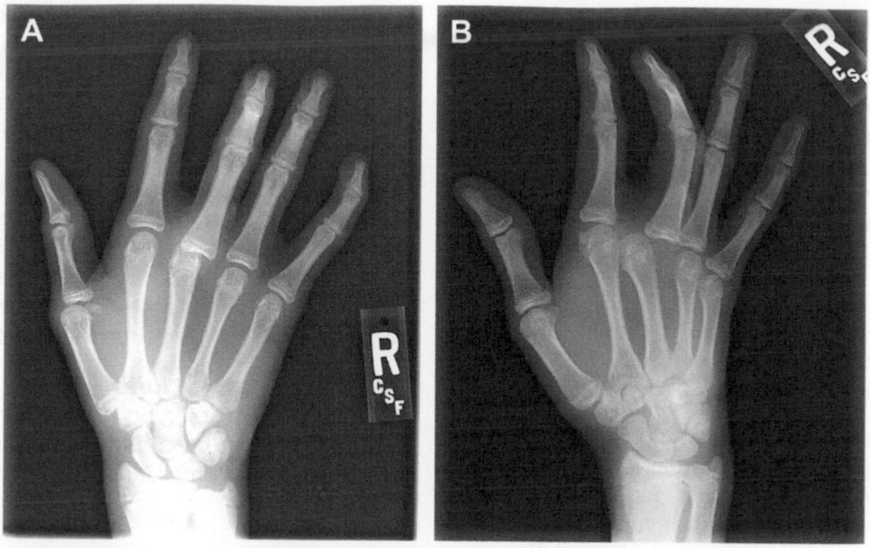

Fig. 5. (*A, B*) Metacarpophalangeal dislocation of the middle finger. These typically require open operative reduction.

are stabilized distally by the deep transverse intermetacarpal ligaments and proximally by the interosseous ligaments. The index and middle finger rays are more rigid than the ring finger and small finger joints. Owing to the cam shape of the metacarpal head, the collateral ligaments are tight in flexion and loose in extension. Excessive hyperextension of the MCP joint is limited by the volar plate, which attaches to the intermetacarpal ligament.

Typical management of metacarpal fractures is conservative. Extraarticular fractures often do not require operative intervention. As long as clinical malrotation causing scissoring is not present, angular deformity and even minor rotational deformity are well-tolerated.[42,43]

Periarticular fractures of the metacarpal are classified by location:

- Head,
- Neck, and
- Base.

Metacarpal head fractures

Typical surgical indications for metacarpal head fractures include:

- Articular step-off of greater than 1 mm;
- Comminution greater than 25%; and
- Involvement of the articular surface.

Typically metacarpal head fractures are treated with open reduction and internal fixation of the small fracture fragments. Headless, countersunk, cannulated screws are often a good option. Complications of these fractures include:

- Stiffness and
- Posttraumatic osteoarthritis.

Stiffness can be prevented by early motion in the stably fixed metacarpal head fracture. If the surgeon is concerned about bony stability, immobilization in the intrinsic plus position is key to maintaining MCP joint flexibility. Arthrolysis can be performed late, if needed, to take down adhesions, but is rarely necessary at the MCP joint, unlike the PIP joint.

Posttraumatic osteoarthritis is a common radiographic outcome, but unless it is symptomatic it is not necessarily a complication. Prevention is achieved by the best anatomic fixation possible; if painful posttraumatic arthritis occurs, this can be addressed by MCP arthroplasty, with material options including silicone, metal/polyethylene, or pyrocarbon materials.

Metacarpal neck fractures

Commonly metacarpal neck fractures present with dorsal angulation and rotational deformity. The index and middle rays, owing to the relative rigidity of their associated carpometacarpal (CMC) joints can only tolerate 10° and 20° degrees of angulation, respectively. The ring and small fingers have more CMC motion can tolerate angulation of up to 40° and 50° degrees and some studies have shown up to 70° without functional deficit.[44] Digital overlap or "scissoring" rotational deformity is an indication for operative fixation.

Typical fixation requires closed reduction and percutaneous pinning (**Fig. 6**). Many methods and configurations have been described. The preferred method is placement of 2 or more intramedullary Kirschner wires in an antegrade fashion from the base across the fracture site and docked in the subchondral bone of the head.

Possible complications of treatment include:

- Malunion (nonoperative treatment);
- Stiffness; and
- Adhesion formation.

Complications from metacarpal neck fractures are rare. For nonoperative treatment, subsequent malunion with symptomatic angulation or rotational deformity is the most common complication. If not addressed acutely, residual angulation can leave a prominent volar metacarpal head that can be painful with gripping, or cause a pseudoclawing and hyperextension of the MCP. Rotational deformity may cause finger overlap and interfere with finger flexion. Metacarpal osteotomy to address either a sagittal or rotational malunion may be necessary.

Although percutaneous fixation decreases the potential for scarring and adhesion formation, immobilization is necessary. Stiffness or adhesions are common. Schädel-Höpfner and associates[45] showed that patients treated with antegrade intramedullary fixation, placed through the base of the metacarpal and avoiding the MCP joint, had better MCP motion when compared with those treated with traditional retrograde crossed pinning, presumably owing to extensor hood scarring. Early motion can prevent stiffness and adhesion formation. Tenolysis can be performed late if necessary.

Metacarpal base fractures

These are most common at the fourth and fifth metacarpal bases, and at the thumb metacarpal. Treatment and complications are addressed in the CMC section.

Carpometacarpal Fractures and Dislocations

The thumb

Fractures and dislocations about the CMC joint most commonly occur at the thumb. In both intraarticular and extraarticular thumb base fractures, the abductor pollicis longus is the main deforming force pulling these fractures into flexion.

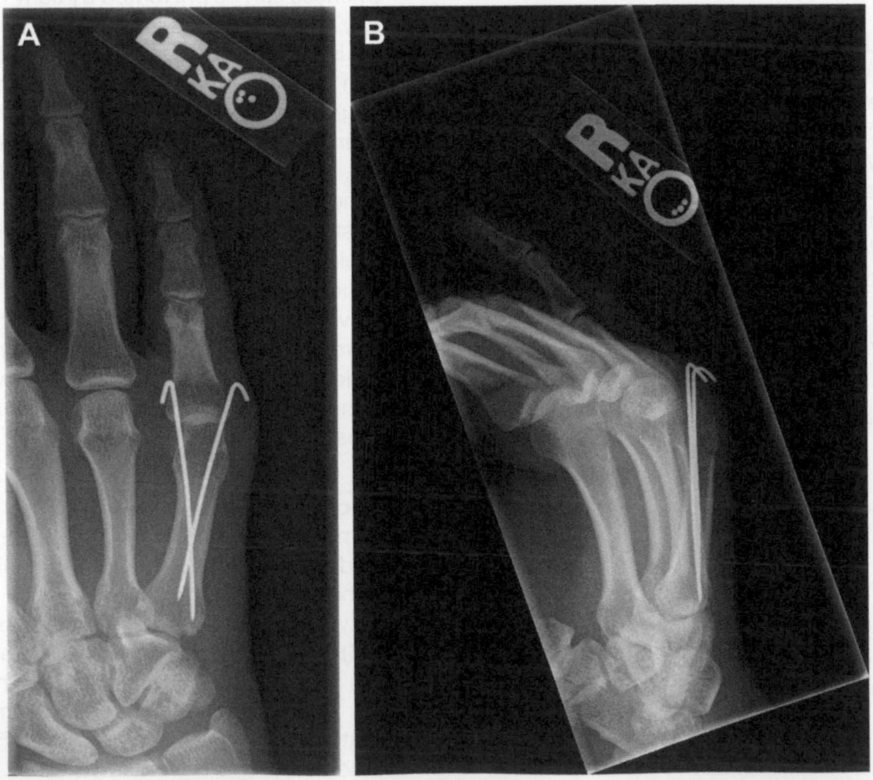

Fig. 6. (*A*, *B*) Typical fixation requires closed reduction and percutaneous pinning.

Fractures at the thumb CMC joint can be divided into:

- Bennett fractures (2-part fractures involving the volar ulnar corner of the metacarpal and the remaining metacarpal base);
- Rolando fractures (T-type or Y-type articular split fractures; **Fig. 7**); and
- Extraarticular or epibasilar fractures.

Although the mainstay of treatment for extraarticular fractures is closed management, Bennett and Rolando fractures have a tendency to displace during closed treatment.[46] Open or closed reduction and fixation is often necessary for definitive treatment. Bennett fractures can be treated by a variety of methods, including:

- Percutaneous pinning;
- Headless screw fixation; and
- Tension band wire fixation.

Rolando fractures, because of their comminution with risk of irregularity of the joint surface, are often treated by means of open reduction and plate fixation with an inverted T-plate configuration.

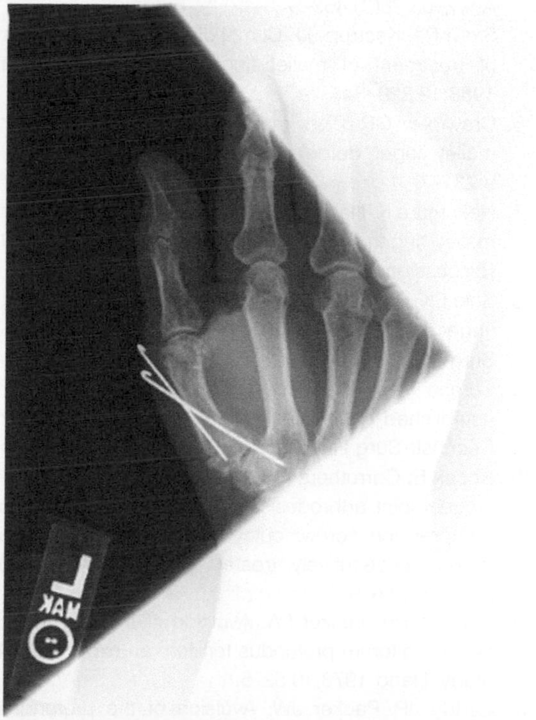

Fig. 7. Rolando type fracture of the first metacarpal base transfixed with two Kirschner wires.

Although most of these treatments result in successful bone healing, complications include:

- Malunion, typically owing to angulation; and
- Posttraumatic osteoarthritis.

Prevention of these complications can be achieved with close follow-up for loss of reduction. Corrective osteotomy and revision open reduction and internal fixation have been described for cases of significant thumb metacarpal malunion.[47,48] The fracture site is easily exposed through a Wagner-type incision. In salvage situations, CMC trapeziectomy and interposition arthroplasty is a good choice to relieve pain from posttraumatic arthritis.

Extraarticular fractures can often be treated closed, because up to approximately 25° of flexion angulation can be tolerated in extraarticular fractures. When metacarpal deformities exceed 30°, compensatory MCP hyperextension is likely to occur and operative reduction and fixation should be performed.

Ring and small finger metacarpal base fractures

Although relatively rare, metacarpal base fractures of the fourth and fifth digits can occur with axial loading and flexion causing impaction of the volar base into the hamate. Fractures of the fifth metacarpal base are often the result of direct trauma to the metacarpal base, experienced during a fall or as a result of the patient's striking a hard object with a firmly clenched fist.[49–51] The extensor carpi ulnaris is the primary deforming force that displaces the fracture fragment causing ulnar displacement. These injuries are often missed on initial review of radiographs.

Radiographic evidence for ring and small CMC fractures include:

- Loss of parallelism and symmetry at the fourth CMC joint; and
- Evidence of overlap at the fifth CMC joint (**Fig. 8**A, B).

Fourth and fifth metacarpal base fractures are best viewed with a lateral radiograph in 30° pronation.[52] In the acute setting, these fractures can be immobilized in a dorsal and volar splint with the wrist in 30° of extension and the MCP joints unimpeded. Traction in 30° of extension assists in reduction of these fractures by minimizing the deforming dorsal ulnar pole of the extensor carpi ulnaris on the displaced metacarpal base.[53] Many treatments have been proposed, including cast immobilization, open reduction and internal fixation, or percutaneous Kirschner wire fixation (see **Fig. 8**C).[53,54]

The CMC joints of the fourth and fifth ray have inherently more motion than the second and third

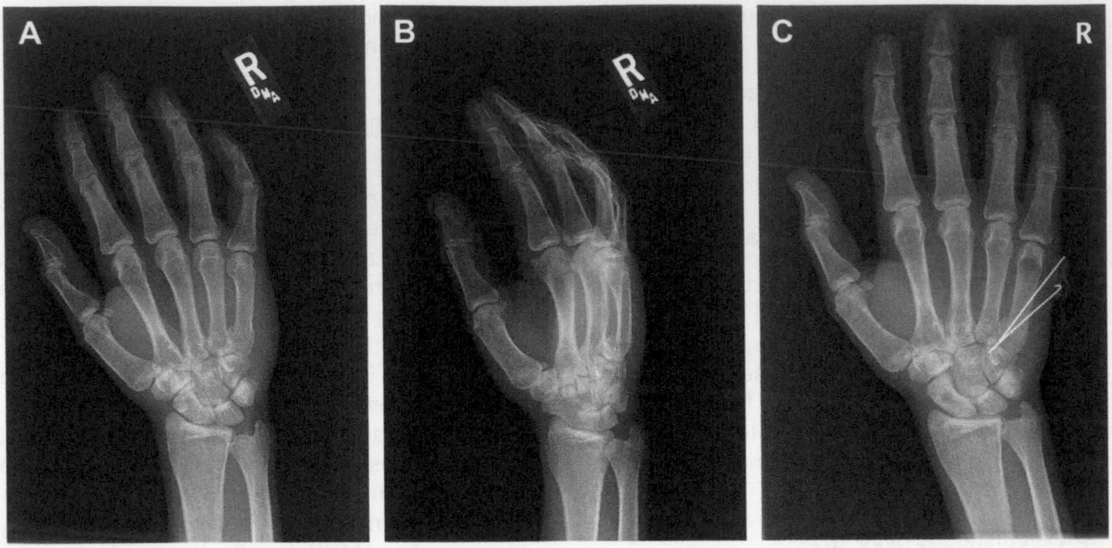

Fig. 8. (*A,B*) Displaced and angulated fracture of the base of the small finger metacarpal. (*C*) Closed reduction and pinning of the fracture using Kirschner wires.

rays. This fact, coupled with the deforming force of the extensor carpi ulnaris, decreases the ability to maintain an anatomic reduction of these fractures. Complications include:

- Painful malunion;
- Nonunion; and
- Posttraumatic arthritis.

Freeland and Lindley[55] recommended corrective osteotomy if needed for issues of function, or capsulolysis if soft tissue release is sufficient. Additionally, CMC fusion can be considered for persistent painful osteoarthritis at the ring and small finger bases.

SUMMARY

Fractures about the hand are one of the most common injuries. Many of these injuries can be successfully treated nonoperatively. However, complications do arise and most commonly include stiffness and osteoarthritis. The soft tissues are damaged by the initial trauma, and any surgical intervention to restore bony anatomy or soft tissue repair can produce scarring and motion deficits. Early mobilization is vital to support recovery of joint motion, which in the case of hand fractures is challenged by the need for immobilization for healing.

REFERENCES

1. Van Onselen EB, Karim RB, Hage J, et al. Prevalence and distribution of hand fractures. J Hand Surg Am 2003;28B:491–5.
2. Alla SR, Deal ND, Dempsey IJ. Current concepts: mallet finger. Hand (N Y) 2014;9(2):138–44.
3. Mazurek MT, Hofmeister EP, Shin AY, et al. Extension-block pinning for treatment of displaced mallet fractures. Am J Orthop (Belle Mead NJ) 2002; 31(11):652–4.
4. Hofmeister EP, Mazurek MT, Shin AY, et al. Extension block pinning for large mallet fractures. J Hand Surg Am 2003;28(3):453–9.
5. Stern PJ, Kastrup JJ. Complications and prognosis of treatment of mallet finger. J Hand Surg Am 1988;13:329–34.
6. Crawford GP. The molded polythene splint for mallet finger deformities. J Hand Surg Am 1984; 9:231–7.
7. Nakamura K, Nanjyo B. Reassessment of surgery for mallet finger. Plast Reconstr Surg 1994;93:141–9 [discussion: 150–1].
8. Shin EK, Bae DS. Tenodermodesis for chronic mallet finger deformities in children. Tech Hand Up Extrem Surg 2007;11:262–5.
9. Sorene ED, Goodwin DR. Tenodermodesis for established mallet finger deformity. Scand J Plast Reconstr Surg Hand Surg 2004;38:43–5.
10. Kocak E, Carruthers KH, Kobus RJ. Distal interphalangeal joint arthrodesis with the Herbert headless compression screw: outcomes and complications in 64 consecutively treated joints. Hand (N Y) 2011;6(1):56–9.
11. Manske PR, Lesker PA. Avulsion of the ring finger flexor digitorum profundus tendon: an experimental study. Hand 1978;10:52–5.
12. Leddy JP, Packer JW. Avulsion of the profundus tendon insertion in athletes. J Hand Surg Am 1977; 2(1):66–9.

13. Trumble TE, Vedder NB, Benirschke SK. Misleading fractures after profundus tendon avulsions: a report of six cases. J Hand Surg Am 1992;17:902–6.
14. Tuttle HG, Olvey SP, Stern PJ. Tendon avulsion injuries of the distal phalanx. Clin Orthop Relat Res 2006;445:157–68.
15. Elfar J, Mann T. Fracture-dislocations of the proximal interphalangeal joint. J Am Acad Orthop Surg 2013; 21:88–98.
16. Calfee RP, Sommerkamp TG. Fracture-dislocation about the finger joints. J Hand Surg Am 2009;34: 1140–7.
17. Shah CM, Sommerkamp TG. Fracture dislocation of the finger joints. J Hand Surg Am 2014;39(4): 792–802.
18. Mangelson JJ, Stern PJ, Abzug JM, et al. Complications following dislocations of the proximal interphalangeal joint. Instr Course Lect 2014;63:123–30.
19. Khouri JS, Bloom JM, Hammert WC. Current trends in the management of proximal interphalangeal joint injuries of the hand. Plast Reconstr Surg 2013; 132(5):1192–204.
20. Blazar PE, Steinberg DR. Fractures of the proximal interphalangeal joint. J Am Acad Orthop Surg 2000;8(6):383–90.
21. Hamilton SC, Stern PJ, Fassler PR, et al. Mini-screw fixation for the treatment of proximal interphalangeal joint dorsal fracture-dislocations. J Hand Surg Am 2006;31(8):1349–54.
22. Ruland RT, Hogan CJ, Cannon DL, et al. Use of dynamic distraction external fixation for unstable fracture-dislocations of the proximal interphalangeal joint. J Hand Surg Am 2008;33:19–25.
23. Ellis SJ, Cheng R, Prokopis P, et al. Treatment of proximal interphalangeal dorsal fracture-dislocation injuries with dynamic external fixation: a pins and rubber band system. J Hand Surg Am 2007;32: 1242–50.
24. Masden DL, Iorio ML, Higgins JP. Small joint reconstruction of the hand. Clin Plast Surg 2011;38: 751–60.
25. Eaton RG, Malerich MM. Volar plate arthroplasty of the proximal interphalangeal joint: a review of ten years' experience. J Hand Surg Am 1980;5:260–8.
26. Williams RM, Hastings H, Kiefhaber TR. PIP fracture/dislocation treatment technique: use of a hemi-hamate resurfacing arthroplasty. Tech Hand Up Extrem Surg 2002;6:185–92.
27. Calfee RP, Kiefhaber TR, Sommerkamp TG, et al. Hemi-hamate arthroplasty provides functional reconstruction of acute and chronic proximal interphalangeal fracture-dislocations. J Hand Surg Am 2009;34:1232–41.
28. Beekman RA, Abbot AE, Taylor NL, et al. Extensor mechanism slide for the treatment of proximal interphalangeal joint extension lag: an anatomic study. J Hand Surg Am 2004;29(6):1063–8.
29. Viegas SF. Extension block pinning for proximal interphalangeal joint fracture dislocations: preliminary report of a new technique. J Hand Surg Am 1992;17:896–901.
30. Posner MA, Green SM. Diagnosis and treatment of finger deformities following injuries to the extensor tendon mechanism. Hand Clin 2013;29:269–81.
31. Zhang X, Yang L, Shao X, et al. Treatment of bony boutonniere deformity with a loop wire. J Hand Surg Am 2011;36:1080–5.
32. Griffin M, Hindocha S, Jordan D, et al. Management of extensor tendon injuries. Open Orthop J 2012;6: 36–42.
33. Eberlin KR, Babushkina A, Neira JR, et al. Outcomes of closed reduction and periarticular pinning of base and shaft fractures of the proximal phalanx. J Hand Surg Am 2014;39:1524–8.
34. Pun WK, Chow SP, So YC, et al. A prospective study on 284 digital fractures of the hand. J Hand Surg Am 1989;14(3):474–81.
35. Duncan RW, Freeland AE, Jabaley ME, et al. Open hand fractures: an analysis of the recovery of active motion and of complications. J Hand Surg Am 1993; 18(3):387–94.
36. Jupiter JB, Goldfarb CA, Nagy L, et al. Posttraumatic reconstruction in the hand. Instr Course Lect 2007;56:91–9.
37. Light TR. Salvage of intraarticular malunions of the hand and wrist. The role of realignment osteotomy. Clin Orthop Relat Res 1987;(214):130–5.
38. Pellegrini VD, Burton RI. Osteoarthritis of the proximal interphalangeal joint of the hand: arthroplasty or fusion? J Hand Surg Am 1990;15:194–209.
39. Bales JG, Wall LB, Stern PJ. Long-term results of Swanson silicone arthroplasty for proximal interphalangeal joint osteoarthritis. J Hand Surg Am 2014;39: 455–61.
40. Sweets TM, Stern PJ. Pyrolytic carbon resurfacing arthroplasty for osteoarthritis of the proximal interphalangeal joint of the finger. J Bone Joint Surg Am 2011;93(15):1417–25.
41. Barry K, McGee H, Curtin J. Complex dislocation of the metacarpo-phalangeal joint of the index finger: a comparison of the surgical approaches. J Hand Surg Br 1988;13:466–8.
42. Burkhalter WE, Reyes FA. Closed treatment of fractures of the hand. Bull Hosp Jt Dis Orthop Inst 1984;44:145–62.
43. Ashkenaze DM, Ruby LK. Metacarpal fractures and dislocations. Orthop Clin North Am 1992;23:19–33.
44. Hunter JM, Cowen NJ. Fifth metacarpal fractures in a compensation clinic population. A report on one hundred and thirty-three cases. J Bone Joint Surg Am 1970;52(6):1159–65.
45. Schädel-Höpfner M, Wild M, Windolf J, et al. Antegrade intramedullary splinting or percutaneous retrograde crossed pinning for displaced neck fractures

of the fifth metacarpal? Arch Orthop Trauma Surg 2007;127(6):435–40.
46. Livesley PJ. The conservative management of Bennett's fracture-dislocation: a 26-year follow-up. J Hand Surg Am 1990;15B:291–4.
47. Giachino AA. A surgical technique to treat a malunited symptomatic Bennett's fracture. J Hand Surg Am 1996;21(1):149–51.
48. Jebson PJ, Blair WF. Correction of malunited Bennett's fracture by intra-articular osteotomy: a report of two cases. J Hand Surg Am 1997;22:441–4.
49. Schortinghuis J, Klasen HJ. Open reduction and internal fixation of combined fourth and fifth carpometacarpal (fracture) dislocations. J Trauma 1997; 42:1052–5.
50. Kjaer-Petersen K, Jurik AG, Petersen LK. Intra-articular fractures at the base of the fifth metacarpal. A clinical and radiographical study of 64 cases. J Hand Surg Br 1992;17(2):144–7.
51. Lundeen JM, Shin AY. Clinical results of intraarticular fractures of the base of the fifth metacarpal treated by closed reduction and cast immobilization. J Hand Surg Br 2000;25(3):258–61.
52. Bora FW, Didizian NH. The treatment of injuries to the carpometacarpal joint of the little finger. J Bone Joint Surg Am 1974;56(7):1459–63.
53. Bushnell BD, Draeger RW, Crosby CG, et al. Management of intra-articular metacarpal base fractures of the second through fifth metacarpals. J Hand Surg Am 2008;33(4):573–83.
54. Petrie PW, Lamb DW. Fracture-subluxation of base of fifth metacarpal. Hand 1974;6(1):82–6.
55. Freeland AE, Lindley SG. Malunions of the finger metacarpals and phalanges. Hand Clin 2006;22(3): 341–55.

Management of Complications of Wrist Fractures

R. Glenn Gaston, MD*, R. Christopher Chadderdon, MD

KEYWORDS

• Carpal fracture • Complications • Nonunion • Scaphoid

KEY POINTS

- The scaphocapitate syndrome is uncommon but easily missed on standard radiographs.
- Trapezial ridge fractures can also be overlooked with standard radiographs. Hook of hamate fractures are conspicuous on standard radiographs, and delayed diagnosis can lead to prolonged patient impairment, tendon rupture, and neurologic symptoms.
- Conservative treatment of scaphoid fractures can result in prolonged immobilization, time out of work, and ultimately nonunions.
- Scaphoid fractures are the second most common fracture of the upper extremity, and complications of both nonoperative and operative management are common.

INTRODUCTION

Scaphoid fractures account for nearly two-thirds of all carpal fractures and are second only to fractures of the distal radius in incidence of all upper-extremity fractures.[1] Complications of scaphoid fractures are numerous and include wrist stiffness, weakness, nonunion, malunion, avascular necrosis, and degenerative change. Fractures of the scaphoid are at times associated with even more complicated wrist injuries including fractures of the capitate and distal radius as well as greater arc injuries of the wrist.

Fractures of the other carpal bones are much less common; however, all share in common the potential for significant morbidity should complications in management arise. Because of the rarity of nonscaphoid carpal fractures, the diagnosis of many of these fractures can be easily overlooked if the clinician is not particularly astute.

Although a robust body of literature exists concerning the management and outcomes of carpal fractures, there is a paucity of evidence published on the complications of carpal fractures with the exception of scaphoid nonunions. The literature's attention to complications is sparse likely because of authors' reluctances to publish negative outcomes, especially those that are caused by poor surgical technique, although it is critically important to learn from our mistakes.

This chapter considers complications in the context of those occurring with surgery and those from nonoperative treatment. Furthermore, complications are considered in the context of modifiable and nonmodifiable factors (both by the patient and surgeon).

COMPLICATIONS OF SCAPHOID FRACTURES

Complications of Nonoperative Treatment

Many of the complications encountered in the management of scaphoid fractures can be avoided by the treating physician and are thus modifiable. The single most important modifiable complication is failure to diagnose. Delay in diagnosis and missed diagnoses can increase the risk of

OrthoCarolina, 1915 Randolph Road, Charlotte, NC 28207, USA
* Corresponding author.
E-mail address: glenn.gaston@orthocarolina.com

Hand Clin 31 (2015) 193–203
http://dx.doi.org/10.1016/j.hcl.2015.01.001

secondary complications including nonunion, avascular necrosis, posttraumatic arthritis, and flexor and extensor tendon ruptures.[2–4] Myriad factors can contribute to a delayed or missed diagnosis of a scaphoid fracture.

Failure to diagnose

Patients with scaphoid fractures often present for medical attention in a delayed fashion, as the injury can be minimally painful and is often dismissed as a simple sprain. Of patients who do seek medical attention, the clinical examination has is found to have a high sensitivity but a specificity of only 75% to 80% for scaphoid fracture.[5,6] The variables of male sex, sports injury, scaphoid tubercle tenderness, and anatomic snuffbox pain with wrist ulnar deviation are found to be independently significant positive factors for scaphoid fracture, and all 4 combined factors are 91% predictive of fracture.[7] When fracture is suspected, plain radiographs are routinely ordered but also have a sensitivity of only 65% to 70%.[8–10] When radiographs are normal but clinical suspicion is high, the physician has 2 options: either immobilize the wrist for 2 weeks then repeat x-rays or obtain advanced imaging, most often MRI scanning. Traditionally, it is taught that immobilization for 2 weeks and allowing some slight bone resorption to occur adjacent to the fracture site will make the fracture line visible on subsequent films.[11] It is our practice, based in part on our own complications, that when clinical suspicion is high, advanced imaging should be obtained. Two cases highlight this need. The first case is that of a teenage boy whose 2-week postinjury radiographs were still normal, but then he returned 9 months later with the obvious missed scaphoid nonunion (**Fig. 1**). Pediatric scaphoid fractures are reported to have a higher rate of false-negative radiographs, and, in this case, additional views at the 2-week visit could have potentially aided in the diagnosis.

Even in adults with appropriate films, however, missed injuries can occur. The second case is that of a 40-year-old-man with wrist pain after a fall whose radiographs remained normal even 6 weeks after injury. An MRI at 6 weeks found the extreme proximal pole fracture, and surgery followed (**Fig. 2**). Although there is an obvious financial cost to obtaining an MRI scan, the socioeconomic burden of immobilization or delayed diagnosis must be considered. Studies have found the cost of radiographs, immobilization, time off work, and office visits for an occult scaphoid fracture to be similar to or exceeding the cost of advanced imaging.[12–14] Advantages of MRI scanning versus other imaging modalities include its high sensitivity (95%–100%) and specificity (almost 100%) for detecting scaphoid fractures[15–17] and its ability to detect other soft tissue injuries in the differential diagnosis of similar wrist pain. Furthermore, in subacute or chronic cases of scaphoid fracture, MRI has utility in assessment of the vascularity of the proximal pole of the scaphoid, which may alter the surgical decision making.[18] One recent study challenged the notion that MRI should be the reference standard for suspected scaphoid fractures because of the higher-than-anticipated false-positive rate in healthy volunteers.[19] The utility of healthy volunteers without wrist pain or injury as a reference standard is debatable, however, and we continue to use MRI as our imaging modality of choice for suspected occult fractures.

Our algorithmic approach to the patient presenting with a clinical examination for scaphoid fracture is to obtain 4-view plain radiographs of the scaphoid (wrist posterior-anterior [PA], lateral, ulnar deviation, and pronated oblique). If radiographs are normal but clinical suspicion is high,

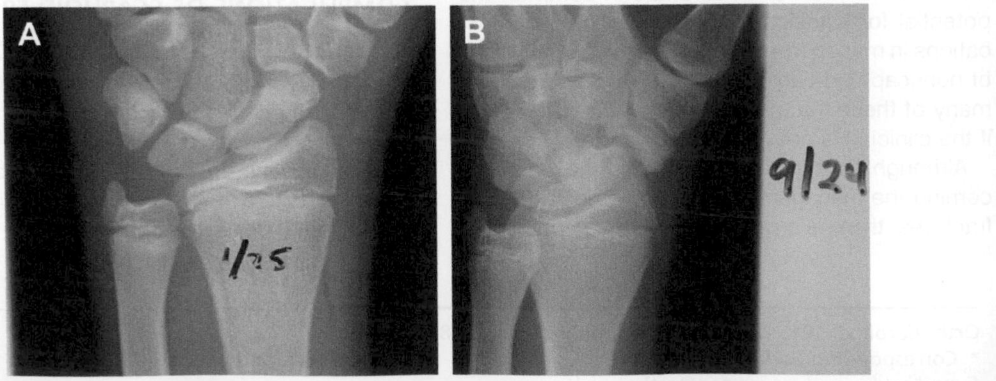

Fig. 1. (*A*) Wrist PA view 2 weeks postinjury shows no evidence of scaphoid fracture. (*B*) Wrist oblique radiograph 9 months postinjury shows scaphoid nonunion.

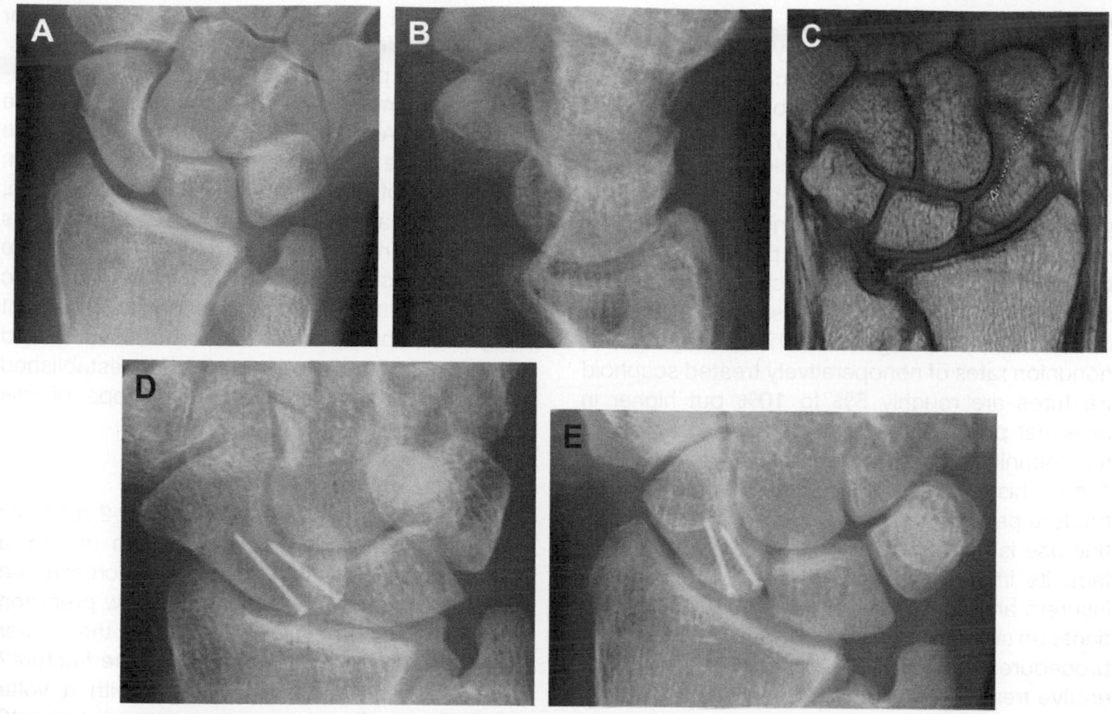

Fig. 2. (*A, B*) 6 week postinjury ulnar deviation and lateral wrist radiographs fail to show a fracture. (*C*) MRI 6 weeks postinjury shows a proximal pole scaphoid fracture (*arrow*). (*D, E*) Oblique and PA wrist radiographs status post screw fixation of the proximal pole fracture.

MRI is usually obtained to avoid delayed or missed injuries and unnecessary immobilization. Once the diagnosis of a scaphoid fracture has been made, one must embark on either operative or nonoperative care, both of which have potential complications. This decision is often based on perceived fracture stability and, thus, runs the risk of nonunion.

Guesstimating fracture stability

Because fracture displacement is the most critical factor in determining the risk of nonunion, our ability to determine fracture stability on imaging is paramount. Radiographic classifications such as the Mayo and Russe classifications[11,20] are based on the anatomic planes of the scaphoid, not considering fracture stability, and also are found to have low interobserver agreement.[21,22] The Herbert classification was designed to address fracture stability by separating perceived stable fractures (tubercle [A1] and incomplete waist [A2]), from potentially unstable fractures (oblique distal third [B1], displaced waist [B2], proximal pole [B3], fracture dislocations [B4], and comminuted fractures [B5]).[23] Recently, however, our traditional thinking of scaphoid fracture stability is called into further question. An important study by Buijze and colleagues[24] found radiographs and computed tomography (CT) scans to be unreliable in assessing scaphoid fracture stability compared with arthroscopy. This study used arthroscopy in 44 patients, half of whom had displaced fractures preoperatively and half of whom had nondisplaced fractures. At the time of arthroscopy, assessment of stability and displacement of the fracture was made. The sensitivity, specificity, and accuracy of plain radiographs in determining stability was 34%, 93%, and 55%, respectively, and CT scanning was found to be 62%, 87%, and 70%, respectively. The authors have found in their practice that seemingly nondisplaced stable fractures can prove to be unstable once directly visualized in the operating room. Although it remains unknown whether these radiographically inaccurately perceived stable nondisplaced fractures are at higher risk of nonunion compared with other truly stable nondisplaced fractures, it certainly seems that our ability to predict fracture stability is lower than previously thought. The decision of when to choose surgery and when cast immobilization alone will suffice is thus made even more difficult now. The decision is key in avoiding the most common complication of nonoperative treatment, nonunion.

Nonunion

The precarious blood supply is the primary impetus for scaphoid complications, especially nonunion and avascular necrosis. A retrograde blood flow from the radial artery into the nonarticular dorsal ridge of the scaphoid at its waist renders the proximal aspect of the scaphoid particularly vulnerable to nonunion and avascular necrosis.[25,26] The superficial palmar branch of the radial artery provides a much more rich blood supply to the distal pole, increasing the probability of union in the region of the bone. Overall, nonunion rates of nonoperatively treated scaphoid fractures are roughly 5% to 10% but higher in proximal pole fractures.[22] Additional risk factors for nonunion include displacement of more than 1 mm, history of osteonecrosis, vertical oblique fracture pattern, and nicotine use.[1] Of these, nicotine use is the only modifiable risk factor, and, in fact, its importance now is well appreciated by insurers and physicians alike and counseling patients on smoking cessation is now a billable office procedure. The final nonmodifiable risk of nonoperative treatment is avascular necrosis (AVN).

Avascular necrosis

AVN is reported to occur in up to 13% to 50% of all scaphoid fractures with an incidence increasing with more proximal fractures. Proximal one-fifth fractures have been shown to have rates approaching 100% in some studies.[23,26–28] Given the higher risk of both nonunion and AVN in proximal pole fractures, the authors favor surgical fixation of even nondisplaced proximal pole fractures. Waist fractures are more controversial.

Meta-analyses show that surgical treatment results in higher rate of union, less time off work, and higher improved functional outcomes but is associated with greater complication rates when compared with casting for nondisplaced and minimally displaced scaphoid waist fractures.[2] It is the authors' current practice to discuss the risks and benefits of surgery and casting with patients who have nondisplaced fractures to offer percutaneous screw fixation as an option for all patients. The primary risks of nonoperative treatment include prolonged healing time (which can increase time out of work or sport and disuse atrophy of the arm) and higher rate of nonunion. The complications associated with surgery, however, are more frequent.

Complications of Operative Treatment

Overall published complication rates of surgical fixation of scaphoid fractures vary widely from 0% to 29% with most studies reporting very low complication rates.[1,29] One recent report by Bushnell and colleagues[29] found a 21% major complication rate (nonunion, misplaced screws, and proximal pole fracture) and 8% minor complication rate (intraoperative screw and guide wire breakages). Although some complications have nonmodifiable risk factors (fracture location, some cases of nonunion/AVN, smoking cessation, hardware breakage), most surgical complications are in the control of the surgeon. These include surgical precision with screw placement, anatomic fracture alignment, iatrogenic tendon and ligament injury, and appropriate selection of vascularized versus nonvascularized grafts for established nonunions (which is beyond the scope of this article).

Screw placement

Precise screw placement is critical for 2 reasons: to minimize iatrogenic injuries and to maximize biomechanical strength (and thus increase the likelihood of union). Questions of screw precision include, should the screw be down the center axis of the bone or perpendicular to the fracture? Should the trapezium be violated with a volar approach to allow a proper screw placement? Should a volar or dorsal approach be preferred? McCallister and colleagues[30] showed biomechanically that a centrally placed screw provides 43% greater stiffness and 39% increased load to failure compared with an eccentrically placed screw, suggesting screws should ideally be placed down the central axis of the scaphoid. To obtain central screw placement from a volar approach, some surgeons prefer a transtrapezial approach to allow more accurate screw placement down the central aspect of the proximal and distal poles.[31] Central screw placement has remained the prevailing approach to scaphoid fracture management; however, in some cases this may not be the ideal or even practical method. In another biomechanical study, Luria and colleagues[32] found that screw placement perpendicular to the fracture site placed through the scaphoid tuberosity with a volar approach had similar stability to a screw placed down the central axis of the bone while avoiding placement of the screw across the scaphotrapeziotrapezoidal joint. In some extreme proximal pole fractures, screw placement perpendicular to the fracture site to gain purchase in the fragment may be necessary without central axis placement (see **Fig. 2**).

In terms of a volar or dorsal approach, there are sufficient clinical and biomechanical data to support both approaches as safe and effective.[33,34] Generally speaking, volar approaches are preferred for distal fractures and dorsal approaches for proximal fractures. Each approach carries its own unique complications. Volar approaches are at increased risk of scaphotrapeziotrapezoidal arthritis, although reported incidence is lower than previously suspected (less than 3% in one recent study),[35] whereas the dorsal approach places the extensor pollicis longus and the blood supply to the bone at higher risk. Other technical errors are likely far more common than the literature would suggest. We have experienced and have been referred cases of errant screw placement necessitating revision surgery. Despite multiple studies reporting additional fluoroscopic views as helpful in preventing misplaced screws,[36–38] improper screw placement still occurs, although the exact incidence remains unknown (**Fig. 3**). A final complication not reported, but one that the authors have seen, is propagation of a fracture at the site of screw insertion. In the authors' experience, the variable pitch cannulated headless Acutrak screw placed without the use of the second drill bit (termed *profile drill*), especially in proximal pole fractures, is particularly vulnerable. The trailing diameter of the micro and mini screws are 2.8 mm and 3.6 mm, respectively. By contrast, the standard long drill bit diameters are only 1.9 mm and 2.7 mm, respectively. Simply placing the screw after drilling with the standard long drill bit can generate excessive hoop stresses leading to iatrogenic fracture line propagation from the screw entry point during the insertional torque (**Fig. 4**). The profile drill bits are 2.9 mm and 3.4 mm (1 mm larger than the trailing screw diameter of each screw) and are recommended to minimize this risk of iatrogenic fracture of the proximal pole.

Malunion

The scaphoid fails in a predictable pattern of shortening, flexion, and at times rotationally as well producing the so-called humpback deformity. When the scaphoid unites either with or without surgery in a malunited position, the following are observed: the potential for altered carpal kinematics, ongoing pain, loss of motion, and degenerative change.[39,40] Although malunion is typically radiographically defined as an intrascaphoid angle of greater than 35°[40] the degree of clinical acceptability remains unknown. It appears that milder malunions are well tolerated,[41] but more severe malunions may remain symptomatic, although the literature is conflicting.

Forward and colleagues[42] found no correlation between the degree of malunion and patient outcomes (range of motion, grip strength, pain scores, and DASH scores) at 1-year follow-up in 42 cases. In contrast, Amadio and colleagues[40] reported on 46 scaphoid fractures (20 united with normal alignment and 26 with malunion). They found that those fractures healing in proper alignment had 83% satisfactory outcomes versus only 27% satisfactory outcomes in those healing with a malunion.[40] Similarly, Lynch and Linscheid[43] prospectively followed up with 13 patients who had symptomatic malunion with persistent pain, weakness, and limited wrist function necessitating osteotomy. All cases united with osteotomy and had a commensurate improvement in radiographic and functional outcomes at 42-month follow-up.[43] Jiranek and colleagues[44] reports the only long-term follow-up study on scaphoid malunions compared with properly aligned union cases that had undergone surgery with volar wedge grafting

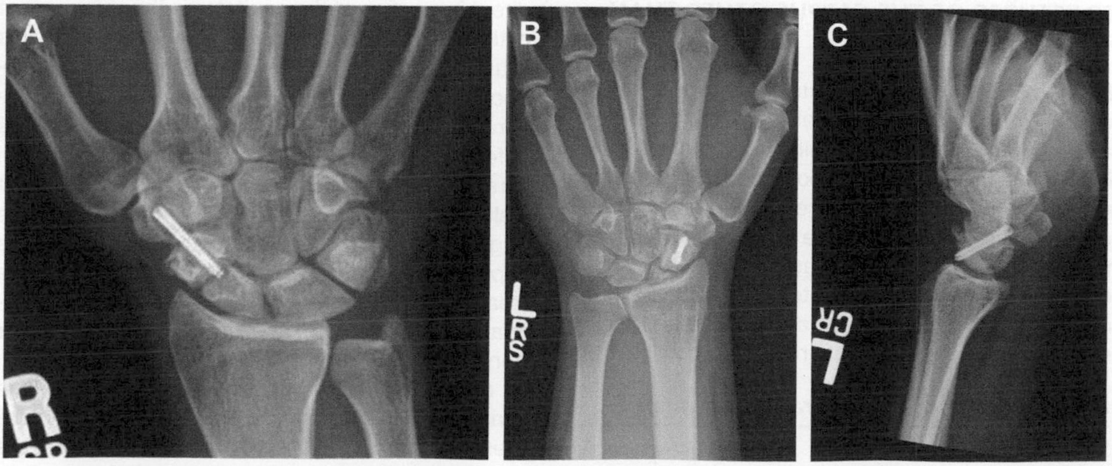

Fig. 3. (*A*) An erroneously placed screw across the scaphotrapezoid joint rather than the scaphoid nonunion. (*B*) A dorsal screw that failed to engage the proximal fragment. (*C*) A volar screw penetrating the proximal dorsal cortex.

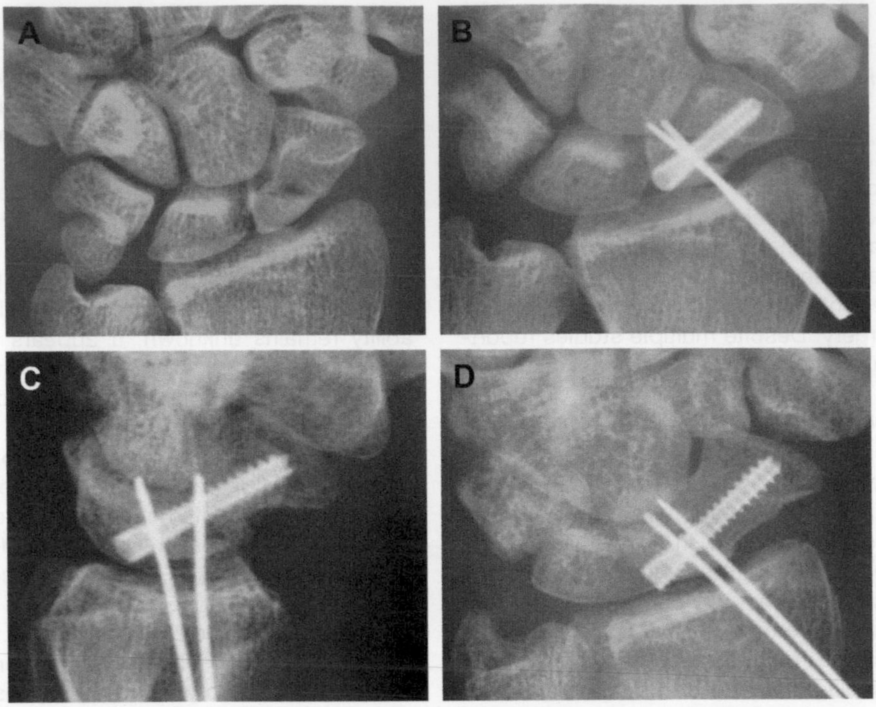

Fig. 4. (*A*) Preoperative wrist PA view shows a proximal third scaphoid fracture. (*B–D*) Postoperative PA, lateral, and oblique images show dorsal screw placement with additional K-wire fixation through the iatrogenic fracture of the proximal pole through the screw entry site.

for symptomatic nonunion as an index procedure. Interestingly, objective results were better in the properly aligned group (radiographic findings, range of motion, and strength); however, there was no difference in patient-rated subjective outcomes (pain, subjective function, satisfaction) at 11-year follow-up. When symptomatic malunion does develop, there is ample literature to support corrective osteotomy as an effective treatment option.[40,43,45]

FRACTURES OF THE CARPUS OTHER THAN THE SCAPHOID

Even though scaphoid fractures comprise most carpal fractures, injuries to all other carpal bones are also encountered. As with the scaphoid, it is imperative that a hand surgeon be familiar with the many fracture patterns, presentations, and appropriate treatments to minimize the risk of complications. Most complications associated with other carpal fractures seem to stem from delayed or missed diagnosis, but there are specific avoidable surgical complications that are also discussed.

Complications of Nonoperative Treatment

Scaphocapitate syndrome

An uncommon but easily misdiagnosed injury is the scaphocapitate fracture syndrome, originally described and referred to as naviculocapitate fracture syndrome by Fenton.[46] This injury pattern involves a fracture of the scaphoid along with a fracture of the proximal capitate; the proximal fragment may remain nondisplaced but can also be rotated 90° or 180°. There has been debate about the mechanism of injury. Most reports propose a wrist hyperextension mechanism, whereby either the radial styloid or dorsal lip of the radius directly impacts the capitate. However, extreme volar flexion of the wrist has also been implicated, resulting in direct impaction of the capitate on the volar aspect of the radius.[47] There is general consensus that this injury pattern includes a combination of transscaphoid and transcapitate perilunar fracture dislocation.[48–53] Vance and colleagues[47] described 6 different scaphocapitate patterns, including transverse fractures of the scaphoid and capitate without dislocation (type I), an inverted proximal capitate fragment that remains in articulation with the lunate (type II), a dorsal perilunate dislocation (type III), a volar perilunate dislocation of the carpus and proximal capitate (type IV), and isolated volar (type V) or dorsal (type VI) dislocation of the proximal capitate. As noted by Kim and colleagues,[54] these multiple variations can be more broadly categorized into 2 presentations—a transverse fracture of the scaphoid and capitate without dislocation (with or without proximal capitate fragment rotation) or dorsal perilunar dislocation variants. A hand surgeon may only encounter these injuries a handful of times in their career, and plain radiograph findings may be quite subtle (**Fig. 5**). Thus, a full awareness of the multiple presentations of the scaphocapitate fracture syndrome is critical to avoid a missed diagnosis. Indeed, there are several reports of delayed diagnosis, which can result in avascular necrosis or nonunion with resultant carpal arthritis and collapse. If a complex injury or sufficient mechanism presents and plain radiographs do not adequately elucidate the fracture pattern, then 3-dimensional imaging (CT scan) should be considered to detect these rare fractures.

Fractures of the trapezium

Fracture of the palmar trapezial ridge is another underrecognized and likely underdiagnosed injury pattern. Originally described by McClain and Boyes in 1966,[55] this rare carpal fracture typically occurs during a fall onto an outstretched hand resulting in either direct trauma to the ridge or an avulsion caused by a tension load applied via the insertion of the transverse carpal ligament as the trapezium and hypothenar eminence diverge.[56] Patients typically present with localized pain and tenderness at the base of the thenar eminence but may also have concordant median nerve symptoms. Pain may be elicited by wrist flexion against resistance, as this loads the flexor carpi radialis in its path over the trapezial ridge. As with hook of hamate fractures, standard hand radiographs do not adequately image the trapezial ridge. Hart and Gaynor[57] described the carpal tunnel view, and this places the palmar trapezial ridge in profile, typically allowing for adequate visualization. Alternatively, 3-dimensional imaging is definitive. Palmer[56] defined a type I fracture as a fracture of base of the ridge and noted that, if diagnosed early and treated with thumb spica immobilization, it will typically lead to fracture. Type II fractures involve the tip of the ridge and are more likely to lead to symptomatic nonunions, and Palmer[56] notes that consideration can be given to primary or delayed surgical fragment excision. Surgeons cognizant of this entity will obtain appropriate imaging and can avoid the potential complications of delayed diagnosis, including nonunion and prolonged hand dysfunction. An additional complication that the authors and others[58] have encountered is tendinitis and rupture of the flexor carpi radialis secondary to a missed diagnosis of a trapezial ridge fracture (**Fig. 6**).

Fractures of the hamate hook

Fractures of the hook of the hamate are common among athletes who participate in "ball and stick" sports, but can also occur with non–sports-related trauma, including falls onto an outstretched hand and motor vehicle collisions (direct impact of the hamulus or hook against the steering wheel).

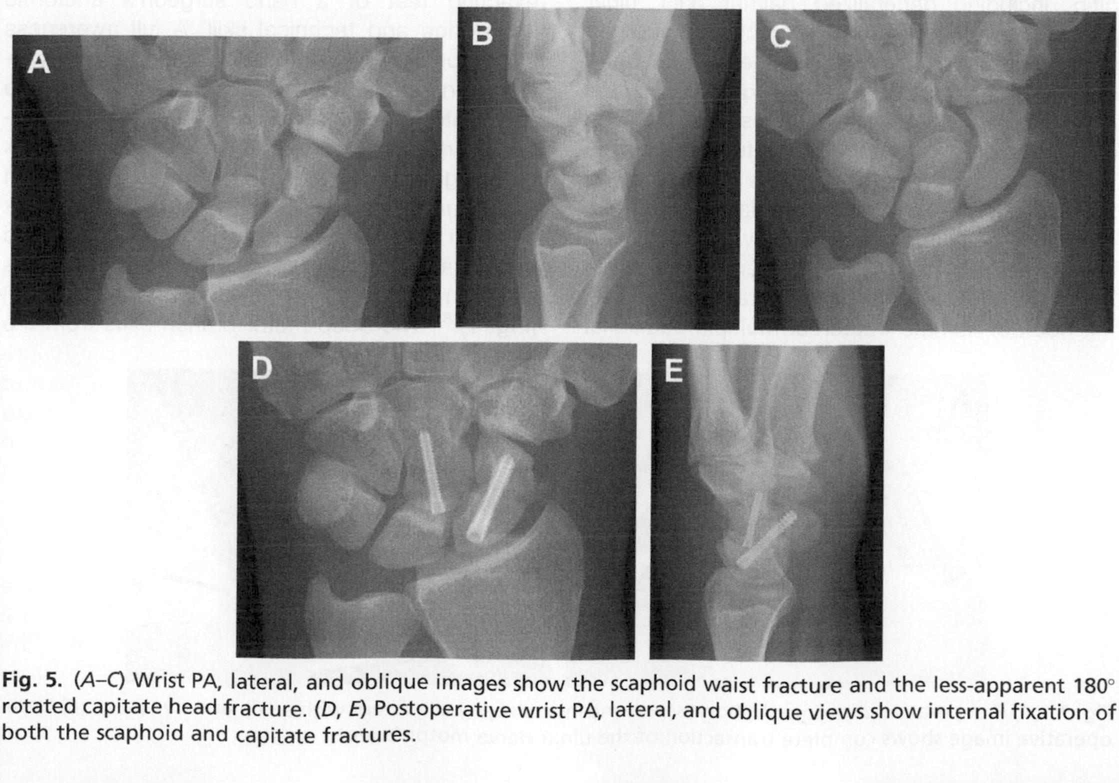

Fig. 5. (*A–C*) Wrist PA, lateral, and oblique images show the scaphoid waist fracture and the less-apparent 180° rotated capitate head fracture. (*D, E*) Postoperative wrist PA, lateral, and oblique views show internal fixation of both the scaphoid and capitate fractures.

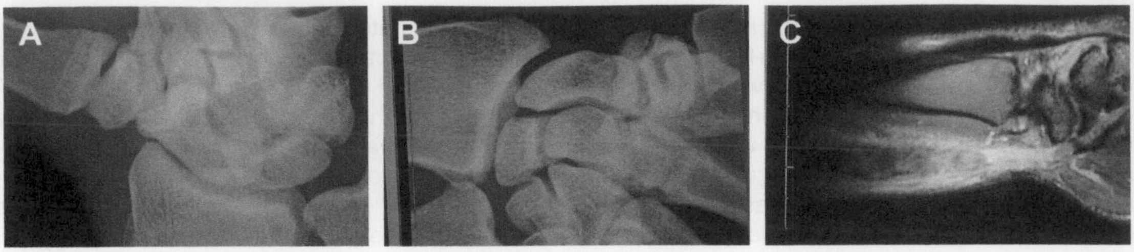

Fig. 6. (*A*) Thumb carpo-metacarpal view fails to show the trapezium fracture. (*B*) Wrist PA radiograph 1-year postinjury shows a trapezial ridge nonunion. (*C*) MRI sagittal view shows an flexor carpi radialis rupture.

Nondisplaced acute fractures can at times be treated successfully with immobilization if promptly addressed; however, this treatment is seldom chosen in the athlete population because of demands of rapid return to sport and a relatively high nonunion rate. Most investigators agree that the treatment for symptomatic patients is to excise the hook. Thus, a delay in diagnosis (or missed diagnosis) may not alter this ultimate treatment. Nonetheless, a missed diagnosis can significantly impact a patient's functional level, including time to return to work or sports. Moreover, a delay in diagnosis can result in ulnar neuritis, ulnar artery thrombosis, and rupture of the extrinsic flexor tendons (typically small or ring finger flexor digitorum profundus, as these tendons' excursions are intimate with the radial aspect of the hook).[59] Despite fairly wide recognition of this entity, missed hook of hamate fractures are well described.[60,61] Symptoms of hook of hamate fractures can be nonspecific, including generalized palmar pain, ulnar sided wrist and hand pain, subjective diminished grip strength, or symptoms of either median or ulnar neurapraxia. Standard plain radiographs of the hand typically do not adequately visualize the hook of the hamate, as the hook is obfuscated by the hamate body on a PA view and is overshadowed by the capitate and other radial-sided carpal bones on a standard lateral view. In suspected cases, additional radiographs can increase the sensitivity of conventional radiography in detecting hook of hamate fractures. Multiple additional projections have been described, including specific oblique views (ie, 15° reverse oblique view, 45° supination position with slight extension, and radial deviation with the tube tilted distally to proximally 30°) and a carpal tunnel view (keeping in mind that pain caused by the hyperextension required for the carpal tunnel view may limit this study). Andresen and colleagues[62] evaluated the sensitivity of conventional radiographic views in a cadaveric model, comparing these with CT scan as the standard. Collectively, multiple conventional radiographic projections increase the sensitivity to 90%. However, with appropriate suspicion and in the absence of definitive findings on plain films, 3-dimensional imaging should be obtained to prevent a missed fracture.

Complications of Operative Management

Excision of the hook of the hamate can be an exacting test of a hand surgeon's anatomic knowledge and technical skill. A full awareness of neurovascular and musculotendinous relationships and meticulous dissection are needed to avoid intraoperative and postoperative complications. Arguably the most critical structure at risk of iatrogenic injury is the deep motor branch of the ulnar nerve. The complication rate of hook excision is reported to be as low as 3%,[63] and specifically injury to the deep motor branch has been reported (and likely underreported) (**Fig. 7**).[64] The deep motor branch exits from the

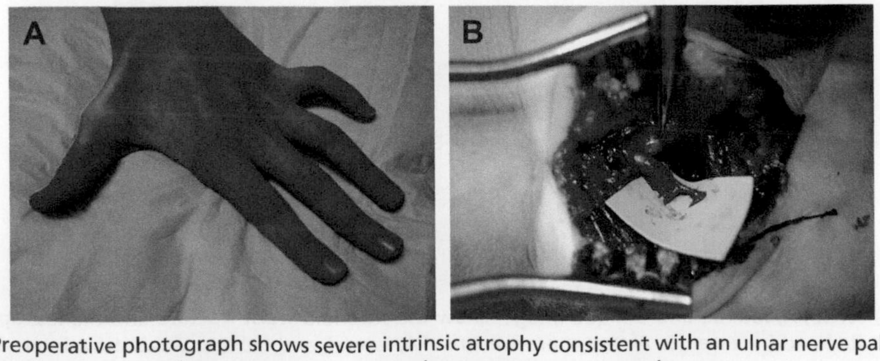

Fig. 7. (*A*) Preoperative photograph shows severe intrinsic atrophy consistent with an ulnar nerve palsy. (*B*) Intraoperative image shows complete transaction of the ulnar nerve motor branch.

ulnar nerve from its dorsal ulnar aspect and courses dorsally and radially behind the ulnar nerve and flexor digiti minimi before passing just distal and adjacent to the hook. With initial exposure of the ulnar nerve through Guyon's canal, this deep motor branch is not immediately visible. It is only after gentle radial retraction of the ulnar nerve and release of the tendinous leading edge of the hypothenar musculature from the hook that the deep motor branch is exposed. By fully exposing and gently protecting the deep motor branch during excision of the hook, iatrogenic injury to this critical nerve becomes an avoidable complication. The authors have noted occasional transient partial palsies of the deep motor branch after hook excision, but the patients can be reassured of motor recovery if meticulous technique is used.

SUMMARY

Both nonoperative and surgical treatment of carpal fractures can have complications. Missed diagnoses are common, as these fractures are easily overlooked if one is not aware. Meticulous detail to surgical technique can help avoid many of the reported and underreported complications of screw misplacement and iatrogenic injury to nearby structures. It is found that 7.6% of the peer-reviewed literature on scaphoid fractures has misquoted the referenced articles; hopefully, in an effort to synthesize the current literature available, this article exceeds this benchmark![65]

REFERENCES

1. Haisman JM, Rohde RS, Weiland AJ, et al. Acute fractures of the scaphoid. J Bone Joint Surg Am 2006;88(12):2750–8.
2. Buijze GA, Doornberg JN, Ham JS, et al. Surgical compared with conservative treatment for acute nondisplaced or minimally displaced scaphoid fractures: a systematic review and meta-analysis of randomized controlled trials. J Bone Joint Surg Am 2010;92:1534–44.
3. Wacker J, McKie S, MacLean JG. Delayed sequential ruptures of the index and thumb flexor tendons due to an occult scaphoid nonunion. J Hand Surg Br 1999;26:741–3.
4. Saitoh S, Hata Y, Murakami N, et al. Scaphoid nonunion and flexor pollicis longus rupture. J Hand Surg 1999;24:1211–9.
5. Parvizi J, Wayman J, Kelly P, et al. Combining the clinical signs improves diagnosis of scaphoid fractures. A prospective study with follow-up. J Hand Surg Br 1998;23(3):324–7.
6. Grover R. Clinical assessment of scaphoid injuries and the detection of fractures. J Hand Surg Br 1996;21(3):341–3.
7. Duckworth AD, Buizje GA, Moran M, et al. Predictors of fracture following suspected injury to the scaphoid. J Bone Joint Surg Br 2012;94:961–8.
8. Mittal RL, Dargan SK. Occult scaphoid fracture: a diagnostic enigma. J Orthop Trauma 1989;3(4): 306–8.
9. Gabler C, Kukla C, Breitenseher MJ, et al. Diagnosis of occult scaphoid fractures and other wrist injuries. Are repeated clinical examinations and plain radiographs still state of the art? Langenbecks Arch Surg 2001;386(2):150–4.
10. Brismar J. Skeletal scintigraphy of the wrist in suggested scaphoid fracture. Acta Radiol 1988; 29(1):101–7.
11. Linscheid RL, Weber ER. Scaphoid fracture and nonunion. In: Cooney WP, Linscheid RL, Dobyns JH, editors. The Wrist: diagnosis and operative treatment. St Louis (MO): Mosby; 1998. p. 385–430.
12. Pillai A, Jain M. Management of clinical fractures of the scaphoid: results of an audit and literature review. Eur J Emerg Med 2005;12(2):47–51.
13. Dorsay TA, Major NM, Helms CA. Cost-effectiveness of immediate MR imaging versus traditional followup for revealing radiographically occult scaphoid fractures. AJR Am J Roentgenol 2001;177(6): 1257–63.
14. Brooks S, Cicuttini FM, Lim S, et al. Cost effectiveness of adding magnetic resonance imaging to the usual management of suspected scaphoid fractures. Br J Sports Med 2005;39(2):75–9.
15. Raby N. Magnetic resonance imaging of suspected scaphoid fractures using a low field dedicated extremity MR system. Clin Radiol 2001;56(4):316–20.
16. Amrani KK. Diagnosing radiographically occult scaphoid fractures: what's the best second test? J Am Soc Surg Hand 2005;5(3):134–8.
17. Breitenseher MJ, Metz VM, Gilula LA, et al. Radiographically occult scaphoid fractures: value of MR imaging in detection. Radiology 1997;203(1):245–50.
18. Perlik PC, Guilford WB. Magnetic resonance imaging to assess vascularity of scaphoid nonunions. J Hand Surg Am 1991;16(3):479–84.
19. De Zwart AD, Beeres FJ, Ring D, et al. MRI as a reference standard for suspected scaphoid fractures. Br J Radiol 2012;85:1098–101.
20. Russe O. Fracture of the carpal navicular. Diagnosis, non-operative treatment, and operative treatment. J Bone Joint Surg Am 1960;42:759–68.
21. Desai VV, Davis TR, Barton NJ. The prognostic value and reproducibility of the radiological features of the fractured scaphoid. J Hand Surg Br 1999;24(5): 586–90.
22. Adams JE, Steinman SP. Acute scaphoid fractures. Hand Clin 2010;26:97–103.

23. Herbert TJ, Fisher WE. Management of the fractured scaphoid using a new bone screw. J Bone Joint Surg Br 1984;66(1):114–23.
24. Buijze GA, Jorgsholm P, Thomsen NO, et al. Diagnostic performance of radiographs and computed tomography for displacement and instability of acute scaphoid waist fractures. J Bone Joint Surg Am 2012;94:1967–74.
25. Gelberman RH, Menon J. The vascularity of the scaphoid bone. J Hand Surg Am 1980;5(5):508–13.
26. Freedman DM, Botte MJ, Gelberman RH. Vascularity of the carpus. Clin Orthop Relat Res 2001;(383):47–59.
27. Cooney WP, Dobyns JH, Linscheid RL. Fractures of the scaphoid: a rational approach to management. Clin Orthop Relat Res 1980;(149):90–7.
28. Szabo RM, Manske D. Displaced fractures of the scaphoid. Clin Orthop Relat Res 1988;(230):30–8.
29. Bushnell BD, McWilliams AD, Messer TM. Complications in dorsal percutaneous cannulated screw fixation of nondisplaced scaphoid waist fractures. J Hand Surg 2007;32:827–33.
30. McCallister WV, Knight J, Kaliappan R, et al. Central placement of the screw in simulated fractures of the scaphoid waist: a biomechanical study. J Bone Joint Surg Am 2003;85:72–7.
31. Meermans G, Van Glabbeek F, Braem MJ, et al. Comparison of two percutaneous volar approaches for screw fixation of scaphoid waist fractures: radiographic and biomechanical study of an osteotomy-simulated model. J Bone Joint Surg Am 2014;96:1369–76.
32. Luria S, Lenart L, Lenart B, et al. Optimal fixation of oblique scaphoid fractures: a cadaveric model. J Hand Surg 2012;37:1400–4.
33. Soubeyrand M, Biau D, Monsour C, et al. Comparison of percutaneous dorsal versus volar fixation of scaphoid waist fractures using a computer model in cadavers. J Hand Surg 2009;34:1838–44.
34. Levanthal EL, Wolfe SW, Walsh EF, et al. A computer approach to "optimal" screw axis location and orientation in the scaphoid bone. J Hand Surg 2009;34:677–84.
35. Guerts G, Van Riet R, Meermans G, et al. Incidence of scaphotrapezial arthritis following volar percutaneous fixation of nondisplaced scaphoid waist fractures using a transtrapezial approach. J Hand Surg 2011;36:1753–8.
36. Slade JF 3rd, Grauer JN, Mahoney JD. Arthroscopic reduction and percutaneous fixation of scaphoid fractures with a novel technique. Orthop Clin North Am 2001;32:247–61.
37. Zlotolow DA, Knutsen E, Yao J. Optimization of volar percutaneous screw fixation for scaphoid waist fractures using traction, positioning, imaging, and an angiocatheter guide. J Hand Surg 2011;36:916–21.
38. Geissler WB. Arthroscopic management of scaphoid fractures in athletes. Hand Clin 2009;25:356–69.
39. Saffir P. Scaphoid malunion. Chir Main 2008;27:65–75.
40. Amadio PC, Berquist TH, Smith DK, et al. Scaphoid malunion. J Hand Surg 1999;14:679–87.
41. Dias JJ, Singh HP. Displaced fractures of the waist of the scaphoid. J Bone Joint Surg Br 2011;93:1433–9.
42. Forward DP, Singh HP, Dawson S, et al. The clinical outcome of scaphoid malunion at 1 year. J Hand Surg Br 2009;34:40–6.
43. Lynch NM, Linscheid RL. Corrective osteotomy for scaphoid malunion: technique and long term follow up. J Hand Surg Am 1997;22:35–43.
44. Jiranek WA, Ruby LK, Millender LB, et al. Long-term results after Russe bone grafting: the effect of malunion of the scaphoid. J Bone Joint Surg Am 1992;74:1217–28.
45. Fernandez DL, Martin CJ, Gonzalez Del Pino J. Scaphoid malunion: the significance. J Hand Surg Br 1998;23:771–5.
46. Fenton RL. The naviculo-capitate fracture syndrome. J Bone Joint Surg Am 1956;38:681–4.
47. Vance RM, Gelberman RH, Evans EF. Scaphocapitate fractures. Patterns of dislocation, mechanisms of injury, and preliminary results of treatment. J Bone Joint Surg Am 1980;62:271–6.
48. Andreasi A, Coppo M, Danda F. Trans-scapho-capitate perilunar dislocation of the carpus. Ital J Orthop Traumatol 1986;12:461–6.
49. Johnson RP. The acutely injured wrist and its residuals. Clin Orthop Relat Res 1980;(149):33–44.
50. Jones GB. An unusual fracture dislocation of the carpus. J Bone Joint Surg Br 1955;37:146–7.
51. Milliez PY, Dallaserra M, Thomine JM. An unusual variety of scapho-capitate syndrome. J Hand Surg Br 1993;18:53–7.
52. Resnik CS, Gelberman RH, Resnick D. Transscaphoid, transcapitate, perilunar fracture dislocation (scaphocapitate syndrome). Skeletal Radiol 1983;9:192–4.
53. Weseley MS, Barenfeld PA. Trans-scaphoid, transcapitate, transtriquetral, perilunate fracture-dislocation of the wrist. J Bone Joint Surg Am 1972;54:1073–8.
54. Kim YS, Lee HM, Kim JP. The scaphocapitate fracture syndrome: a case report and literature analyis. Eur J Orthop Surg Traumatol 2013;23(Suppl 2):S207–12.
55. McClain EJ, Boyes JH. Missed fractures of the greater multangular. J Bone Joint Surg Am 1966;48:1525–8.
56. Palmer AK. Trapezial ridge fractures. J Hand Surg Am 1981;6(6):561–4.
57. Hart VL, Gaynor V. Roentgenographic study of the carpal canal. J Bone Joint Surg 1941;23:382–3.
58. Soejima O, Iida H, Naito M. Flexor carpi radialis tendinitis caused by malunited trapezial ridge fracture in a professional baseball player. J Orthop Sci 2002;7(1):151–3.

59. O'Shea K, Weiland AJ. Fractures of the hamate and pisiform bones. Hand Clin 2012;28(3):287–300.
60. Nisenfield FG, Neviaser RJ. Fracture of the hook of the hamate: a diagnosis easily missed. J Trauma 1974;14(7):612–6.
61. Terrono A, Ferenz CC, Nalebuff EA. Delayed diagnosis in non-union of the body of the hamate: a case report. J Hand Surg Br 1989;14(3):329–31.
62. Andreson R, Radmer S, Sparmann M, et al. Imaging of hamate bone fractures in conventional x-rays and high-resolution computed tomography. An in vitro study. Invest Radiol 1999;34:46–50.
63. Smith P 3rd, Wright TW, Wallace PF, et al. Excision of the hook of the hamate: a retrospective survey and review of the literature. J Hand Surg Am 1988;13A:612–5.
64. Fredericson M, Kim BJ, Date ES, et al. Injury to the deep motor branch of the ulnar nerve during hook of hamate excision. Orthopedics 2006;29(5):456–8.
65. Buijze GA, Weening AA, Poolman RW. Predictors of the accuracy of quotation of references in peer-reviewed orthopaedic literature in relation to publications of the scaphoid. J Bone Joint Surg Br 2012;94:276–80.

Management of Complications of Distal Radius Fractures

Alexandra L. Mathews, BS[a], Kevin C. Chung, MD, MS[b,*]

KEYWORDS

• Preventive • Complications • Early diagnosis • CRPS • Malunion • Infection • Extensor tendon • Flexor tendon

KEY POINTS

- Prevention of the possible complications associated with a fracture of the distal radius should be the treating surgeon's primary concern.
- Complication type may vary depending on the method of treatment.
- Complication rates can depend on patient factors including patient lifestyle, age, social support, and medical comorbidities.
- Early diagnosis and treatment is important to avoid possible long-term consequences.

INTRODUCTION

Fractures occurring at the distal end of the radius are seen frequently in emergency departments, representing approximately one-sixth of all fractures.[1] Based on decades of extensive research, surgeons have developed multiple approaches for the treatment of distal radius fractures, including conservative and nonconservative options. These options include closed reduction and casting, closed reduction and percutaneous pinning, external fixation, and open reduction with internal fixation (ORIF).[2] The conservative treatment of closed reduction and casting has historically been the mainstay of treatment of distal radius fractures. However, because of the increased complication rate associated with this treatment, such as fracture collapse, surgical options, specifically ORIF, are becoming more common.[1,3]

Overall, distal radius fracture complication rates have been found to vary between 6% and 80% of patients, depending on the definition of complication.[4] Complications after distal radius fractures occur for many reasons, and often vary depending on the method of treatment.[2] When deciding on a treatment option, it is important that surgeons focus on recognition, management, and prevention of known associated complications to achieve a good outcome.[5] Patient factors must also be taken into account when considering treatment methods. Factors including patient lifestyle, age, mental attitude, social support, comorbid conditions, and compliance with treatment can influence the likelihood for complications.[1] For example, a prospective cohort study designed to identify predictors of hand outcomes after distal radius fracture treatment found that increased

Research reported in this publication was supported by the National Institute of Arthritis and Musculoskeletal and Skin Diseases of the National Institutes of Health under Award Number 2 K24-AR053120-06. The content is solely the responsibility of the authors and does not necessarily represent the official views of the National Institutes of Health.

[a] Section of Plastic Surgery, Department of Surgery, The University of Michigan Health System, 1500 East Medical Center Drive, Ann Arbor, MI 48109–5340, USA; [b] Section of Plastic Surgery, Department of Surgery, The University of Michigan Health System, 1500 East Medical Center Drive, 2130 Taubman Center, SPC 5340, Ann Arbor, MI 48109–5340, USA
* Corresponding author.
E-mail address: kecchung@med.umich.edu

Hand Clin 31 (2015) 205–215
http://dx.doi.org/10.1016/j.hcl.2014.12.002
0749-0712/15/$ – see front matter

hand.theclinics.com

age and lower income led to a significantly worse long-term outcome 1 year after successful surgery using a volar locking plating system.[6] Awareness of potential risk factors can aid in the prevention of possible complications. This article focuses on the prevention and management of complex regional pain syndrome (CRPS), malunions, infections, and tendon complications after distal radius fracture treatment.

COMPLEX REGIONAL PAIN SYNDROME

Characterized by autonomic dysfunction, trophic changes, and impaired function, CRPS can occur after operative and nonoperative treatments of a distal radius fracture.[7] The rate of incidence of CRPS after a fracture of the distal radius has been found to vary (1%–37%)[8–10] and often rises with increasing severity of the fracture.[11] There is no definitive cause or treatment of this syndrome; however, many association factors have been discovered. For operatively treated fractures, excessive distraction with an external fixator can raise the risk of CRPS development.[12] For fractures treated nonoperatively, a correlation was found between an increased incidence of CRPS and an increase in pressure under the cast.[13] There are also several theories for the pathophysiologic mechanism leading to the development of CRPS; however, the true cause remains unclear. Possible involvement of the sympathetic nervous system, abnormal inflammatory reactions, sequelae of nerve injury, and psychological disturbances have all been considered.[14]

CRPS can be categorized into two different types depending on the presence or absence of nerve trauma. Formerly known as reflex sympathetic dystrophy, CRPS type I is defined as chronic pain without an identifiable nerve injury.[7] Conversely, CRPS type II is characterized by nerve involvement. It has been reported that women, the elderly, and individuals with a psychological predisposition have a higher likelihood of developing CRPS type I.[15] For example, Roh and colleagues[11] recently evaluated potential factors influencing the rate of CRPS type I after the surgical treatment of a distal radius fracture, and found female patients to be 2.2 times more likely to develop CRPS type I compared with male patients. Additionally, incidences of CRPS have been shown to be higher in smokers compared with nonsmokers.[16]

Early diagnosis is important for ensuring the best possible recovery. Patients with suspected CRPS can begin to show symptoms 2 weeks after surgery, but symptoms can also develop several weeks after surgery.[14] Early diagnosis and treatment of CRPS has been shown to result in recovery in 80% to 90% of cases.[14] However, diagnosing CRPS can prove to be difficult because there are no formal, standardized diagnostic criteria available to date. Zyluk and Puchalski[14] highlighted the recent increase in use of the International Association for the Study of Pain criteria of diagnosis in many scientific studies. The International Association for the Study of Pain criteria involve four categories for diagnosing CRPS: (1) sensory, (2) vasomotor, (3) sudomotor/edema, and (4) motor trophic.[17]

In a clinical setting, patients with possible symptoms of CRPS usually present with pain, swelling, and changes in color, temperature, and perspiration of the affected limb.[14] Pain is normally described as a tearing or burning sensation and is often intensified by exposure to cold.[18] We often observe a shiny appearance of the upper extremity as an indication of CRPS (**Fig. 1**). The absence of pain relief after narcotic use is also a good indication for possible CRPS, because patients with this condition are typically unresponsive to this form of pain medication.[18] Other indications that require careful consideration of possible CRPS include patients with unexpected intense pain, stiffness, sleep difficulties, or slower than anticipated recovery.[18]

Certain diagnostic tests have been found to aid in the diagnosis of CRPS. Radiographic images can display irregularities in patients with CRPS; however, changes may not be visible until 2 or more weeks post injury.[18] Radiographs may show osteopenic bone with subchondral and periarticular resorption, but normal results may be found in 30% of patients with CRPS symptoms.[18] Additionally, phase I and phase II bone scans may show hyperperfusion (hot or warm hand) and hypoperfusion (cold, stiff hand), which are common symptoms of patients with CRPS.[7] Three-phase

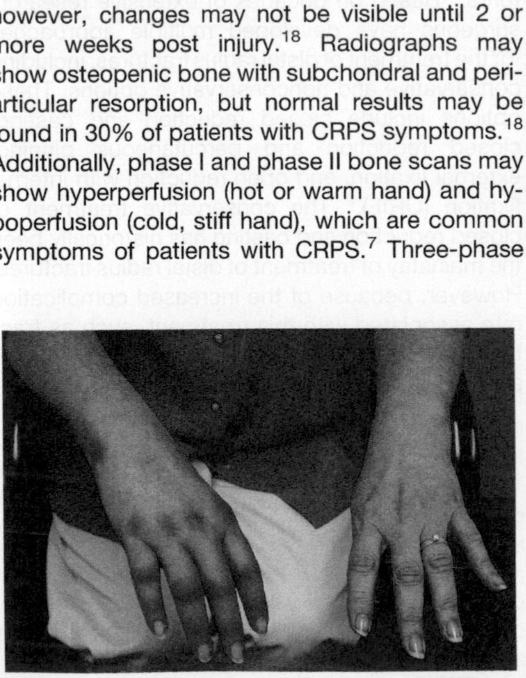

Fig. 1. Patient diagnosed with complex regional pain syndrome presenting with a shiny appearance of the right hand.

bone scans demonstrate a high specificity and are useful when confirming a positive diagnosis of CRPS; however, a poor correlation between three-phase bone scans and CRPS has been described because of a reported sensitivity of only 50%.[19]

Given the high prevalence of CRPS after fractures of the wrist, researchers have studied possible prevention techniques including the use of vitamin C. Two studies by Zollinger and colleagues[20,21] assessed the relationship between vitamin C use and the incidence of CRPS for patients with nonoperatively treated wrist fractures and concluded that vitamin C reduced the prevalence of CRPS. A more recent double-blind prospective randomized study of patients treated operatively and nonoperatively for distal radius fractures provided further support for the use of vitamin C.[22] Shah and colleagues[22] found that 500 mg of vitamin C taken daily for 50 days after a distal radius fracture lowered the risk of CRPS from 10% to 2%. The use of vitamin C was found to have no effect on patients given a dose of 200 mg or less per day or greater than 500 mg per day. Researchers suggested that 500 mg should be the recommended amount and that typical dietary intake without the addition of a vitamin C supplement may be insufficient in the prevention of CRPS.[22] Excessive amounts of vitamin C can result in side effects, including diarrhea, abdominal cramping, and kidney stone formation.[22] Vitamin C should be given with caution, especially to patients who have been diagnosed with hyperoxaluria or hyperuricosuria, because of the risk of renal calculi development.[5,22]

These studies[20–22] influenced the decision by the American Academy of Orthopedic Surgeons in 2009 to recommend the use of vitamin C in the prevention and management of CRPS following distal radial fractures.[23] However, a recent randomized controlled trial by Ekrol and colleagues[24] contradicted this recommendation after finding no significant difference in the incidence of CRPS with the use of vitamin C after a distal radius fracture. Based on these results, the use of vitamin C may not have strong scientific evidence to endorse its use.

After a positive diagnosis of CRPS following a distal radius fracture, a multidisciplinary treatment approach is recommended. A combination of psychiatric therapy, occupational therapy, and pain management therapy has been shown to produce the best recovery outcome.[18] Passive and active range of motion, splinting, and contrast baths may be performed along with oral medication as a first line of treatment.[18] Based on clinical experience, specific classes of oral agents are recommended, such as antidepressants, adrenergic agents, anticonvulsants, and membrane-stabilizing agents.[7] Li and colleagues[7] recently explained how treatment of CRPS can often depend on the patient's presentation of symptoms. For a hot, swollen hand, the investigators recommend an antidepressant in combination with an anticonvulsant. Conversely, for patients presenting with cold, stiff hands, a mild antidepressant in combination with a calcium channel blocker is suggested.[7] Other possible treatments for early forms of CRPS include calcitonin, physiotherapy, or free radical scavengers. Researchers developed a free radical scavenger treatment using the assumption that CRPS is caused by an exaggerated inflammatory response to trauma, medicated by an overproduction of toxic oxygen and hydroxyl free radicals.[25] When diagnosed early, patients may expect a significant reduction in pain within 1 month of treatment.[14]

Intravenous agents have also been used to treat CRPS following a distal radius fracture; however, there is controversy in recent literature on the effectiveness of such agents as guanethidine, cortisone, reserpine, lidocaine, and bretylium.[7] Livingstone and Atkins[26] studied this relationship by randomizing 57 patients diagnosed with CRPS type I 9 weeks after an isolated closed distal radius fracture to receive either serial intravenous regional blockade with guanethidine or a normal saline solution. They found no significant analgesic advantage for the treatment of early CRPS type I after a distal radius fracture and concluded that this treatment may even delay the resolution of vasomotor instability.[26] Paraskevas and colleagues[27] found results conflicting with Livingston and Atkins[26] after evaluating the efficacy of guanethidine and lidocaine in the treatment of CRPS of the hand. A total of 17 of the 28 patients evaluated reported excellent pain relief and full restoration of function and range of motion of the affected hand.[27] Further studies should be performed on the use of intravenous regional blockade in patients diagnosed with CRPS following a distal radius fracture to clarify this discrepancy.

MALUNION

A malunion is the most common complication that occurs following a fracture of the distal radius.[28] A malunited distal radius fracture can be extra-articular, intra-articular, or both[29] and occurs when a fracture heals with improper alignment, articular incongruity, incorrect length, or a combination of these elements.[30] Extra-articular malunions are commonly characterized by a loss of the normal palmar tilt of the articular surface in the sagittal plane, a loss of ulnar inclination in the frontal plane, and a loss of length relative to the ulna.[29] Conversely, an intra-articular malunion is frequently associated with a step-off or a gap at the radiocarpal joint and/or the distal radioulnar joint.[29]

Researchers have found many indications for the development of distal radius fracture malunions. Fractures treated conservatively are a common cause of malunions. For example, a recent study comparing the outcomes and complications of distal radius fractures between volar plating and nonoperative treatment found that 35% of the patients treated conservatively developed a malunion.[31] Patients treated with volar plate fixation, however, reported no incidence of malunion.[31] In 2010, the American Academy of Orthopedic Surgeons aimed to prevent possible distal radius fracture complications associated with conservative treatment by publishing guidelines for operative fixation. According to these guidelines, distal radius fractures displaying a postreduction dorsal tilt of greater than 10 degrees, radial shortening of greater than 3 mm, or intra-articular displacement or step-off of greater than 2 mm indicate a need for surgical fixation.[23] Malunions can also be anticipated in patients with a dorsally displaced fracture when the strongest portion of the metaphysis, the volar cortex, is not in contact.[30]

Malunited distal radius fractures are associated with a variety of symptoms including decreased grip strength, decreased wrist mobility, increased pain, and worsened cosmetic appearance.[29,32] Patients may also present with pain over the ulnar wrist, caused by either a distal radioulnar joint incongruity or an ulna impaction.[30] Patients treated in our facility commonly complain of decreased motion at the wrist, specifically pronation and supination, in addition to chronic pain. Pronation and supination deformities can be seen in dorsally and palmarly angulated malunions.[33]

A suspected malunion should be confirmed with radiographic images and verified with specific criteria used to define a malunion of the distal radius. The criteria used in our facility involve[30]

1. Radial inclination less than 10 degrees
2. Volar tilt greater than 20 degrees, dorsal tilt greater than 20 degrees
3. Radial height less than 10 mm
4. Ulnar variance greater than 2+
5. Intra-articular step or gap greater than 2 mm

Evidence recommends surgeons take into account the patient's motivation, functional demands, and the anatomy of the deformity before deciding on a treatment option for a distal radius malunion.[29] Surgical correction should be strongly considered for patients presenting with both clinical and radiographic symptoms of a malunion.[30] Fernandez recommended a corrective osteotomy if the angulation of the distal articular surface of the radius became greater than 25 degrees in the sagittal plane.[34]

If surgical correction is agreed on by the patient and surgeon, preoperative planning should be executed. Preoperative anteroposterior, lateral, and oblique radiographs of the wrists are used to determine the specific fracture pattern (**Fig. 2**). The malunited distal radius fracture should be compared with the contralateral normal wrist, allowing the surgeon to identify the proper length, angle extent, and type of osteotomy needed.[28] Additionally, computed tomography scans and three-dimensional imaging can be helpful in determining malunion alignment and aid in the reconstructive planning, and are used in our facility. Researchers have noted the successful use of computer-assisted techniques in the evaluation, deformity modeling, preoperative planning, and intraoperative execution of osteotomies.[35–37]

A corrective osteotomy should be performed as soon as possible after the diagnosis to correct the biomechanics of the wrist and prevent or minimalize possible soft tissue contracture.[30] By using an osteotomy to adjust the alignment of the distal end of the radius in relation to the wrist and the distal end of the ulna, preliminary reduction can be achieved. Corrective osteotomies have also been shown to improve wrist and forearm motion and patient pain levels.[38] Jupiter and Ring retrospectively compared patients treated with either early or late osteotomies, documenting considerable positive results after early reconstruction and a decrease in the overall period of disability.[39]

The key factor of the surgical technique for corrective osteotomies is placing the wedge osteotomy through the fracture to recreate the initial fracture pattern.[30] Two types of osteotomies are used, each offering specific advantages and disadvantages. A closing wedge osteotomy allows direct bone-to-bone contact and offers more stability, preventing the need for bone grafting and the potential for nonunions.[28] However, this technique can cause the distal radius to become shortened relative to the ulna. Closing wedge osteotomies are often paired with an additional osteotomy, shortening the ulna to maintain the distal radioulnar joint. Wada and colleagues[40] presented encouraging results using a radial closing wedge osteotomy when correcting a dorsal tilt deformity of the distal radius, simultaneously pairing the procedure with an ulnar-shortening osteotomy. However, if the shortened distal radius

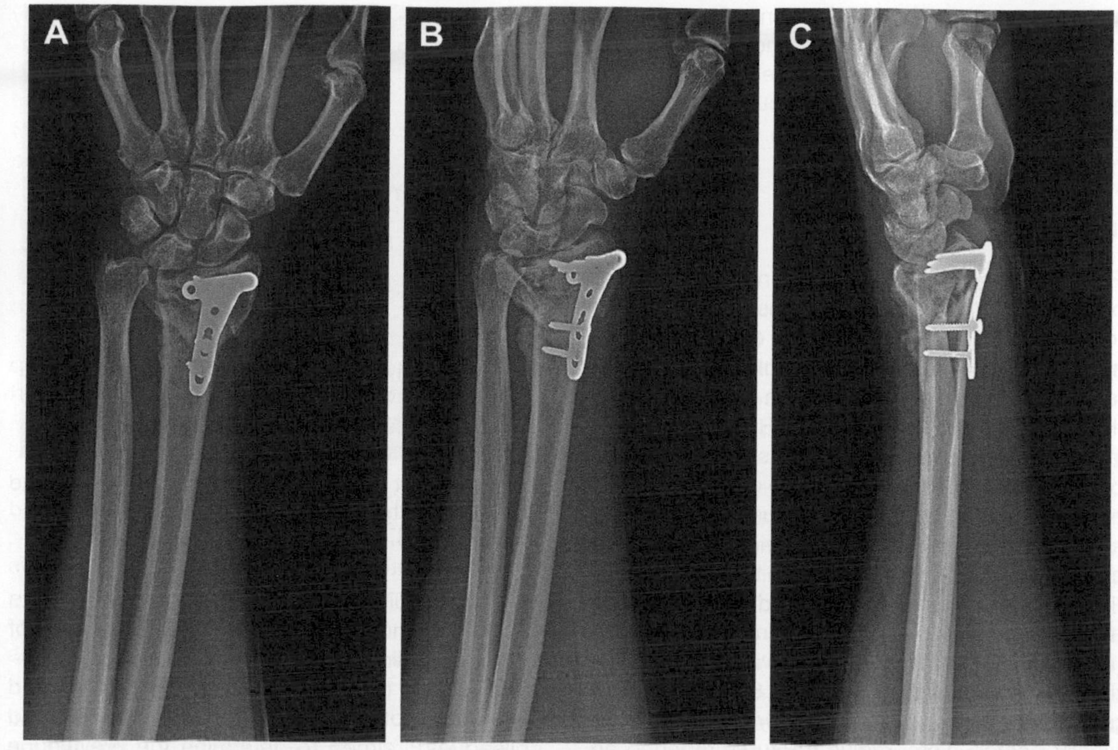

Fig. 2. (*A*) Anteroposterior, (*B*) lateral, and (*C*) oblique preoperative radiographs of a patient who sustained a left intra-articular distal radius fracture. The fracture was fixated at an outside hospital; however, the articular surface collapsed causing distal radioulnar joint incongruity.

is not addressed, ulnar abutment can occur, resulting in impaction of the ulnar head against the carpus and gradual development of triangular fibrocartilage complex lesions and ulnocarpal arthrosis.[41]

Opening wedge osteotomies are more popular because they restore the radial length preventing the need for a distal ulna procedure.[28] This technique can also correct angular deformities in the frontal and sagittal planes. The disadvantage of opening wedge osteotomies is the risk of increased instability of the construct before it has healed completely.[28] There is also a possibility of construct failure from axial loading associated with early wrist motion.[28]

After the biomechanics of the wrist have been corrected with an osteotomy, the distal radius fracture must be fixated. The surgical fixation approach depends greatly on the fracture pattern and the preference of the surgeon. However, the use of a volar approach has increased recently as an alternative to dorsal plate fixation and external fixation.[42,43] The volar approach was introduced to promote prevention of complications related to the dorsal approach, especially extensor tendon injuries.[44] Approaching the fracture from a volar aspect permits more space for plate fixation and the concave surface protects the flexor tendons from hardware irritation.[45–47] The flexor tendons are located far from the volar surface and placement of the pronator quadratus over the volar plate has been suggested to prevent irritation.[44] Volar plate fixation has also been found to result in a shorter period of immobilization and an earlier return to previous activity level.[31]

Additional advantages of volar locking plates include the decreased requirement for bone grafting. Traditionally, the use of an iliac crest structural bone graft and fixation with a dorsal plate has been recommended for substantial bone gaps greater than 1 cm.[48] However, donor-site morbidity has been reported in up to 20% of cases, along with other minor complications.[49] Researchers began to study the use of dorsal plate fixation without the addition of bone grafting. This was found to be an effective technique[48]; however, the high incidence of plate removal because of painful hardware, tendon irritation, or tendon rupture led to the increased use of volar plates.[50] Haase and Chung[30] have shown that the volar approach restores a sturdy volar cortex where a distal plate can be placed, avoiding the need for a large bone graft. Tarallo and colleagues[51] and Mahmoud and colleagues[52] have also reported effective results associated with volar plate fixation without the use of bone grafting. Tarallo and colleagues[51] concluded that this should be the preferred technique when correcting extra-articular distal radius fracture malunions, especially in elderly patients with poor bone quality.

INFECTION

Patients suspected of an infection after a fracture of the distal radius normally present with symptoms of redness, erythema, drainage, pain, swelling, tenderness, or a combination of these factors. Infection can occur as a result of k-wire fixation, external fixation, or ORIF. The rate of infection after k-wire fixation has been found to be higher compared with the rate of infection after external fixation of a distal radius fracture, 33% and 21%, respectively.[53,54] Recent literature has also reported a large difference in the rate of infection between external fixation and ORIF. Esposito and colleagues[55] reported a pin tract infection rate of 9.8% in patients treated with external fixation, compared with a rate of 2.8% in the ORIF group. Furthermore, a meta-analysis of 1520 surgically treated distal radius fractures reported an infection rate of 11% for fractures treated with external fixation, and only a 0.8% infection rate in patients treated with internal fixation.[56] Before choosing a distal radius fracture treatment method, it is important to take these infection rates into consideration.

In addition to careful consideration of the possible treatment options, certain preventive measures can be taken to ensure patients do not develop an infection following treatment of a distal radius fracture. If possible, all pins and k-wires should be buried under the skin. A study performed by Hargreaves and colleagues[53] demonstrated a significantly higher pin tract infection rate in k-wires that were left percutaneously compared with those buried under the skin. The rate of infection was found to be 34% for pins left out of the skin, compared with only 7% when the k-wires were buried beneath the skin.[53] Most infection complications seen in our facility after treatment of a distal radius fracture resulted from percutaneous pinning of the fracture (**Fig. 3**). One specific case of pin infection observed after percutaneous pinning resulted in further complication requiring an additional surgery. The patient's pins were removed prematurely because of the infection, and as a result the patient experienced dorsal angulation of the distal radius fragment and a loss of the radial and ulnar tilt. A corrective osteotomy was performed along with the placement of a plate to promote accurate bone reformation. If the infection requires the removal of the pin, patients should be monitored closely for symptoms of further complications.

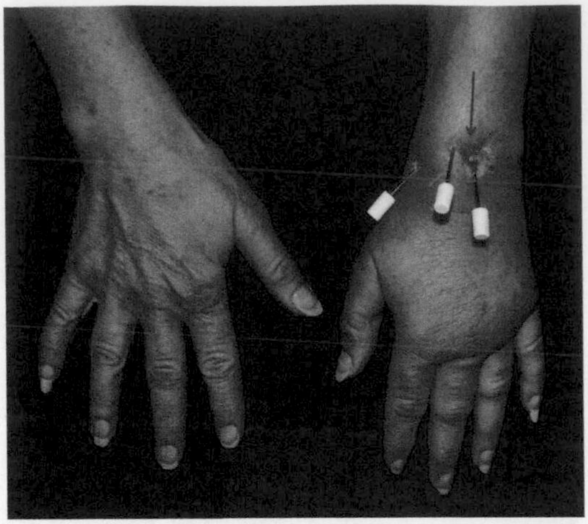

Fig. 3. Patient presenting with purulent drainage from one of the dorsal pins (*arrow*), which resulted in pin removal.

Preventive measures have also been studied with the use of external fixation devices. Egol and colleagues[57] aimed to determine the prevalence of pin-track infection associated with external fixation for the treatment of distal radius fractures. They tested the ability of a chlorhexidine-impregnated disk to provide a significant reduction in pin-track infection compared with traditional methods of pin-site care. After noting a pin-track infection rate of 19% without a significant difference between pin-site care protocols, researchers concluded that the use of hydrogen peroxide care or chlorhexidine-impregnated dressings does not reduce the rate of infection.[57] Additional wound care beyond the use of dry, sterile dressings for pin-track care is not recommended. They also noted an increased risk of pin-track complications associated with an increase in age.[57] This factor should be considered carefully when deciding on a treatment option after a fracture of the distal radius.

Open distal radius fractures can also predispose patients to infection; however, the rate of occurrence is not as common compared with other factors. Glueck and colleagues[58] aimed to identify factors associated with infection after open distal radius fractures and found that contamination, rather than absolute wound size, was significantly associated with infection development. Researchers recommended that physicians include contamination as a factor for prognosis and that open distal radius fractures be treated with multiple debridements as part of the initial treatment plan.[58] Multiple debridements can prevent the development of infection by clearing all possible sources of wound contamination.

Researchers have tested the use of prophylactic antibiotics before distal radius fracture treatment; however, the value of antibiotics for elective clean cases is uncertain. Subramanian and colleagues[59] conducted a recent study on the use prophylactic antibiotics before k-wire fixation for a distal radius fracture, and concluded that they do not advocate the use of prophylactic antibiotics because it does not affect the rate of infection. Further analysis should be done to investigate the benefits of prophylactic antibiotics to clarify the use of this prevention measure.

Infection is a common complication following a distal radius fracture. Treatment methods may vary depending on the severity of the infection. For minor infections consisting of a slight discharge and redness around the pin site, pin removal is not normally required.[60,61] The pins and wound should be cleaned and monitored for the addition of symptoms of tenderness in the soft tissue. Patients with an infection involving the soft tissue should be given antibiotics and pins should be removed if the infection fails to improve.[60,61] Patients must be monitored closely with frequent follow-up and radiographic images should be taken to rule out a possible osteomyelitis involving the bone. In the case of osteomyelitis, surgical intervention is required.[41]

TENDON COMPLICATIONS

Surgical fixation after a distal radius fracture can result in flexor and extensor tendon complications. Complications may be minor, such as simple irritation, adhesion formation, or tenosynovitis, or more severe including laceration or rupture.[5] Tendon ruptures normally occur at a mean of 7 weeks, but can also occur within the first few weeks of a distal radius fracture.[62] Rupture complication rates can vary, and often depend on the surgical fixation technique. Margaliot and colleagues[56] compared the risk of tendon complications between internal fixation and external fixation devices, finding a six-fold higher risk of tendon rupture associated with internal fixation after a distal radius fracture. Volar plate fixation was developed as an alternative to external fixation and dorsal plating. Studies have demonstrated a lower rate of tendon complications associated with volar plating, but rates have still been reported as high as 16%.[63]

Extensor Tendon Complications

Extensor tendon complications can result from volar and dorsal fixation of a distal radius fracture. The incidence of extensor tendon injuries after volar plate fixation specifically has been reported to be between 3% and 5%.[63,64] Complications with volar plating are likely to occur because of drill-bit penetration or dorsal screw prominence and most commonly affect the extensor pollicis longus (EPL) tendon, especially at the location of the Lister tubercle.[65–67] This is because the Lister tubercle is a watershed area of blood supply to the tendon.[66,67]

If tendon irritation is suspected, removal of the plate is recommended to prevent further damage. In cases of EPL rupture, to restore thumb function the extensor indicis proprius may be transferred to the EPL or free tendon graft reconstruction may be performed.[5] Both are acceptable methods to treat EPL ruptures, as shown in a recent study by Schaller and colleagues[68] comparing the two techniques. At a mean of 4.3 years after the surgery, the investigators noted very good to good Geldmacher scores in 86% of patients treated with extensor indicis proprius to EPL transfer (N = 28), and 77% of patients treated with free tendon graft reconstruction (N = 17). To avoid extensor tendon injuries after the use of volar locking plates, drilling should reach the dorsal cortex but not extend through it, and shorter, unicortical screws or small pegs should be used (**Fig. 4**).[5,65]

Extensor tendon irritation or rupture after a distal radius fracture treated with dorsal plate fixation is likely to occur because of screw-head or plate prominence.[65] Rozental and colleagues[69] studied 19 patients treated with dorsal plate fixation, noting seven cases of extensor tendon irritation and one rupture of the extensor digitorum communis to the ring finger. After immediate removal of the hardware, the investigators discovered complete resolution of the tendon irritation and that function was fully recovered in the affected digit after extensor digitorum communis tendon reconstruction.[69] The use of local tissue interposition flaps has been proposed as a preventive

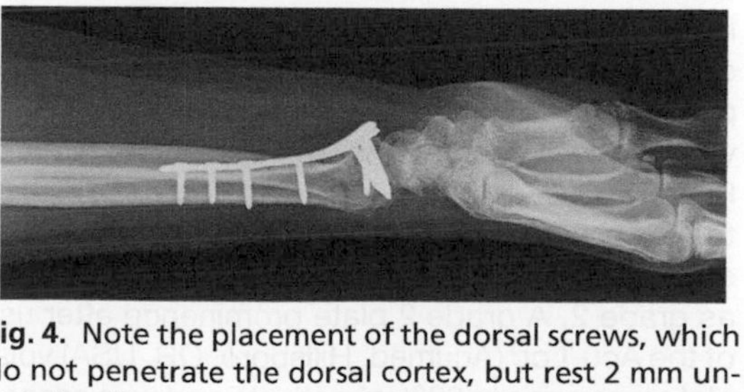

Fig. 4. Note the placement of the dorsal screws, which do not penetrate the dorsal cortex, but rest 2 mm under the dorsal cortex to prevent tendon injury. Also note the placement of the volar plate distally over the watershed line, which can cause irritation and possible rupture of the flexor pollicis longus.

technique to minimize the risk of extensor tendon complications associated with dorsal plate fixation.[5] The flaps serve to protect the overlying tendons from the dorsal plate, preventing any contact. Althausen and Szabo studied the use of local tissue interposition flaps, specifically the elevation of the dorsal distal radius periosteum with the third and fourth extensor compartments and subsequent reapproximation of the periosteum over the dorsal plate.[70] The investigators recommended the use of this technique after reporting no incidence of tenosynovitis, tendon adhesions, or tendon ruptures.[70] Use of the extensor retinaculum to cover the dorsal hardware has also been proposed as a possible prevention technique.[71] However, symptoms of continued dorsal wrist pain were reported in 12 of 20 patients studied by Chiang and colleagues[71] after implementing this technique.

Flexor Tendon Complications

Flexor tendon injuries are thought to be caused primarily by hardware irritation resulting from distally placed volar locking plates.[63] The flexor pollicis longus (FPL) is the most commonly injured tendon; however, the flexor digitorum superficialis, flexor digitorum profundus, and flexor carpi radialis are also at risk.[72] To avoid flexor tendon complications, volar plates should be placed in alignment with the transverse ridge along the distal volar surface of the radius between the pronator quadratus and volar radiocarpal ligaments called the watershed line.[63,65,73] Arora and colleagues[63] recommend the use of a plate system with two distal rows of screw holes permitting screw fixation at various angles to help place the plate proximal to this line.

Plates placed distal to the watershed line may result in direct plate or screw head contact with the deep flexor tendons causing damaging complications.[47,73] Soong and colleagues[74] recently studied the variation in volar plate placement around the watershed line and its association with flexor tendon ruptures. Through this study they developed a system for categorizing volar plate placement. For example, plates that did not extend volar to the watershed line were labeled as grade 0. Plates volar to the watershed line but proximal to the volar rim were labeled as grade 1, and plates directly on or distal to the volar rim were labeled as grade 2. A grade 2 plate prominence after use of the Acu-Loc (Acumed, Hillsboro, OR, USA) volar plate was seen in 63% of patients and was associated with two of the three reported cases of flexor tendon ruptures.[74] Researchers concluded that direct visualization may be beneficial to avoid improper plate position, loss of reduction, and screw head prominence, factors directly responsible for tendon complications.[74]

A study performed by Arora and colleagues[63] on the complications associated with volar plate fixation reported 11 patients with plates placed distal to the watershed line. All of the patients presented with tendon injuries including nine cases of flexor tendon synovitis and two FPL ruptures. To prevent possible tendon complications, volar plates should be removed early if they are found to be placed distal to this line, or if the distal edge of the plate becomes prominent because of collapse of the fracture site.[75] Tada and colleagues[76] performed early plate removal in 9 out of 12 patients complaining of FPL tendon irritation, and concluded that volar plate removal may prevent FPL rupture.

Early removal after volar plate fixation has also been recommended for patients using steroids.[75] Bell and colleagues[75] experienced four patients with FPL ruptures after volar plating of a distal radius fracture and noted that all four of the patients were taking steroids. In the case of FPL rupture, reconstruction can be performed using direct repair, tendon transfer, or interposition grafting.[5] Reconstruction is often performed using a palmaris longus tendon graft.[63] In the absence of the palmaris longus, however, the plantaris or long toe extensor tendons may be used.[77]

To prevent the risk of flexor tendon injuries, Orbay recommends covering the volar plate with the pronator quadratus muscle.[44] Restoration of the pronator quadratus to its original position can prevent irritation of the flexor tendons by disallowing the plate from coming in contact with the tendons. However, a recent study performed by Brown and Lifchez contradicts Orbay's recommendation. The authors reported a partial-thickness laceration of the FPL 2.5 years after volar plating of a distal radius fracture, despite the restoration of the pronator quadratus to its native position.[78] They concluded that even after coverage of the volar plate with the pronator quadratus, irritation can still occur and that this technique does not protect the overlying flexor tendons.[78] Further investigation should be performed to clarify the use of this prevention method.

SUMMARY

Prevention of the possible complications that can occur following treatment of a distal radius fracture should be the surgeon's foremost concern. Patients should be well informed about the symptoms associated with these complications and monitored closely with follow-up appointments.

Complications that do arise should be treated as early as possible to prevent further long-term consequences. This article discusses the prevention and management of common complications; however, the surgeon should be aware of all possible complications including those that are not referenced in this article.

REFERENCES

1. Ilyas AM, Jupiter JB. Distal radius fractures: classification of treatment and indications for surgery. Orthop Clin North Am 2007;38(2):167–73, v.
2. Davis DI, Baratz M. Soft tissue complications of distal radius fractures. Hand Clin 2010;26(2):229–35.
3. Schneppendahl J, Windolf J, Kaufmann RA. Distal radius fractures: current concepts. J Hand Surg Am 2012;37(8):1718–25.
4. McKay SD, MacDermid JC, Roth JH, et al. Assessment of complications of distal radius fractures and development of a complication checklist. J Hand Surg Am 2001;26(5):916–22.
5. Rhee PC, Dennison DG, Kakar S. Avoiding and treating perioperative complications of distal radius fractures. Hand Clin 2012;28(2):185–98.
6. Chung KC, Kotsis SV, Kim HM. Predictors of functional outcomes after surgical treatment of distal radius fractures. J Hand Surg Am 2007;32(1):76–83.
7. Li Z, Smith BP, Tuohy C, et al. Complex regional pain syndrome after hand surgery. Hand Clin 2010;26(2): 281–9.
8. Jellad A, Salah S, Ben Salah Frih Z. Complex regional pain syndrome type I: incidence and risk factors in patients with fracture of the distal radius. Arch Phys Med Rehabil 2014;95(3):487–92.
9. Atkins RM, Duckworth T, Kanis JA. Features of algodystrophy after Colles' fracture. J Bone Joint Surg Br 1990;72(1):105–10.
10. Dijkstra PU, Groothoff JW, ten Duis HJ, et al. Incidence of complex regional pain syndrome type I after fractures of the distal radius. Eur J Pain 2003;7(5):457–62.
11. Roh YH, Lee BK, Noh JH, et al. Factors associated with complex regional pain syndrome type I in patients with surgically treated distal radius fracture. Arch Orthop Trauma Surg 2014;134(12):1775–81.
12. Combalia A. Over-distraction of the radiocarpal and midcarpal joints with external fixation of comminuted distal radial fractures. J Hand Surg Br 1996;21(2):289.
13. Field J, Protheroe DL, Atkins RM. Algodystrophy after Colles fractures is associated with secondary tightness of casts. J Bone Joint Surg Br 1994; 76(6):901–5.
14. Zyluk A, Puchalski P. Complex regional pain syndrome of the upper limb: a review. Neurol Neurochir Pol 2014;48(3):200–5.
15. Zyluk A. Complex regional pain syndrome type I. Risk factors, prevention and risk of recurrence. J Hand Surg Br 2004;29(4):334–7.
16. An HS, Hawthorne KB, Jackson WT. Reflex sympathetic dystrophy and cigarette smoking. J Hand Surg Am 1988;13(3):458–60.
17. Galer BS, Bruehl S, Harden RN. IASP diagnostic criteria for complex regional pain syndrome: a preliminary empirical validation study. International Association for the Study of Pain. Clin J Pain 1998; 14(1):48–54.
18. Patterson RW, Li Z, Smith BP, et al. Complex regional pain syndrome of the upper extremity. J Hand Surg Am 2011;36(9):1553–62.
19. Lee GW, Weeks PM. The role of bone scintigraphy in diagnosing reflex sympathetic dystrophy. J Hand Surg Am 1995;20(3):458–63.
20. Zollinger PE, Tuinebreijer WE, Breederveld RS, et al. Can vitamin C prevent complex regional pain syndrome in patients with wrist fractures? A randomized, controlled, multicenter dose-response study. J Bone Joint Surg Am 2007; 89(7):1424–31.
21. Zollinger PE, Tuinebreijer WE, Kreis RW, et al. Effect of vitamin C on frequency of reflex sympathetic dystrophy in wrist fractures: a randomised trial. Lancet 1999;354(9195):2025–8.
22. Shah AS, Verma MK, Jebson PJ. Use of oral vitamin C after fractures of the distal radius. J Hand Surg Am 2009;34(9):1736–8.
23. Lichtman DM, Bindra RR, Boyer MI, et al. Treatment of distal radius fractures. J Am Acad Orthop Surg 2010;18(3):180–9.
24. Ekrol I, Duckworth AD, Ralston SH, et al. The influence of vitamin C on the outcome of distal radial fractures: a double-blind, randomized controlled trial. J Bone Joint Surg Am 2014;96(17):1451–9.
25. Goris RJ. Treatment of reflex sympathetic dystrophy with hydroxyl radical scavengers. Unfallchirurg 1985;88(7):330–2.
26. Livingstone JA, Atkins RM. Intravenous regional guanethidine blockade in the treatment of post-traumatic complex regional pain syndrome type 1 (algodystrophy) of the hand. J Bone Joint Surg Br 2002;84(3):380–6.
27. Paraskevas KI, Michaloglou AA, Briana DD, et al. Treatment of complex regional pain syndrome type I of the hand with a series of intravenous regional sympathetic blocks with guanethidine and lidocaine. Clin Rheumatol 2006;25(5):687–93.
28. Bushnell BD, Bynum DK. Malunion of the distal radius. J Am Acad Orthop Surg 2007;15(1):27–40.
29. Prommersberger KJ, Pillukat T, Mühldorfer M, et al. Malunion of the distal radius. Arch Orthop Trauma Surg 2012;132(5):693–702.
30. Haase SC, Chung KC. Management of malunions of the distal radius. Hand Clin 2012;28(2):207–16.

31. Sharma H, Khare GN, Singh S, et al. Outcomes and complications of fractures of distal radius (AO type B and C): volar plating versus nonoperative treatment. J Orthop Sci 2014;19(4):537–44.
32. Jenkins NH, Mintowt-Czyz WJ. Mal-union and dysfunction in Colles' fracture. J Hand Surg Br 1988;13(3):291–3.
33. Prommersberger KJ, Froehner SC, Schmitt RR, et al. Rotational deformity in malunited fractures of the distal radius. J Hand Surg Am 2004;29(1):110–5.
34. Fernandez DL. Malunion of the distal radius: current approach to management. Instr Course Lect 1993; 42:99–113.
35. Jupiter JB, Ruder J, Roth DA. Computer-generated bone models in the planning of osteotomy of multidirectional distal radius malunions. J Hand Surg Am 1992;17(3):406–15.
36. Athwal GS, Ellis RE, Small CF, et al. Computer-assisted distal radius osteotomy. J Hand Surg Am 2003; 28(6):951–8.
37. Miyake J, Murase T, Moritomo H, et al. Distal radius osteotomy with volar locking plates based on computer simulation. Clin Orthop Relat Res 2011; 469(6):1766–73.
38. Sato K, Nakamura T, Iwamoto T, et al. Corrective osteotomy for volarly malunited distal radius fracture. J Hand Surg Am 2009;34(1):27–33, 33.e1.
39. Jupiter JB, Ring D. A comparison of early and late reconstruction of malunited fractures of the distal end of the radius. J Bone Joint Surg Am 1996; 78(5):739–48.
40. Wada T, Tsuji H, Iba K, et al. Simultaneous radial closing wedge and ulnar shortening osteotomy for distal radius malunion. Tech Hand Up Extrem Surg 2005;9(4):188–94.
41. Turner RG, Faber KJ, Athwal GS. Complications of distal radius fractures. Orthop Clin North Am 2007; 38(2):217–28, vi.
42. Koval KJ, Harrast JJ, Anglen JO, et al. Fractures of the distal part of the radius. The evolution of practice over time. Where's the evidence? J Bone Joint Surg Am 2008;90(9):1855–61.
43. Chung KC, Shauver MJ, Birkmeyer JD. Trends in the United States in the treatment of distal radial fractures in the elderly. J Bone Joint Surg Am 2009; 91(8):1868–73.
44. Orbay JL. The treatment of unstable distal radius fractures with volar fixation. Hand Surg 2000;5(2): 103–12.
45. Fernandez DL. Should anatomic reduction be pursued in distal radial fractures? J Hand Surg Br 2000;25(6):523–7.
46. Baratz ME, Des Jardins JD, Anderson DD, et al. Displaced intra-articular fractures of the distal radius: the effect of fracture displacement on contact stresses in a cadaver model. J Hand Surg Am 1996;21(2):183–8.
47. Orbay J. Volar plate fixation of distal radius fractures. Hand Clin 2005;21(3):347–54.
48. Tiren D, Vos DI. Correction osteotomy of distal radius malunion stabilised with dorsal locking plates without grafting. Strategies Trauma Limb Reconstr 2014;9(1):53–8.
49. Dimitriou R, Mataliotakis GI, Angoules AG, et al. Complications following autologous bone graft harvesting from the iliac crest and using the RIA: a systematic review. Injury 2011;42(Suppl 2):S3–15.
50. Simic PM, Robison J, Gardner MJ, et al. Treatment of distal radius fractures with a low-profile dorsal plating system: an outcomes assessment. J Hand Surg Am 2006;31(3):382–6.
51. Tarallo L, Mugnai R, Zambianchi F, et al. Volar plate fixation for the treatment of distal radius fractures: analysis of adverse events. J Orthop Trauma 2013; 27(12):740–5.
52. Mahmoud M, El Shafie S, Kamal M. Correction of dorsally-malunited extra-articular distal radial fractures using volar locked plates without bone grafting. J Bone Joint Surg Br 2012;94(8):1090–6.
53. Hargreaves DG, Drew SJ, Eckersley R. Kirschner wire pin tract infection rates: a randomized controlled trial between percutaneous and buried wires. J Hand Surg Br 2004;29(4):374–6.
54. Ahlborg HG, Josefsson PO. Pin-tract complications in external fixation of fractures of the distal radius. Acta Orthop Scand 1999;70(2):116–8.
55. Esposito J, Schemitsch EH, Saccone M, et al. External fixation versus open reduction with plate fixation for distal radius fractures: a meta-analysis of randomised controlled trials. Injury 2013;44(4): 409–16.
56. Margaliot Z, Haase SC, Kotsis SV, et al. A meta-analysis of outcomes of external fixation versus plate osteosynthesis for unstable distal radius fractures. J Hand Surg Am 2005;30(6):1185–99.
57. Egol KA, Paksima N, Puopolo S, et al. Treatment of external fixation pins about the wrist: a prospective, randomized trial. J Bone Joint Surg Am 2006;88(2): 349–54.
58. Glueck DA, Charoglu CP, Lawton JN. Factors associated with infection following open distal radius fractures. Hand (N Y) 2009;4(3):330–4.
59. Subramanian P, Kantharuban S, Shilston S, et al. Complications of Kirschner-wire fixation in distal radius fractures. Tech Hand Up Extrem Surg 2012; 16(3):120–3.
60. Hargreaves DG, Pajkos A, Deva AK, et al. The role of biofilm formation in percutaneous Kirschner-wire fixation of radial fractures. J Hand Surg Br 2002;27(4): 365–8.
61. Santy J. A review of pin site wound infection assessment criteria. Int J Orthop Trauma Nurs 2010;14(3): 125–31.

62. Bonatz E, Kramer TD, Masear VR. Rupture of the extensor pollicis longus tendon. Am J Orthop (Belle Mead NJ) 1996;25(2):118–22.
63. Arora R, Lutz M, Hennerbichler A, et al. Complications following internal fixation of unstable distal radius fracture with a palmar locking-plate. J Orthop Trauma 2007;21(5):316–22.
64. Soong M, van Leerdam R, Guitton TG, et al. Fracture of the distal radius: risk factors for complications after locked volar plate fixation. J Hand Surg Am 2011;36(1):3–9.
65. Meyer C, Chang J, Stern P, et al. Complications of distal radial and scaphoid fracture treatment. J Bone Joint Surg Am 2013;95(16):1517–26.
66. Kozin SH, Wood MB. Early soft-tissue complications after fractures of the distal part of the radius. J Bone Joint Surg Am 1993;75(1):144–53.
67. Owers KL, Lee J, Khan N, et al. Ultrasound changes in the extensor pollicis longus tendon following fractures of the distal radius: a preliminary report. J Hand Surg Eur Vol 2007;32(4):467–71.
68. Schaller P, Baer W, Carl HD. Extensor indicis-transfer compared with palmaris longus transplantation in reconstruction of extensor pollicis longus tendon: a retrospective study. Scand J Plast Reconstr Surg Hand Surg 2007;41(1):33–5.
69. Rozental TD, Beredjiklian PK, Bozentka DJ. Functional outcome and complications following two types of dorsal plating for unstable fractures of the distal part of the radius. J Bone Joint Surg Am 2003;85-A(10):1956–60.
70. Althausen PL, Szabo RM. Coverage of distal radius internal fixation and wrist fusion devices with AlloDerm. Tech Hand Up Extrem Surg 2004;8(4):266–8.
71. Chiang PP, Roach S, Baratz ME. Failure of a retinacular flap to prevent dorsal wrist pain after titanium Pi plate fixation of distal radius fractures. J Hand Surg Am 2002;27(4):724–8.
72. Oren TW, Wolf JM. Soft-tissue complications associated with distal radius fractures. Operat Tech Orthop 2009;19(2):100–6.
73. Orbay JL, Touhami A. Current concepts in volar fixed-angle fixation of unstable distal radius fractures. Clin Orthop Relat Res 2006;445:58–67.
74. Soong M, Earp BE, Bishop G, et al. Volar locking plate implant prominence and flexor tendon rupture. J Bone Joint Surg Am 2011;93(4):328–35.
75. Bell JS, Wollstein R, Citron ND. Rupture of flexor pollicis longus tendon: a complication of volar plating of the distal radius. J Bone Joint Surg Br 1998;80(2):225–6.
76. Tada K, Ikeda K, Shigemoto K, et al. Prevention of flexor pollicis longus tendon rupture after volar plate fixation of distal radius fractures. Hand Surg 2011;16(3):271–5.
77. Unglaub F, Bultmann C, Reiter A, et al. Two-staged reconstruction of the flexor pollicis longus tendon. J Hand Surg Br 2006;31(4):432–5.
78. Brown EN, Lifchez SD. Flexor pollicis longus tendon rupture after volar plating of a distal radius fracture: pronator quadratus plate coverage may not adequately protect tendons. Eplasty 2011;11:e43.

Management of Complications of Forearm Fractures

Albert V. George, MD[a], Jeffrey N. Lawton, MD[b,*]

KEYWORDS

• Fractures • Forearm • Galeazzi • Monteggia • Essex–Lopresti

KEY POINTS

- Optimal outcomes in the treatment of forearm fracture–dislocations depend on early recognition and management.
- Restoration and maintenance of anatomic alignment are the key principles in managing forearm fracture–dislocations.
- When missed, correction of complication needs to consider the anatomic region in each section.
- Children are managed typically with nonoperative treatment except in certain circumstances, whereas adults are always managed surgically.

INTRODUCTION

Forearm fractures may be complicated by the disruption of the distal radioulnar, proximal radioulnar, or radiocapitellar joints. The forearm is truly a component of both the wrist and the elbow with pathology in one area potentially affecting other areas as well. Careful history, physical examination, and radiographic evaluation of the wrist, forearm, and elbow is necessary in all forearm fractures to recognize this unique subset of injuries. Historically, these forearm fracture-dislocations have had poor outcomes, but early recognition of these injuries and advances in fixation techniques have led to much improved results. This article discusses radial diaphyseal fractures with distal radioulnar joint disruption, proximal ulnar fractures with radiocapitellar disruption, and disruption of the forearm longitudinal axis and how to properly recognize and manage these forearm fracture-dislocations to avoid these problems, and how to treat these complications as they arise.

RADIAL DIAPHYSEAL FRACTURE WITH DISTAL RADIOULNAR JOINT DISRUPTION

A Galeazzi fracture is defined as a fracture of the shaft of the radius with an associated disruption of the distal radioulnar joint (DRUJ; **Fig. 1**).[1,2] Sir Astley Cooper was the first to describe this fracture pattern in 1822,[3,4] but Galeazzi reported a series of 18 patients in 1934 with this injury and was the first to recognize the connection between the fracture of the radial shaft and the dislocation of the DRUJ, as well as the importance of addressing these injuries together.[3,5,6] It is also known as a reverse Monteggia fracture, a Piedmont fracture, a Darrach–Hughston–Milch fracture, and a fracture of necessity.[3] Nearly 7% of all adult forearm fractures are radial diaphyseal fractures with associated DRUJ disruption.[7] There are also other injuries that are considered Galeazzi's equivalents. In children, this is a fracture of the shaft of the radius with an associated separation of the distal ulnar epiphysis but without disruption of DRUJ.[2,3] In adults, this is a both bone forearm

[a] Department of Orthopedic Surgery, University of Michigan Hospital, University of Michigan, 1500 Medical Center Drive, Taubman Center – Orthopedic Surgery Office, Ann Arbor, MI 48109, USA; [b] Hand and Microsurgery, Department of Orthopedic Surgery, University of Michigan, 2098 South Main Street, Ann Arbor, MI 48103, USA
* Corresponding author.
E-mail address: jeflawto@med.umich.edu

Hand Clin 31 (2015) 217–233
http://dx.doi.org/10.1016/j.hcl.2015.01.010
0749-0712/15/$ – see front matter

A

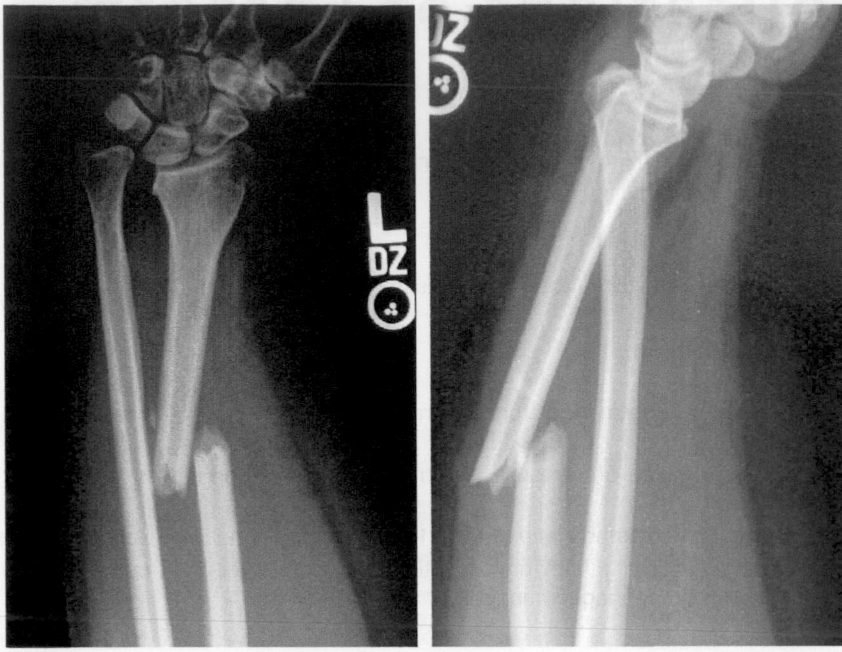

Fig. 1. (*A*) Posteroanterior and lateral radiographs demonstrating a Galeazzi fracture of the left forearm of a 62-year-old, right hand–dominant nurse. (*B*) Follow-up images and clinical pictures of forearm rotation.

fracture with an associated disruption of the DRUJ.[2,3]

Anatomy and Classification

To help understand the mechanics of forearm fracture dislocations, the radius, ulna, proximal radioulnar joint (PRUJ), and DRUJ can be thought of as stable ring. An injury to more than 1 component of the ring makes it unstable and all components must be addressed properly to restore function.[3] At the DRUJ, the radius and ulna are connected by the triangular fibrocartilage complex (TFCC), including the volar and dorsal radioulnar ligaments, and at the PRUJ they are connected by the annular and quadrate ligaments. The interosseous membrane (IOM) connects the intermediate area with the central one-third sometimes referred to as the interosseous ligament.

The ulna is a fixed structure at the elbow with disruption of the DRUJ, resulting in displacement of the radius relative to the ulna. Historically, dislocations at the DRUJ have been described in terms of the position of the ulna at the wrist, "the ulna being dorsally dislocated." This nomenclature is anatomically incorrect. The literature has shifted recently toward describing DRUJ dislocations in the anatomically correct manner of the position of the radius relative to the fixed ulna. In this article, we are careful to define clearly the direction of the radius/carpus/hand at the DRUJ dislocation to minimize any confusion.

The DRUJ is stabilized primarily by the TFCC, which is composed of the triangular fibrocartilage or articular disc, the ulnocarpal meniscal homologue, the dorsal and volar radioulnar ligaments, the ulnar collateral ligament, and the sheath of the extensor carpi ulnaris tendon.[8,9] Secondary stabilizers of the DRUJ include the pronator quadratus, IOM, joint capsule, and extensor carpi ulnaris.[10]

The mechanism of injury in a radial diaphyseal fracture with associated DRUJ disruption is theorized to be caused by a fall on an outstretched hand with a hyperpronated forearm.[2] Other mechanisms of injury that have been reported include motor vehicle accidents and gunshot wounds.[11,12] The fractured radius shortens, leading to a disruption of the TFCC or an ulnar styloid fracture.[13] The disruption of the TFCC is the key factor causing instability of the DRUJ.[2] A fracture of the ulnar styloid process can also cause instability of the DRUJ because the separate structures that comprise the TFCC blend and attach at the fovea. If the ulnar styloid process is fractured, it is usually displaced volar to the distal part of the ulna.[13]

Disruption of the DRUJ may be more likely to occur with more distal radial shaft fractures. Rettig and Raskin[14] proposed a classification scheme for Galeazzi fractures with type I fractures located less

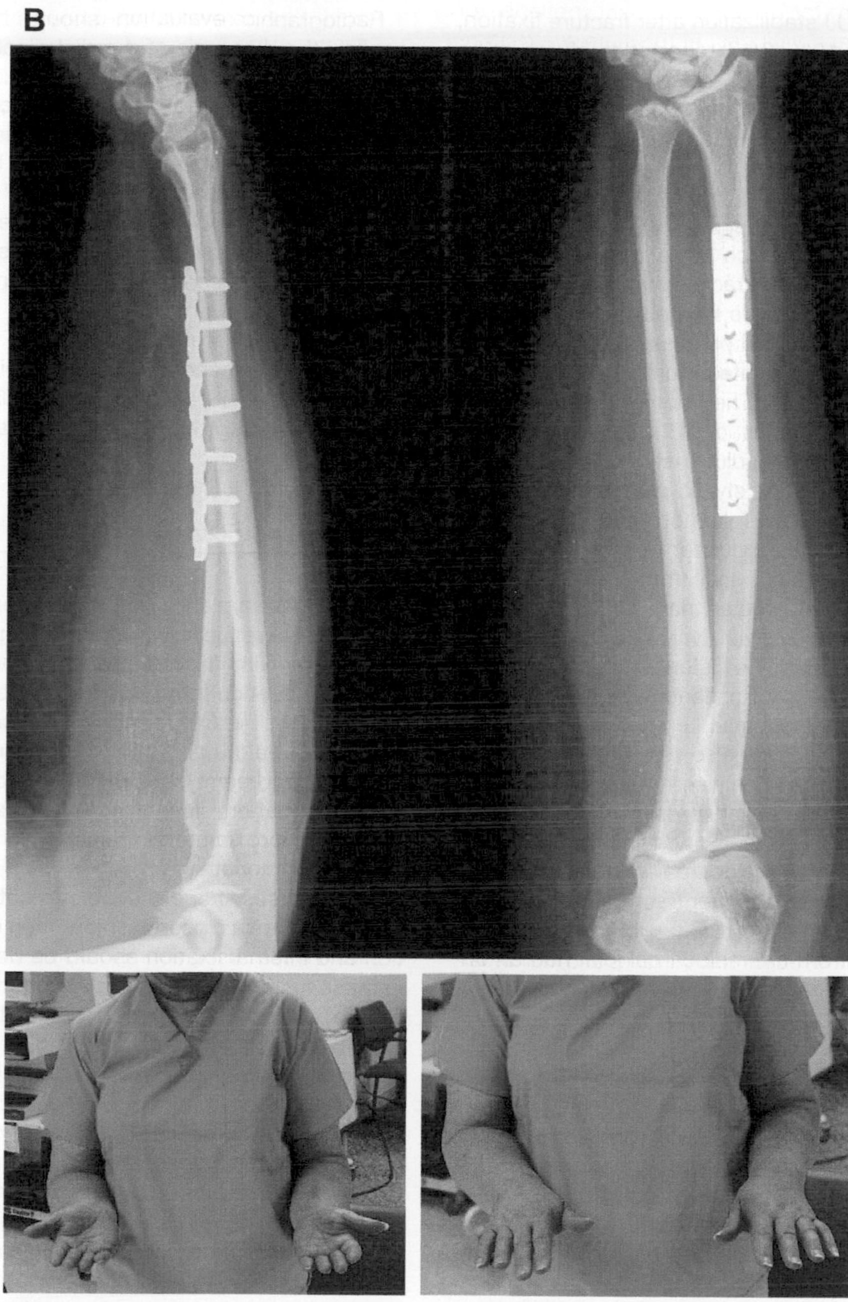

Fig. 1. (*continued*)

than 7.5 cm from the midarticular surface of the distal radius and type II fractures located more than 7.5 cm from the midarticular surface of the distal radius. They found that the risk of persistent DRUJ instability after radial shaft fracture fixation was significantly greater in type I Galeazzi fractures with 55% of these fractures (12/22) having persistent DRUJ instability, whereas only 6% of type II Galeazzi fractures (1/18) had persistent DRUJ instability.[14]

Alternatively, a more recent study by Korompilias and colleagues[15] proposed a different classification scheme for Galeazzi fractures, with type I fractures located in the distal one-third of the radial shaft, type II fractures located in the middle one-third of the radial shaft, and type III fractures located in the proximal one-third of the radial shaft. They found similar results to Rettig and Raskin[14] in their series of patients, with 54% (37/69) reporting fractures in the distal one-third of the radius requiring DRUJ stabilization after fracture fixation, whereas only 12% (2/17) reported fractures in the middle one-third of the radius and only 11% (1/9) reporting fractures in the proximal one-third of the radius requiring DRUJ stabilization after fracture fixation.

Maculé Beneyto and colleagues[11] divided Galeazzi fractures, in their series of patients, into type I fractures, which were located between 0 and 10 cm from the radial styloid process; type II fractures, which were located between 10 and 15 cm from the styloid process; and type III fractures, which were located more than 15 cm from the styloid process. They noted the worst outcomes in their series of 33 Galeazzi fractures with fractures of the radius that occurred between 0 and 10 cm from the styloid process.

A recent study by Takemoto and colleagues[16] found that the only predictor of persistent DRUJ instability after radial shaft fracture fixation was ulnar variance of greater than ±2 mm on injury films. Of patients with variance greater than 2 mm, 79% had persistent DRUJ instability, whereas only 21% of patients with an ulnar variance between less than 2 mm had persistent DRUJ instability. They also reported no association, in their series, between the location of the radial shaft fracture and persistent instability of the DRUJ. Of patients with fractures within 7.5 cm from the radiocarpal joint, 41% (7/17) had an unstable DRUJ after fracture fixation; similarly, 39% of patients (13/33) with fractures more than 7.5 cm from the radiocarpal joint had an unstable DRUJ after fracture fixation.

Presentation and Workup

A fracture of the forearm should always trigger a careful examination of the wrist and elbow joints. Functionally, the forearm should be considered a single unit and although an isolated diaphyseal fracture, such as a nightstick fracture, is possible, the diagnosis should be one of exclusion. DRUJ disruption is a common but often subtle complication of displaced radial shaft fractures.[17,18] When DRUJ disruption is present, the wrist is typically deformed, swollen, and painful and forearm rotation may be limited.[13] In a dislocation where the radius is displaced volar to the ulna, the ulnar head is prominent dorsally on physical examination.[13,14] This prominence may be difficult to identify in an edematous and contused forearm.[19] In a dislocation where the radius is displaced dorsal to the ulna, which is much less common, the wrist may seem narrow and a depression may be noted where the ulnar head is normally located.[13] Neurovascular injury is rare.[17]

Radiographic evaluation should be used to confirm the diagnosis of a radial diaphyseal fracture with associated DRUJ disruption. Anteroposterior (AP) and lateral radiographs of the wrist, forearm, and elbow should be obtained. Radiographs of the contralateral wrist may be obtained for comparison. Radiographic signs of DRUJ injury include widening of the DRUJ space on the AP radiograph, dislocation of the radius relative to the ulna on the lateral radiograph, 5 mm or more of ulnar-positive variance, or a base of the ulnar styloid fracture.[7] If it is unclear from plain radiographs whether there is an associated DRUJ injury, CT may be used to aid evaluation of the joint.[9] Additionally, MRI may discern the status of the TFCC.[9]

Treatment and Outcomes

Children

Children are typically managed nonoperatively with closed reduction performed under general anesthesia with fluoroscopic guidance followed by immobilization in an above-the-elbow cast for 4 to 6 weeks. The DRUJ should be assessed under anesthesia before and after reduction of the fracture.[20] The forearm should be immobilized in full supination after closed reduction as the torn TFCC is approximated in this position, allowing it to heal appropriately.[21]

In rare cases, if one is unable to obtain or maintain reduction in closed fashion, then open reduction and internal fixation should be done. Options in these instances include open reduction without internal fixation; open reduction with Kirschner wire fixation, intramedullary nailing, or dorsal plate fixation of the radius; or open reduction with radioulnar transfixation.[1,2,11,22] Owing to the relatively small number of pediatric Galeazzi fractures that are managed surgically, the outcomes of these different techniques have not been compared adequately.

In a series of 26 children with Galeazzi fractures by Eberl and colleagues,[22] 22 patients were treated with closed reduction and cast immobilization; 90% of patients (20/22) had excellent results, whereas the remaining 10% of patients (2/22) had good results with none of the patients having long-term instability of the DRUJ. Notably, 14 of these patients had their associated DRUJ injury initially unrecognized, but they still had good-to-excellent outcomes.

Walsh and colleagues[20] conducted a study of 41 children with Galeazzi fractures; 93% of these patients (38/41) had fair-to-excellent results with closed reduction and cast immobilization and only 2 patients required open reduction and internal fixation owing to an inability to achieve an acceptable closed reduction. Worse outcomes were found with more distal fractures located in the distal one-third of the radius.

Galeazzi equivalent fractures in children are managed in the same manner, with closed reduction followed by immobilization in an above-the-elbow cast.[23] In rare cases, if one is unable to obtain or maintain reduction, then open reduction and internal fixation should be done. It is important to treat this injury properly because it can lead to growth plate arrest of the distal ulnar physis if unrecognized or unreduced.[23]

Adults

Radial diaphyseal fractures with associated DRUJ disruption are managed in adults with open reduction and internal fixation. Nonoperative treatment of adult Galeazzi fractures has been attempted in the past with consistently unsatisfactory outcomes. In a study by Hughston,[24] 92% of Galeazzi fractures (35/38) failed closed reduction and immobilization. In a series by Mikić,[2] 80% of patients (16/20) treated with closed reduction and immobilization had a poor result, whereas 83% of patients (10/12) treated with open reduction and plate-and-screw fixation had fair-to-excellent results. Although they were able to obtain proper reduction initially in most of the cases treated with closed reduction, slippage of the fracture fragments and subluxation or dislocation of the DRUJ usually occurred 7 to 10 days after reduction.[2] In another series by Reckling,[18] 63% of patients (7/11) treated with closed reduction and immobilization had a poor result with the remainder having a fair result, whereas all 17 of the patients treated with open reduction and plate-and-screw fixation had a good result.

There are several factors that contribute to the loss of reduction with nonoperative treatment. The weight of the hand provides a strong volar displacing force on the distal radial fragment. The pronator quadratus inserts on the distal fracture fragment, rotating the fragment toward the ulna and pulling it in a volar and proximal direction. The brachioradialis shortens the distal radial fragment relative to the ulna. Thumb abductors and extensors shorten the radial side of the wrist, leading to relaxation of the radial collateral ligament.[24] If reduction is lost, then there may be malalignment of the fracture fragments, causing recurrent dislocation and loss of forearm motion.[18]

The guiding principles in the treatment of radial diaphyseal fractures with associated DRUJ disruption in adults is the restoration and maintenance of anatomic alignment of the radius with intraoperative assessment of the DRUJ and repair of associated soft tissue damage. If these principles are followed, then Galeazzi fractures have been noted to have the same results as isolated radial shaft fractures without DRUJ injury. Van Duijvenbode and colleagues[25] found no difference in long-term outcomes including DRUJ stability between 10 patients who had isolated radial shaft fractures and 7 patients who had radial shaft fractures with associated DRUJ dislocation at 19-year follow-up with treatment of all fractures with near-anatomic open reduction and plate and screw fixation.

Plate and screw fixation is the preferred method of radial fracture fixation. It is best done with a 3.5-mm dynamic compression plate, as seen in more recent series, or a 4.5-mm dynamic compression plate, as seen in older series, applied through a volar approach.[7,16,18,25,26]

After internal fixation of the radial shaft fracture, stability of the DRUJ should be assessed intraoperatively. AP and lateral radiographs of the DRUJ should be obtained. The DRUJ should then be tested clinically. This testing is done by holding the radius and ulna with separate hands and then moving the distal radius in a dorsal–volar direction. This motion can be done with the forearm in the neutral, fully supinated, and fully pronated positions. The contralateral DRUJ should be evaluated for comparison before surgical scrub. The DRUJ of the injured wrist is then able to be compared with a standard on that patient and classified as stable, unstable but reducible, or irreducible.[16,25]

If the DRUJ is stable, then all that is required is immobilization in an above-the-elbow cast. The arm can be immobilized in supination for 4 weeks or in neutral for 2 weeks followed by functional bracing. A recent study by Park and colleagues[27] found no difference in outcomes when patients with Galeazzi fractures found to have a stable DRUJ after radius fixation were treated with immobilization in supination for 4 weeks compared with immobilization in neutral for 2 weeks followed by functional bracing.

If the DRUJ is unstable but reducible, the DRUJ should be manually reduced and one or two 0.62-inch Kirschner wires should be used to temporarily stabilize the joint for 4 weeks. The pin(s) should be inserted just proximal to the DRUJ and parallel to the radiocarpal joint in an ulnar to radial direction for ease of placement. They should penetrate the radial border of the radius to make retrieval of the pin(s) easier if they break. The authors favor the use of 2 parallel pins (**Fig. 2**). Transfixation of the DRUJ is contraindicated in a complex dislocation that is defined by Bruckner and colleagues[28] as characterized by obvious irreducibility,

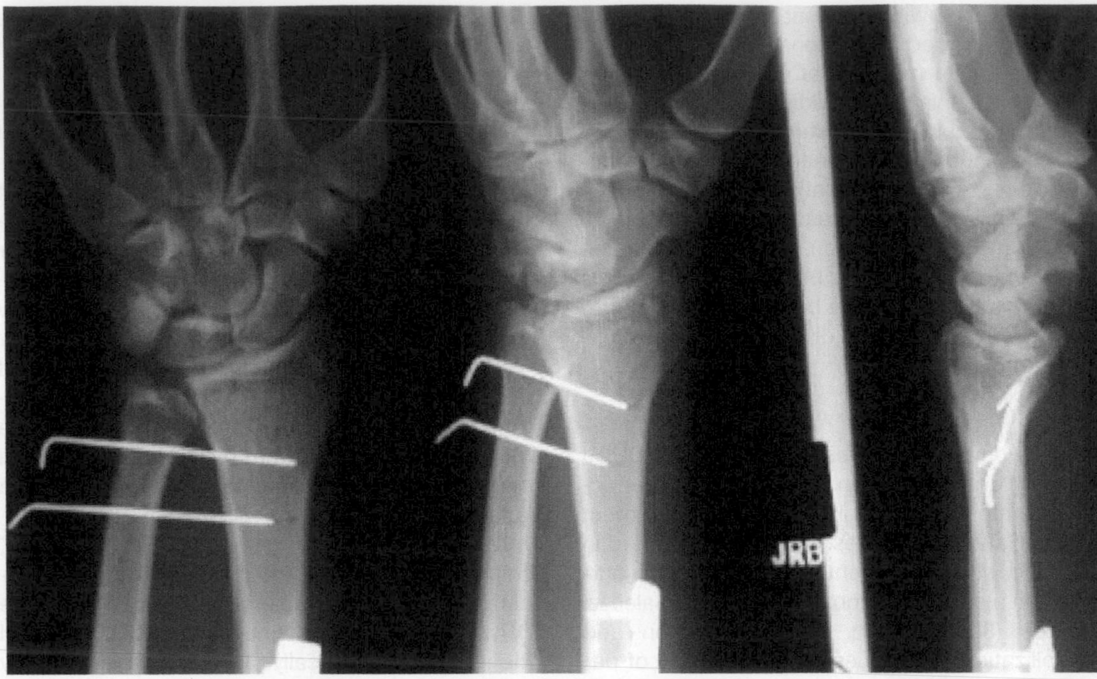

Fig. 2. Posteroanterior (*left*), oblique (*center*), and lateral (*right*) radiographs demonstrating 2 ulnar/radial pins. Note loosening and backing out of the proximal pin.

recurrent subluxations, or a mushy sensation owing to soft tissue or bone interposition. Korompilias and associates[15] reported that 42% of patients (40/95) with Galeazzi fractures in their series of 95 patients required pinning of the DRUJ. At a follow-up of 6 years, none of these patients had persistent DRUJ instability.

If the DRUJ is irreducible, then exploration of the DRUJ through a dorsal approach is indicated, with careful dissection at the dorsal cutaneous branch of the ulnar nerve (**Fig. 3**). Difficulty with reduction of the DRUJ is most commonly caused by interposition of soft tissue, commonly the extensor carpi ulnaris tendon.[1,29] The interposed soft tissue or fracture fragments should be removed to facilitate reduction of the DRUJ. If there is a massive tear of the TFCC, the TFCC should be repaired with suture anchors or sutures passed in mattress fashion through the distal ulna.[10] If there is a fracture of the ulnar styloid process, it should be treated by open reduction and internal fixation with either a cannulated lag screw, pins, or tension band, depending on the size of the fragment (**Fig. 4**).[1] After restoration of these structures, the DRUJ may be transfixed with 0.62-inch Kirschner wire(s) as described.

The forearm should be supported in an above-the-elbow cast in full supination for 4 weeks because in that position the dislocation is reduced and the TFCC is approximated.[18] Moore and colleagues[7] had their series of patients undergo 4 weeks of immobilization with their forearm in 5° to 10° of supination or in neutral position with no late DRUJ subluxations or dislocations noted in

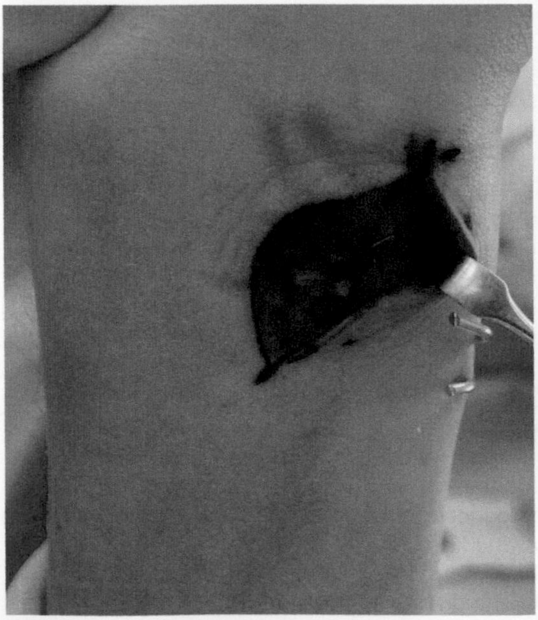

Fig. 3. Dorsal view of right wrist demonstrating approach to distal radioulnar joint with extensor retinaculum repair visible (extensor carpi ulnaris entrapped) and 2 ulnar/radial pins visible.

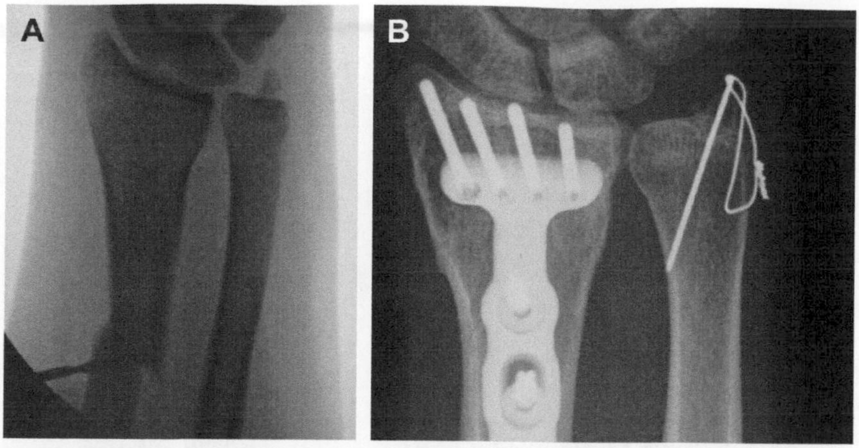

Fig. 4. (*A*) Galeazzi fracture associated with ulnar styloid fracture. (*B*) Tension-band fixation of ulnar styloid fracture.

any their patients. By immobilizing the patient's arm in closer to neutral rotation, they were able to decrease the risk of a disabling supination contracture and still obtain satisfactory long-term soft tissue healing.

Complications of radial diaphyseal fractures with associated DRUJ disruption include delayed union, malunion/nonunion, infection, nerve injury, limited pronation/supination, tendon entrapment, chronic instability of the DRUJ, persistent pain, and loss of grip strength.[1,2,7,13,24]

In chronic cases, the goal is to improve congruency of the DRUJ. This may be accomplished by performing a radial osteotomy with plating and bone graft (**Fig. 5**).[1] If DRUJ congruity is not possible, salvage techniques such as the Darrach procedure,[30,31] Sauve–Kapandji procedure,[32] hemiresection arthroplasty,[33] or implant arthroplasty[34] may be indicated.

Again, it cannot be overstated that the most important method to treat or avoid complications is to not miss this injury. However, the guiding principle for malunion or nonunion remains the restoration of anatomic alignment of the radius and open reduction or salvage of the DRUJ.

PROXIMAL ULNA FRACTURE WITH RADIOCAPITELLAR JOINT DISRUPTION

Monteggia originally described 2 cases of a fracture of the proximal one-third of the ulna associated with an anterior dislocation of the radial head in 1814.[35,36] Bado expanded the definition of a Monteggia lesion to be "a dislocation of the radio-humero-ulnar joint, associated with a fracture of the ulna levels at various or with lesions at the wrist."[35,36] Recently, Ring proposed 2 new definitions for a Monteggia fracture as either a diaphyseal forearm fracture with dislocation of the PRUJ or an ulna fracture with disruption of the radiocapitellar joint.[37] These fractures are relatively rare, accounting for only 1% to 2% of all forearm fractures.[18,38]

Anatomy and Classification

Functionally, dislocation of the PRUJ and/or the radiocapitellar joint is one of the defining features of a Monteggia fracture. The annular and quadrate ligaments stabilize the PRUJ with rupture of these ligaments that disrupts the PRUJ and associated rupture of elbow capsular ligaments cause dissociation of the radiocapitellar joint.[39] The IOM and TFCC remain intact. Thus, the proximal radioulnar joint is restored with anatomic reduction of the ulnar fracture except in the rare instances when there is soft tissue interposition.[39] The mechanism of injury is theorized to be a fall on a pronated and flexed arm or a direct blow to the arm.[17]

Bado proposed a classification scheme for Monteggia fractures that is based on the direction of radial head dislocation and associated angulation of the ulnar fracture. Type I is anterior, type II is posterior, type III is lateral, and type IV is a both bone forearm fracture with radial head dislocation.[35] A fracture of the radial head or coronoid process may be associated with the ulna fracture with both most commonly occurring with type II lesions.[40] The most common Monteggia fracture type in children is type I lesions and in adults it is type II lesions.[38,40–42]

Letts and colleagues[43] proposed an alternate classification scheme for pediatric Monteggia lesions to accommodate plastic deformation and greenstick fractures of the ulna associated with radial head dislocation. These more subtle ulnar

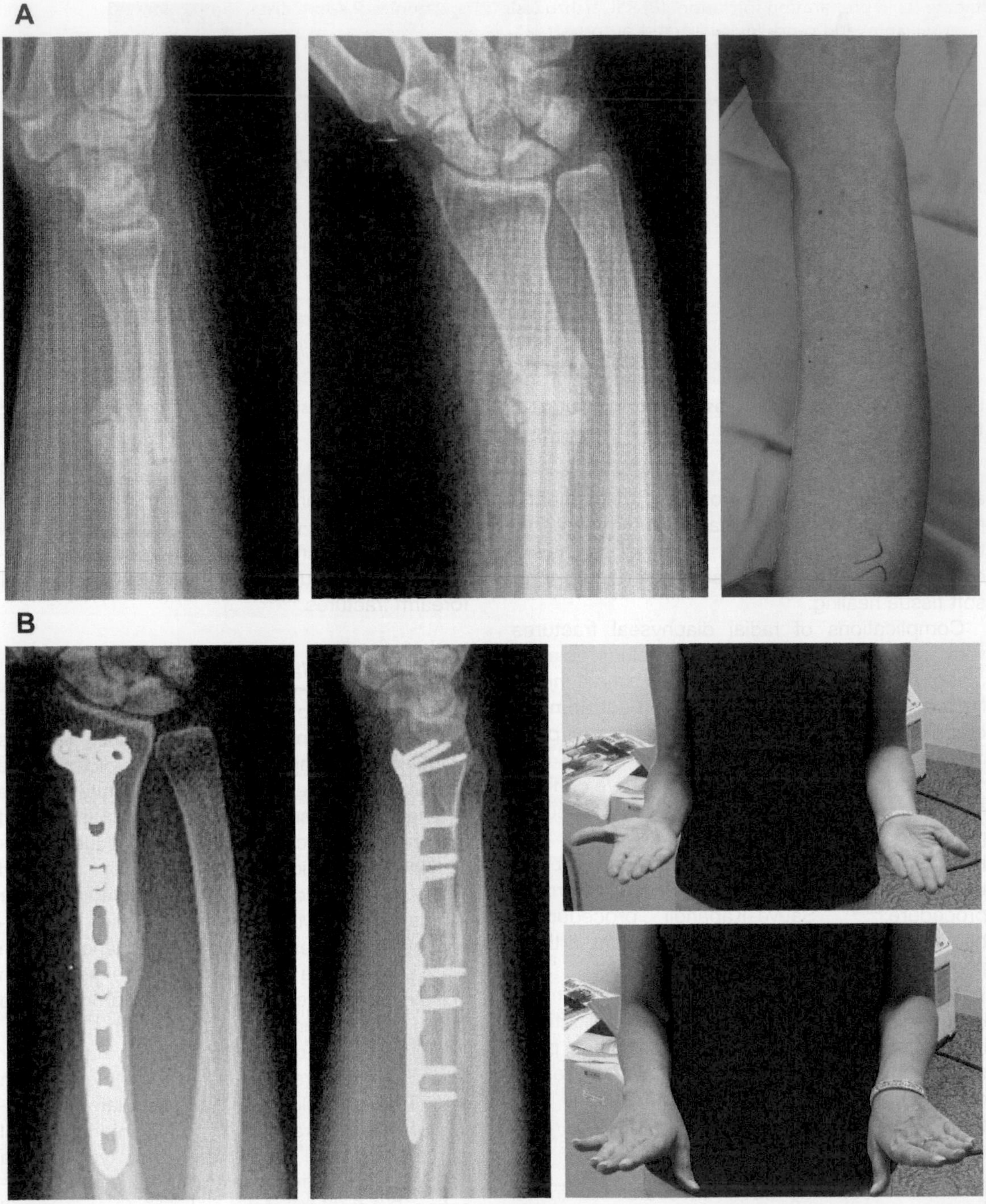

Fig. 5. (*A*) Right Galeazzi malunion of 43-year-old right hand–dominant woman treated conservatively, including a clinical picture demonstrating radial deviation (apex ulnar). (*B*) Follow-up images and clinical pictures of forearm rotation.

fractures often present late and can be more difficult to deal with requiring osteotomy and open reduction of the radiocapitellar joint if missed. Type A is an anterior plastic deformation of the ulna, type B is an anterior greenstick fracture of the ulna, and type C is an anterior complete fracture of the ulna. These are all associated with an anterior radial head dislocation. Type D is a posterior complete fracture with associated radial head dislocation, and type E is a proximal ulnar fracture with lateral radial head dislocation.[43]

Jupiter and colleagues[38] further subclassified Bado type II lesions in adults based on the location and type of ulna fracture. Type IIA involves a fracture of the very proximal ulna and coronoid process; type IIB involves a fracture at the ulna metaphyseal–diaphyseal junction, distal to the coronoid process; type IIIC is a fracture of the ulna diaphysis; and type IIID is a complex ulna fracture that extends from the olecranon to the diaphysis.

Presentation and Workup

Patients may present with considerable pain and swelling at the elbow and elbow flexion and forearm rotation are usually limited and painful.[17] The dislocated radial head may be palpable in the antecubital fossa, posteriorly or laterally, depending on the direction of dislocation.[44] Unlike in Galeazzi fractures, neurovascular injury is not uncommon, especially injury to the posterior interosseous nerve owing to its close anatomic relationship with the radial head.[45,46] This injury may manifest as weakness or paralysis of extension of the thumb or fingers.

Radiographic evaluation should be used to confirm the diagnosis of a proximal ulna fracture with associated PRUJ and/or radiocapitellar joint disruption. AP and lateral radiographs of the wrist, forearm, and elbow should be obtained. Dislocation of the radial head can be recognized by looking for disruption of the normal radiocapitellar relationship. Normally, a line down the center of the radius should intersect the center of the capitellum in any view, but in a Monteggia fracture this line will not intersect the capitellum.[43]

Treatment and Outcomes

Children

The key treatment principles in pediatric proximal ulna fractures with associated PRUJ and/or radiocapitellar joint disruption are early recognition of the injury and restoration of anatomic alignment of the fractured ulna. The ulnar fracture pattern guides treatment with the majority of acute Monteggia fractures in children treated nonoperatively with closed reduction and cast immobilization.[42] Plastic deformation, metaphyseal buckle fractures, and greenstick fractures should be treated with closed reduction of the ulna fracture followed by cast immobilization, whereas complete fractures should be managed operatively. Transverse and short oblique fractures should be treated with intramedullary pin fixation, whereas long oblique and comminuted fractures should be treated with open reduction and plate and screw fixation.[37,42] After closed reduction or operative treatment, cast immobilization should be used for 4 weeks.[37]

In a recent study by Ramski and colleagues[47] of 112 acute pediatric Monteggia fractures with a follow-up of 19 weeks, they found that no failures in 57 patients treated according with closed reduction and immobilization for plastic deformation and greenstick fractures, intramedullary pin fixation for transverse and short oblique fractures, and open reduction and plate fixation for long oblique and comminuted fractures. Twenty-three patients who were treated more rigorously than the strategy described also did not suffer any treatment failures. Treatment failure occurred in 33% of patients (6/18) with complete fractures treated with closed reduction and immobilization as defined by the authors as "failure to maintain an anatomic reduction of the radial head and/or loss of ulnar reduction during follow-up." The only risk factor identified by the authors for failure of treatment was nonoperative treatment of complete fractures.

The treatment of a chronic Monteggia lesion in children is controversial, with several different treatment options described in the literature. These options include open or closed reduction, repair or reconstruction of the annular ligament, ulnar shortening osteotomy, radial shortening osteotomy, or a combination of these techniques.[48–50]

Nakamura and colleagues[51] reported good long-term clinical and radiographic outcomes in a series of 22 pediatric patients with missed Monteggia fractures who were treated by open reduction, ulnar osteotomy, and annular ligament reconstruction if treatment was performed within 3 years of injury or the patient was less than 12 years old.

Closed reduction by ulnar osteotomy followed by gradual lengthening and angulation of the ulna using an external fixator has been described more recently as a less invasive approach to managing chronic pediatric Monteggia lesions.[49,52] Bor and colleagues[49] recently described 4 cases in which they used this method successfully with normal function of the forearm and full movement of the elbow at a follow-up of 3 years. Notably, the average time in the frame was 3.5 months, which may be difficult for some pediatric patients.

Adults

Just like in children, the key treatment principles in adult proximal ulna fractures with associated PRUJ and/or radiocapitellar joint is early recognition of the injury and restoration of anatomic alignment of the fractured ulna. Obtaining adequate alignment of the ulna is important, because inadequate ulnar alignment can lead to residual PRUJ or radiocapitellar joint subluxation.[37,38] Open reduction and internal fixation of the ulna fracture is the treatment of choice for acute Monteggia fractures.[37,39,53] Previous attempts at nonoperative treatment have noted uniformly unsatisfactory results.[18,45,54]

A compression plate should be applied to the dorsal (tension side) of the ulna and should be contoured around the olecranon process. If there is a fracture of the coronoid process, radial head, or injury to the lateral collateral ligament, these should be addressed as well. A fracture of the radial head can be treated with either repair or replacement.[37] If the radial head fracture has 3 or fewer articular fragments, it may be amenable to open reduction and internal fixation.[55] Careful attention is needed to avoid injuring the posterior interosseous nerve while using a lateral approach because it may be encountered beyond 4 cm from the radiocapitellar joint space.[56]

In a study by Konrad and colleagues,[40] the authors reported that 73% of adult patients (35/47) with Monteggia fractures treated by operative fixation had good-to-excellent outcomes at a follow-up of 8 years with Bado type II lesions, Jupiter type IIa lesions, intra-articular radial head fractures, coronoid fractures, and complications requiring additional operations associated with poor outcomes. The authors treated comminuted radial head fractures with either open reduction and internal fixation or radial head excision with no difference in outcomes between these 2 techniques. All Mason type II radial head fractures had good or excellent outcomes with open reduction and internal fixation. Ring and colleagues[57] reported that 83% of adult patients (40/48) with Monteggia fractures in their series had good-to-excellent results at a follow-up of 6 years with plate and screw fixation used for the majority of these patients. Worse outcomes were noted with patients who had a very proximal ulnar fracture, a comminuted radial head fracture, or a coronoid process fracture.

Complications of proximal ulna fracture with associated PRUJ and/or radiocapitellar joint disruption include stiffness, chronic subluxation or dislocation of the PRUJ or radiocapitellar joint, delayed union, malunion or nonunion, proximal radioulnar synostosis, heterotopic ossification, infections, nerve palsy, limitation of forearm pronation or supination, and ulnohumeral instability.[18,37,40,57]

DISRUPTION OF THE FOREARM LONGITUDINAL AXIS

An Essex–Lopresti injury is defined as a fracture of the radial head associated with a rupture of the IOM and disruption of the DRUJ resulting in forearm longitudinal instability.[58–60] Another, more recently described component of this injury is a tear of the TFCC.[61] The first confirmed case of a disruption of the forearm longitudinal axis was reported by Curr and Coe in 1946 and then Essex–Lopresti reported 2 cases in 1951.[58,60,62] Essex–Lopresti demonstrated the importance of examining and imaging the distal radioulnar joint in the case of a radial head fracture, even if the patient has no wrist or forearm symptoms. He also discouraged excision of the radial head and recommended open reduction and internal fixation of the radial head fracture or, if the radial head is severely comminuted, the use of a prosthesis in its place.[58,60] Sixty years later, these principles remain as the foundation for effective management of forearm longitudinal instability and unfortunately are still often violated.

Anatomy and Classification

The radial head abutting the capitellum is the primary forearm stabilizer and the IOM and TFCC function as secondary stabilizers.[61] The central band of the IOM, also known as the interosseous ligament, is the important stabilizer of the IOM. Hotchkiss and colleagues[63] discovered in a cadaveric study that the central band of the IOM was responsible for 71% of longitudinal stiffness after excision of the radial head. Thus, injury to the central band of the IOM may be an important factor for proximal migration of the radius after excision of the radial head. The mechanism of injury is typically a fall onto an outstretched hand. A longitudinal force is transmitted from the wrist to the radial head and, if it is of sufficient magnitude, it results in radial head fracture, IOM disruption, and DRUJ disruption.[61]

Presentation and Workup

The key to an optimal outcome in forearm longitudinal instability is early diagnosis of the injury. Trousdale and colleagues[64] reported in a study that only 25% of patients with a radioulnar dissociation injury were initially diagnosed correctly. For those patients whose diagnosis was delayed, only 20% had a positive outcome with subsequent treatment. In a study by Edwards and Jupiter,[65] the 3 patients with excellent outcomes had surgical restoration of radial length within 5 days of their injury, whereas suboptimal results resulted in the remaining 4 patients in their study who did not have surgery until 4 to 10 weeks after their injury. In a recent study by Grassman and colleagues,[66] 83% of patients (10/12) with Essex–Lopresti injuries who were treated acutely reported being satisfied with the results of their operation at a follow-up of 59 months.

Careful physical examination and radiographs of the wrist and forearm are critical in all cases of radial head fractures. Physical examination signs include tenderness and instability of the DRUJ, excessive prominence over the distal ulnar aspect of the wrist reflecting proximal migration of the radius, painful or limited forearm rotation, and decreased wrist extension.[65–67] One should keep in mind, however, that additional physical examination signs may not be present in the setting of an acute disruption of the forearm longitudinal axis.[59]

Radiographs of the wrist, elbow, and forearm should be done when there is suspicion for forearm longitudinal instability, making sure to obtain a true neutral rotation view of the wrist to accurately measure any variance. Radiographs of the contralateral wrist should also be done for comparison of variance. Initial radiographs may not show any abnormalities indicating IOM or DRUJ injury and thus, if clinical suspicion remains high, further imaging should be considered.[68] MRI and ultrasound have emerged as effective options for the evaluation of ruptures of the IOM.[69] In a cadaver study Fester and colleagues[70] found that MRI had a 96% accuracy rate, 100% positive predictive value, 93% negative predictive value, 93% sensitivity, and 100% specificity in diagnosing disruption of the IOM. Ultrasound showed a 94% accuracy rate, 94% positive predictive value, 100% negative predictive value, 100% sensitivity, and 89% specificity. There was no difference between the 2 modalities. Disadvantages of MRI are it is more expensive and more time consuming to perform, and the main disadvantage of ultrasound is that it is operator dependent.[69]

Intraoperative examination should be done to diagnose suspected IOM and DRUJ injuries when performing operations on a radial head fracture. Smith and colleagues[71] report a cadaveric study that the "radius pull test," which involves intraoperative longitudinal traction of the proximal radius, can be used to assess for disruption of the IOM. Greater than or equal to 3 mm of proximal radial migration with this test this indicates disruption of the IOM (83% sensitivity, 83% specificity), whereas 6 mm or more of proximal radial migration indicates disruption of the IOM and TFCC (100% sensitivity, 100% specificity).

Soubeyrand and colleagues[72] reported another intraoperative test that can be used to assess for disruption of the IOM, which they called the "radius joystick test." It involves applying moderate lateral traction to the radial neck with the forearm in maximal pronation with lateral displacement of the proximal radius indicating rupture of the IOM. In a cadaveric study, they found that the test had a positive predictive value of 90% and negative predictive value of 100% (intraobserver agreement, 77%; interobserver agreement, 97%; sensitivity, 100%; specificity, 88%).

In the setting of chronic forearm longitudinal instability, the patient will have a history of radial head fracture treated with excision and may present with a combination of subsequent chronic wrist pain, limited wrist and forearm motion, and weakness of grip (**Fig. 6**).[59]

Treatment and Outcomes

As is the common theme in this article, the most important principle in the management and avoidance of complications of disruptions of the forearm longitudinal axis is early recognition and management of the injury. Another important principle is restoring radiocapitellar contact, which can be accomplished by either repair or replacement of the radial head.[73] If the radial head can be repaired, it should be treated with open reduction and internal fixation. If there is significant communition of the radial head, it should be treated with radial head excision and prosthetic head replacement with a modular metallic implant. TFCC repair should be considered and the DRUJ should then be temporary stabilized with Kirschner wire(s) for 6 weeks to allow for correct anatomic healing of the IOM.[59,66]

Although radial head excision has been shown to have favorable outcomes for the treatment of uncomplicated radial head fractures, it will result in proximal migration of the radius if used in the setting of a disruption of the forearm longitudinal axis because the TFCC and IOM are not intact and able to resist proximal radial migration.[74,75] In a study by Trousdale and colleagues,[64] all 15 patients with radioulnar dissociation injuries who underwent radial head excision had severe chronic wrist pain with 8 of the patients having 2 mm or more of radial shortening at a follow-up of 113 months.

The most common radial head prostheses used now are metallic radial head implants.[59] Silicone radial head implants are no longer recommended owing to reported long-term complications, including silicone synovitis and an inability to provide longitudinal stability.[76] A biomechanical study by King and colleagues[77] also showed that metallic radial head prostheses provided improved valgus stability compared with silicone radial head prostheses, more closely approximating a native radial head. In a recent study by Grassmann and colleagues,[66] none of the 8 patients with acute Essex-Lopresti injuries who were treated with a cemented bipolar radial head

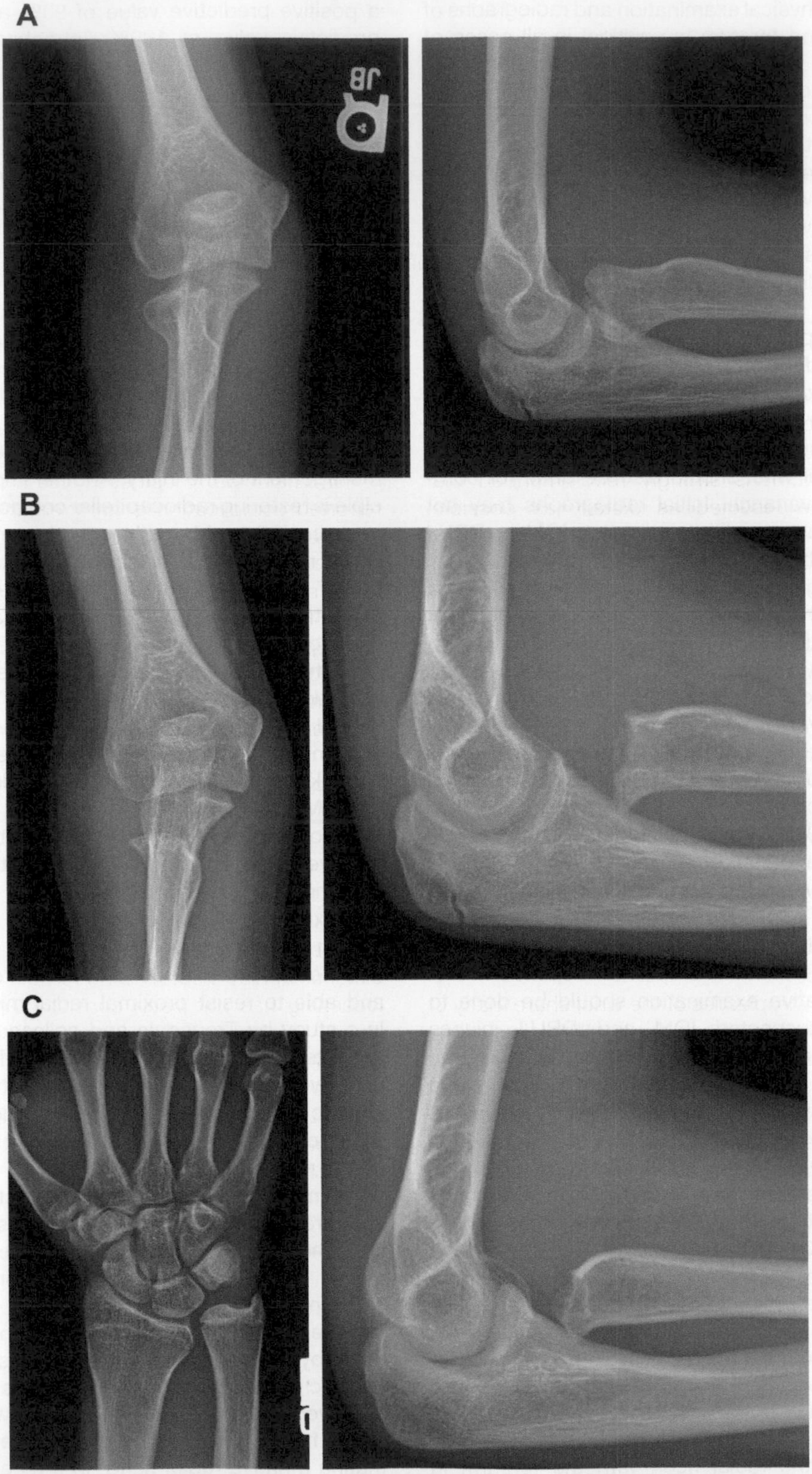

Fig. 6. (*A*) Right radial head/neck malunion in a 14-year-old right hand–dominant boy. (*B*) Right radial head excision that, reportedly, did well initially. (*C*) Two years later, the patient presented with new-onset right wrist pain. Note the significant ulnar positive variance. (*D*) The patient, at age 17, underwent radial head replacement (only partially regained radial subsidence) and concomitant ulnar-shortening osteotomy.

D

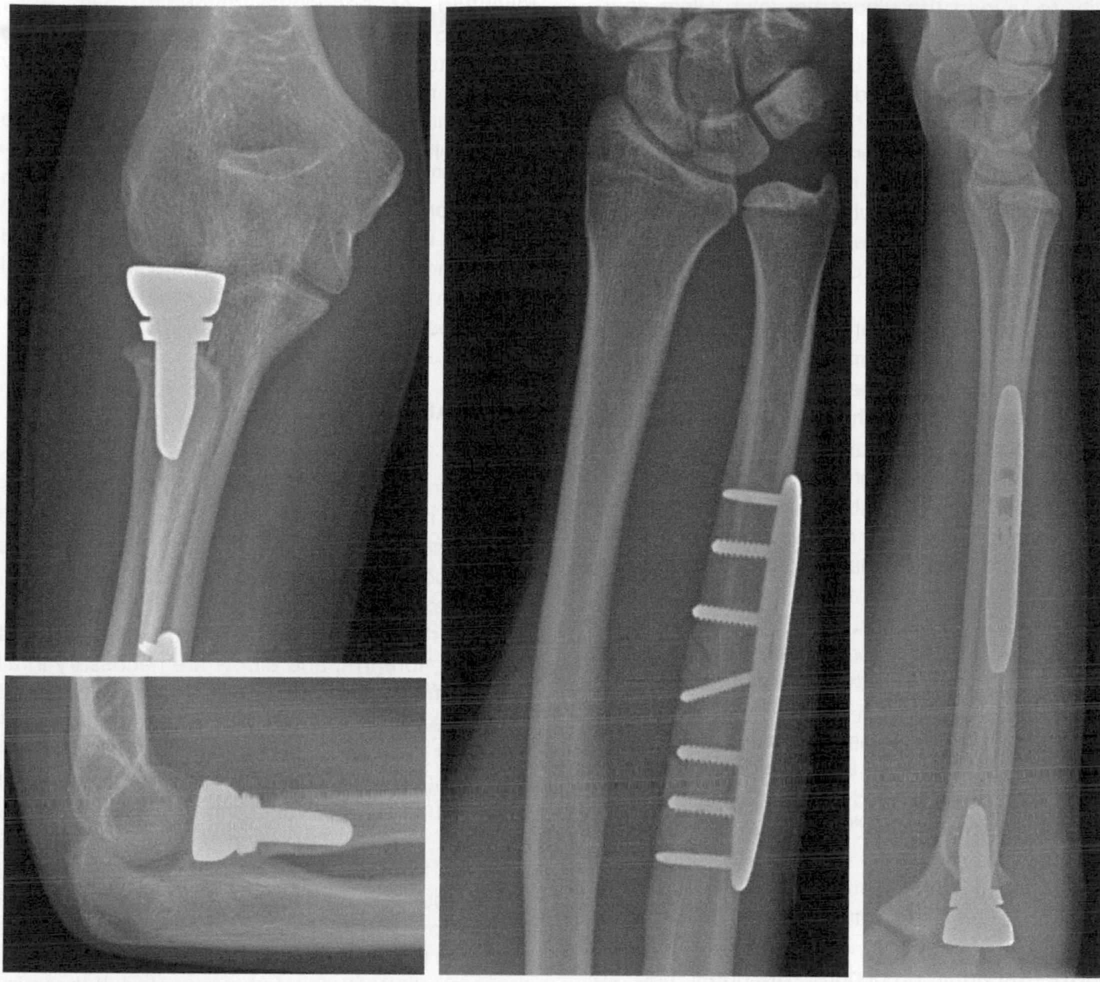

Fig. 6. *(continued)*

prosthesis had loosening of the prosthesis or any significant degenerative change at a follow-up of 59 months.

Pyrocarbon radial head implants have been recently introduced for its theoretically more cartilage-friendly bearing surface. A study by Lamas and colleagues[78] showed that 89% of patients (42/47) with displaced and comminuted radial head fractures having a good-to-excellent result at a follow-up of 4 years.

Both acute and chronic disruptions of the forearm longitudinal axis may be treated by reconstructing the IOM with various tendon grafts along with radial head replacement. Pronator teres,[79] flexor carpi radialis,[80] semitendinosis,[81] palmaris longus,[82] Achilles,[83] and bone–patellar tendon–bone grafts[84] have all been described with varied results reported. In a cadaveric study by Tejwani and colleagues, the authors found that metal radial head replacement combined with reconstructing the IOM with a palmaris longus tendon autograft can reduce distal ulnar force better than metal radial head replacement alone by limiting proximal radial migration, especially in the varus elbow position and thus possibly preventing symptoms from ulnocarpal impaction.[85] In another cadaveric study by Tejwani and colleagues, the authors compared the use of a palmaris longus tendon, flexor carpi radialis tendon, and bone–patellar tendon–bone grafts for IOM reconstruction in cadavers with the radial head excised and reported that the bone–patellar tendon–bone graft had the greatest cross-sectional area and had the least proximal radial displacement among the 3 grafts, although it still allowed significantly more proximal radial displacement compared with the native IOM.[82]

After stabilization of the radius by either prosthetic radial head replacement or IOM reconstruction, ulnar shortening osteotomy may be considered for chronic forearm longitudinal instability to unload the ulnocarpal joint. Ulnar shortening osteotomy should never be done as a stand-alone procedure in cases of forearm longitudinal instability. If a radial stabilization procedure is not done in conjunction with ulnar-shortening osteotomy, further proximal migration of the radius will result, leading to recurrence of ulnocarpal impaction. In addition, ulnar shortening osteotomy is contraindicated if there is DRUJ arthritis. In a series of 7 patients with chronic Essex–Lopresti lesions, Venouziou and colleagues[86] performed radial head replacement and ulnar-shortening osteotomy with improvement in pain and elbow, forearm, and wrist range of motion at a follow-up of 33 months. Ulnar shortening osteotomy may also be done in conjunction with IOM reconstruction. Marcotte and Osterman[87] reported improved wrist pain in 93% of patients (15/16) with chronic longitudinal radioulnar dissociation injuries who were treated with ulnar shortening osteotomy and reconstruction of the IOM using a bone–patellar ligament–bone graft at a follow-up of 78 months and an improvement in grip strength from 59% to 86% of the contralateral limb (see **Fig. 6**).

If the DRUJ continues to remain unstable after proper treatment of an Essex–Lopresti injury, the Sauve–Kapandji procedure may be used. Jungbluth and colleagues[88] reported good results with the treatment of 3 patients with chronic Essex–Lopresti injuries with this technique. Another salvage option is the Aptis (Scheker) DRUJ implant arthroplasty, especially considered after a failed Sauve–Kapandji procedure. Kachooei and colleagues[89] reported recently no prosthesis failures and improvement in activities of daily living, motion, strength, and lifting capacity compared with preoperatively at a follow-up of 60 months in all 13 patients who were treated with the Aptis DRUJ implant arthroplasty for persistent symptoms of pain, instability, and stiffness.

The ultimate salvage procedure for chronic forearm longitudinal instability is the creation of a 1-bone forearm via arthrodesis of the ulna proximally with the radius distally. The goals of this surgery are to treat instability, limit pain, and maintain elbow, wrist, and hand motion, although forearm rotation is sacrificed.[90] Allende and Allende[91] reported all 7 patients who were treated with a 1-bone forearm reconstruction for posttraumatic forearm injuries had a stable and pain-free forearm and were satisfied with the position, function, and appearance of the forearm at a follow-up of 9 years. A study by Peterson and colleagues[92] found more mixed results. Nineteen patients underwent 1-bone forearm surgery owing to radioulnar instability secondary to trauma, tumor resection, or congenital deformity, with 69% achieving good-to-excellent results, 26% having fair results, and 5% having poor results with nearly all of the major complications occurring in the patients who had radioulnar instability secondary to trauma. In a recent study by Jacoby and colleagues[90] of 10 patients who underwent creation of a 1-bone forearm for a chronic Essex–Lopresti injury or isolated DRUJ instability, they reported a 38% nonunion rate and a 40% rate of painful impingement of the proximal radius on nearby structures.

SUMMARY

Forearm fractures may be complicated by the disruption of the distal radioulnar, proximal radioulnar, or radiocapitellar joints. Disruption of these joints in conjunction with a forearm fracture results in the eponymously named Galeazzi, Monteggia, and Essex–Lopresti injuries. Careful history, physical examination, and radiographic evaluation of the wrist, forearm, and elbow are necessary in all forearm fractures to recognize this unique subset of injuries. Historically, these forearm fracture–dislocations have had poor outcomes with conservative management; however, early recognition of these injuries and advances in fixation techniques have led to much improved results. Children are typically treated nonoperatively whereas adults require surgical management. If the principles of restoration and maintenance of anatomic alignment are followed and the injury is treated acutely, then good outcomes can be expected. If these injuries are missed, various salvage options based on the restoration or recreation of anatomy are available depending on the injury, although the outcomes are not as good.

REFERENCES

1. Atesok KI, Jupiter JB, Weiss AP. Galeazzi fracture. J Am Acad Orthop Surg 2011;19:623–33.
2. Mikić ZD. Galeazzi fracture-dislocations. J Bone Joint Surg Am 1975;57(8):1071–80.
3. Sebastin SJ, Chung KC. A historical report on Riccardo Galeazzi and the management of Galeazzi fractures. J Hand Surg Am 2010;35(11):1870–7.
4. Cooper A. Simple fracture of the radius and dislocation of the ulna. In: Cooper A, editor. A treatise on dislocations, and on fractures of the joints. London: Longman; 1825. p. 470–6.
5. Galeazzi R. Di una particolare sindrome traumatica dello scheletro dell 'avambraccio. Atti e memorie della Societa' lombarda di chirurgia 1934;2:663–6.

6. Galeazzi R. Uber ein besonderes syndrom bei verletzungen im bereich der unterarmknochen. Arch Orthop Unfallchir 1935;35:557–62.
7. Moore TM, Klein JP, Patzakis MJ, et al. Results of compression-plating of closed Galeazzi fractures. J Bone Joint Surg Am 1985;67(7):1015–21.
8. Palmer AK, Werner FW. The triangular fibrocartilage complex of the wrist–anatomy and function. J Hand Surg 1981;6(2):153–62.
9. Ahn AK, Chang D, Plate AM. Triangular fibrocartilage complex tears: a review. Bull NYU Hosp Jt Dis 2006;64(3–4):114–8.
10. Zimmerman RM, Jupiter JB. Instability of the distal radioulnar joint. J Hand Surg Eur Vol 2014;39(7):727–38.
11. Maculé Beneyto F, Arandes Renú JM, Ferreres Claramunt A, et al. Treatment of Galeazzi fracture-dislocations. J Trauma 1994;36(3):352–5.
12. Fillingham Y, Hellman M, Haughom B, et al. Report of Galeazzi fracture resulting from a ballistic injury. Pol Orthop Traumatol 2014;79:5–9.
13. Bruckner JD, Alexander AH, Lichtman DM. Acute dislocations of the distal radioulnar joint. Instr Course Lect 1996;45:27–36.
14. Rettig ME, Raskin KB. Galeazzi fracture-dislocation: a new treatment-oriented classification. J Hand Surg Am 2001;26(2):228–35.
15. Korompilias AV, Lykissas MG, Kostas-agnantis IP, et al. Distal radioulnar joint instability (Galeazzi type injury) after internal fixation in relation to the radius fracture pattern. J Hand Surg Am 2011; 36(5):847–52.
16. Takemoto R, Sugi M, Immerman I, et al. Ulnar variance as a predictor of persistent instability following Galeazzi fracture-dislocations. J Orthop Trauma 2014;15(1):41–6.
17. Perron AD, Hersh RE, Brady WJ, et al. Orthopedic pitfalls in the ED: Galeazzi and Monteggia fracture-dislocation. Am J Emerg Med 2001;19(3):225–8.
18. Reckling FW. Unstable fracture-dislocations of the forearm (Monteggia and Galeazzi lesions). J Bone Joint Surg Am 1982;64(6):857–63.
19. Dameron TB. Traumatic dislocation of the distal radio-ulnar joint. Clin Orthop Relat Res 1972;83: 55–63.
20. Walsh HP, Mclaren CA, Owen R. Galeazzi fractures in children. J Bone Joint Surg Br 1987;69(5):730–3.
21. Rodríguez-merchán EC. Pediatric fractures of the forearm. Clin Orthop Relat Res 2005;(432):65–72.
22. Eberl R, Singer G, Schalamon J, et al. Galeazzi lesions in children and adolescents: treatment and outcome. Clin Orthop Relat Res 2008;466(7):1705–9.
23. Letts M, Rowhani N. Galeazzi-equivalent injuries of the wrist in children. J Pediatr Orthop 1993;13(5): 561–6.
24. Hughston JC. Fracture of the distal radial shaft; mistakes in management. J Bone Joint Surg Am 1957; 39-A(2):249–64.
25. Van Duijvenbode DC, Guitton TG, Raaymakers EL, et al. Long-term outcome of isolated diaphyseal radius fractures with and without dislocation of the distal radioulnar joint. J Hand Surg Am 2012;37(3): 523–7.
26. Giannoulis FS, Sotereanos DG. Galeazzi fractures and dislocations. Hand Clin 2007;23(2):153–63, v.
27. Park MJ, Pappas N, Steinberg DR, et al. Immobilization in supination versus neutral following surgical treatment of Galeazzi fracture-dislocations in adults: case series. J Hand Surg Am 2012;37(3):528–31.
28. Bruckner JD, Lichtman DM, Alexander AH. Complex dislocations of the distal radioulnar joint. Recognition and management. Clin Orthop Relat Res 1992;(275):90–103.
29. Cetti NE. An unusual cause of blocked reduction of the Galeazzi injury. Injury 1977;9(1):59–61.
30. Darrach W. Partial excision of lower shaft of ulna for deformity following Colles's fracture. 1913. Clin Orthop Relat Res 1992;(275):3–4.
31. Lau FH, Chung KC. William Darrach, MD: his life and his contribution to hand surgery. J Hand Surg Am 2006;31(7):1056–60.
32. Sauvé L, Kapandji M. Nouvelle technique de traitement chirurgical des luxations récidivantes isolées de l'extrémité inférieure du cubitus. J Chir (Paris) 1936;2:589–94.
33. Bowers WH. Distal radioulnar joint arthroplasty: the hemiresection-interposition technique. J Hand Surg Am 1985;10(2):169–78.
34. Scheker LR. Implant arthroplasty for the distal radioulnar joint. J Hand Surg Am 2008;33(9):1639–44.
35. Bado JL. The Monteggia lesion. Clin Orthop Relat Res 1967;50:71–86.
36. Rehim SA, Maynard MA, Sebastin SJ, et al. Monteggia fracture dislocations: a historical review. J Hand Surg Am 2014;39(7):1384–94.
37. Ring D. Monteggia fractures. Orthop Clin North Am 2013;44(1):59–66.
38. Jupiter JB, Leibovic SJ, Ribbans W, et al. The posterior Monteggia lesion. J Orthop Trauma 1991;5(4): 395–402.
39. Ring D, Jupiter JB, Waters PM. Monteggia fractures in children and adults. J Am Acad Orthop Surg 1998;6(4):215–24.
40. Konrad GG, Kundel K, Kreuz PC, et al. Monteggia fractures in adults: long-term results and prognostic factors. J Bone Joint Surg Br 2007;89(3):354–60.
41. Olney BW, Menelaus MB. Monteggia and equivalent lesions in childhood. J Pediatr Orthop 1989;9(2): 219–23.
42. Ring D, Waters PM. Operative fixation of Monteggia fractures in children. J Bone Joint Surg Br 1996; 78(5):734–9.
43. Letts M, Locht R, Wiens J. Monteggia fracture-dislocations in children. J Bone Joint Surg Br 1985; 67(5):724–7.

44. Beutel BG. Monteggia fractures in pediatric and adult populations. Orthopedics 2012;35(2):138–44.
45. Stein F, Grabias SL, Deffer PA. Nerve injuries complicating Monteggia lesions. J Bone Joint Surg Am 1971;53(7):1432–6.
46. Spar I. A neurologic complication following Monteggia fracture. Clin Orthop Relat Res 1977;(122):207–9.
47. Ramski DE, Hennrikus WP, Bae DS, et al. Pediatric Monteggia fractures: a multicenter examination of treatment strategy and early clinical and radiographic results. J Pediatr Orthop 2015;35(2): 115–20.
48. Hui JH, Sulaiman AR, Lee HC, et al. Open reduction and annular ligament reconstruction with fascia of the forearm in chronic Monteggia lesions in children. J Pediatr Orthop 2005;25(4):501–6.
49. Bor N, Rubin G, Rozen N, et al. Chronic anterior Monteggia lesions in children: report of 4 cases treated with closed reduction by ulnar osteotomy and external fixation. J Pediatr Orthop 2015;35(1): 7–10.
50. Rodgers WB, Waters PM, Hall JE. Chronic Monteggia lesions in children. Complications and results of reconstruction. J Bone Joint Surg Am 1996; 78(9):1322–9.
51. Nakamura K, Hirachi K, Uchiyama S, et al. Long-term clinical and radiographic outcomes after open reduction for missed Monteggia fracture-dislocations in children. J Bone Joint Surg Am 2009;91(6):1394–404.
52. Exner GU. Missed chronic anterior Monteggia lesion. Closed reduction by gradual lengthening and angulation of the ulna. J Bone Joint Surg Br 2001;83(4):547–50.
53. Eathiraju S, Mudgal CS, Jupiter JB. Monteggia fracture-dislocations. Hand Clin 2007;23(2):165–77, v.
54. Bruce HE, Harvey JP, Wilson JC. Monteggia fractures. J Bone Joint Surg Am 1974;56(8):1563–76.
55. Ring D. Open reduction and internal fixation of fractures of the radial head. Hand Clin 2004;20(4): 415–27, vi.
56. Lawton JN, Cameron-Donaldson M, Blazar PE, et al. Anatomic considerations regarding the posterior interosseous nerve at the elbow. J Shoulder Elbow Surg 2007;16(4):502–7.
57. Ring D, Jupiter JB, Simpson NS. Monteggia fractures in adults. J Bone Joint Surg Am 1998;80(12): 1733–44.
58. Essex-Lopresti P. Fractures of the radial head with distal radio-ulnar dislocation; report of two cases. J Bone Joint Surg Br 1951;33B(2):244–7.
59. Loeffler BJ, Green JB, Zelouf DS. Forearm instability. J Hand Surg Am 2014;39(1):156–67.
60. Mcglinn EP, Sebastin SJ, Chung KC. A historical perspective on the Essex-Lopresti injury. J Hand Surg Am 2013;38(8):1599–606.
61. Dodds SD, Yeh PC, Slade JF. Essex-Lopresti injuries. Hand Clin 2008;24(1):125–37.
62. Curr JF, Coe WA. Dislocation of the inferior radio-ulnar joint. Br J Surg 1946;34:74–7.
63. Hotchkiss RN, An KN, Sowa DT, et al. An anatomic and mechanical study of the interosseous membrane of the forearm: pathomechanics of proximal migration of the radius. J Hand Surg Am 1989; 14(2 Pt 1):256–61.
64. Trousdale RT, Amadio PC, Cooney WP, et al. Radio-ulnar dissociation. A review of twenty cases. J Bone Joint Surg Am 1992;74(10):1486–97.
65. Edwards GS, Jupiter JB. Radial head fractures with acute distal radioulnar dislocation. Essex-Lopresti revisited. Clin Orthop Relat Res 1988;(234):61–9.
66. Grassmann JP, Hakimi M, Gehrmann SV, et al. The treatment of the acute Essex-Lopresti injury. Bone Joint J 2014;96-B(10):1385–91.
67. Hotchkiss RN. Injuries to the interosseous ligament of the forearm. Hand Clin 1994;10(3):391–8.
68. Rodriguez-martin J, Pretell-mazzini J, Vidal-bujanda C. Unusual pattern of Essex-Lopresti injury with negative plain radiographs of the wrist: a case report and literature review. Hand Surg 2010;15(1): 41–5.
69. Rodriguez-martin J, Pretell-mazzini J. The role of ultrasound and magnetic resonance imaging in the evaluation of the forearm interosseous membrane. A review. Skeletal Radiol 2011;40(12):1515–22.
70. Fester EW, Murray PM, Sanders TG, et al. The efficacy of magnetic resonance imaging and ultrasound in detecting disruptions of the forearm interosseous membrane: a cadaver study. J Hand Surg Am 2002;27(3):418–24.
71. Smith AM, Urbanosky LR, Castle JA, et al. Radius pull test: predictor of longitudinal forearm instability. J Bone Joint Surg Am 2002;84-A(11):1970–6.
72. Soubeyrand M, Ciais G, Wassermann V, et al. The intra-operative radius joystick test to diagnose complete disruption of the interosseous membrane. J Bone Joint Surg Br 2011;93(10):1389–94.
73. Ring D, Quintero J, Jupiter JB. Open reduction and internal fixation of fractures of the radial head. J Bone Joint Surg Am 2002;84-A(10):1811–5.
74. Rabinowitz RS, Light TR, Havey RM, et al. The role of the interosseous membrane and triangular fibrocartilage complex in forearm stability. J Hand Surg Am 1994;19(3):385–93.
75. Herbertsson P, Josefsson PO, Hasserius R, et al. Uncomplicated mason type-II and III fractures of the radial head and neck in adults. A long-term follow-up study. J Bone Joint Surg Am 2004;86-A(3):569–74.
76. Vanderwilde RS, Morrey BF, Melberg MW, et al. Inflammatory arthritis after failure of silicone rubber replacement of the radial head. J Bone Joint Surg Br 1994;76(1):78–81.
77. King GJ, Zarzour ZD, Rath DA, et al. Metallic radial head arthroplasty improves valgus stability of the elbow. Clin Orthop Relat Res 1999;(368):114–25.

78. Lamas C, Castellanos J, Proubasta I, et al. Comminuted radial head fractures treated with pyrocarbon prosthetic replacement. Hand (N Y) 2011;6(1):27–33.
79. Chloros GD, Wiesler ER, Stabile KJ, et al. Reconstruction of Essex-Lopresti injury of the forearm: technical note. J Hand Surg Am 2008;33(1):124–30.
80. Skahen JR, Palmer AK, Werner FW, et al. Reconstruction of the interosseous membrane of the forearm in cadavers. J Hand Surg Am 1997; 22(6):986–94.
81. Soubeyrand M, Oberlin C, Dumontier C, et al. Ligamentoplasty of the forearm interosseous membrane using the semitendinosus tendon: anatomical study and surgical procedure. Surg Radiol Anat 2006; 28(3):300–7.
82. Tejwani SG, Markolf KL, Benhaim P. Reconstruction of the interosseous membrane of the forearm with a graft substitute: a cadaveric study. J Hand Surg Am 2005; 30(2):326–34.
83. Tomaino MM, Pfaeffle J, Stabile K, et al. Reconstruction of the interosseous ligament of the forearm reduces load on the radial head in cadavers. J Hand Surg Br 2003;28(3):267–70.
84. Adams JE, Culp RW, Osterman AL. Interosseous membrane reconstruction for the Essex-Lopresti injury. J Hand Surg Am 2010;35(1):129–36.
85. Tejwani SG, Markolf KL, Benhaim P. Graft reconstruction of the interosseous membrane in conjunction with metallic radial head replacement: a cadaveric study. J Hand Surg Am 2005;30(2): 335–42.
86. Venouziou AI, Papatheodorou LK, Weiser RW, et al. Chronic Essex-Lopresti injuries: an alternative treatment method. J Shoulder Elbow Surg 2014;23(6): 861–6.
87. Marcotte AL, Osterman AL. Longitudinal radioulnar dissociation: identification and treatment of acute and chronic injuries. Hand Clin 2007;23(2): 195–208, vi.
88. Jungbluth P, Frangen TM, Arens S, et al. The undiagnosed Essex-Lopresti injury. J Bone Joint Surg Br 2006;88(12):1629–33.
89. Kachooei AR, Chase SM, Jupiter JB. Outcome assessment after aptis distal radioulnar joint (DRUJ) implant arthroplasty. Arch Bone Jt Surg 2014;2(3): 180–4.
90. Jacoby SM, Bachoura A, Diprinzio EV, et al. Complications following one-bone forearm surgery for posttraumatic forearm and distal radioulnar joint instability. J Hand Surg Am 2013;38(5):976–82.e1.
91. Allende C, Allende BT. Posttraumatic one-bone forearm reconstruction. A report of seven cases. J Bone Joint Surg Am 2004;86-A(2):364–9.
92. Peterson CA, Maki S, Wood MB. Clinical results of the one-bone forearm. J Hand Surg Am 1995; 20(4):609–18.

Management of Complications of Distal Radioulnar Joint

Kagan Ozer, MD

KEYWORDS

• Arthritis • Convergence • Distal radioulnar joint • Impingement

KEY POINTS

- Removal of the ulnar head permanently changes forearm dynamics, rotation, and stability of the distal radioulnar joint.
- Young ages and moderate to high activity levels are associated with poorer outcomes, resulting in pain and limited motion.
- No direct correlation exists between radioulnar convergence, pain, objective, and subjective outcomes, but stabilization of the ulnar stump seems to alleviate pain and improve forearm rotation and functional outcomes.
- Procedures designed to prevent radioulnar convergence include biological methods (Achilles allograft interposition arthroplasty, tendon strip stabilization), implant arthroplasties, and salvage options (one-bone forearm).

INTRODUCTION

Despite its complex anatomy, distal radioulnar joint (DRUJ) problems can be classified into 3 categories: instability, impingement, and incongruity/arthrosis. Surgical procedures offered to alleviate these problems can sometimes lead to other complications, as seen after resection of the distal ulna. Distal ulnar excision has been performed to treat ulnocarpal impingement and DRUJ arthritis for a century. Despite the overall high satisfaction rate on well-selected patients, the resultant radioulnar convergence is often unavoidable and may result in painful forearm rotation. This article outlines management options for symptomatic radioulnar convergence based on current literature.

ANATOMY AND MECHANICS

Forearm rotation occurs because of mobility at the proximal and DRUJs. Proximally, the axis of rotation passes through the center of the radial head. Distally, it exits through the DRUJ. During rotation the ulna is the pivot point. The radius, carpus, and hand rotate around the ulna. The ulnar head serves as a support for the ulnar side of the wrist by transmitting 20% of the longitudinal load across the wrist.[1] It also helps to stabilize the DRUJ through ligamentous attachments. Articular surfaces of the DRUJ consist of the ulnar head and the sigmoid notch of the radius. Those 2 surfaces are not symmetric. The diameter of the sigmoid notch is 4 to 7 mm greater than the ulnar head. Owing to this difference, osseous stability is limited. Only 20% of DRUJ constraint is provided by articular surfaces; the remaining comes from ligamentous attachments and triangular fibrocartilage complex (TFCC). TFCC provides stability in the volar/dorsal plane but also prevents radioulnar translation. Resection of the ulnar head not only changes the overall axis of rotation in the forearm but also results in instability of the forearm and carpus.[2,3]

Author has no financial interest to disclose.
Department of Orthopedic Surgery, University of Michigan, 2098 South Main Street, Ann Arbor, MI 48103, USA
E-mail address: kozer@umich.edu

Hand Clin 31 (2015) 235–242
http://dx.doi.org/10.1016/j.hcl.2014.12.003
0749-0712/15/$ – see front matter

PHYSICAL EXAMINATION AND DIAGNOSIS

The diagnosis of radioulnar convergence is straightforward. Symptomatic patients often complain about pain while lifting weights as little as a few pounds. In patients with distal ulnar excision, the end of the ulna is usually unstable, which is demonstrated in a positive chuck test. Because radioulnar convergence is a dynamic process, static forearm images, unless taken as stress views, may not show the contact or narrowing of the space between the radius and ulna. Scheker[4,5] described a simple radiographic method and took full-length forearm posteroanterior radiographs when patients were holding 5 pounds of weight (**Fig. 1**). This method is sufficient to demonstrate the problem even in its earliest stage. In later stages, one can also see notching and erosions along the ulnar border of the radius corresponding to the tip of the ulnar stump (**Fig. 2**).

MANAGEMENT OF RADIOULNAR CONVERGENCE AFTER DISTAL ULNAR RESECTION

Resection of the distal end of the ulna was originally described by Malgaigne[6] and Moore,[7] but later attributed to Darrach.[8] The procedure was recommended for treatment of symptomatic DRUJ conditions after distal radius fractures. Later, it was performed for degenerative arthritis of DRUJ with satisfactory results. Using this technique, various authors reported their outcomes.[9–16] Many of these case series had limited follow-up, and lacked patient-rated outcomes and objective evaluation criteria. More recent studies with long-term follow-up indicate satisfactory range of motion (ROM) with minimal to no symptoms of instability.[11,13] Recently, Stern and colleagues[11] conducted a retrospective analysis of distal ulnar resections. Of the 98 patients, 27 were available for follow-up at an average of 13 years and only 15 were available for an in-office follow-up visit. At the final follow-up, the quick DASH (Disabilities of the Arm, Shoulder and Hand) score was 17, and patient-rated wrist evaluation score was 14. Between rest and activity, patients reported a slight increase in pain, from 0.1 to 0.6, based on a visual analog scale (VAS; score range, 0–4), with an average forearm pronation/supination of 85°/78°. However, the average age of the cohort available for final follow-up was 66 years, likely contributing to those exceptionally satisfactory results because of lower-than-average activity levels. Contrary to Stern and colleagues, other investigators reported ongoing clicking, and pain with active forearm rotation, and substantial functional limitations, particularly in patients with moderate to high level of activity.[17–19]

In search of a more stable and less painful forearm and wrist motion, various surgical techniques have been proposed to stabilize the remaining ulnar stump. Although the intensity of pain or the functional outcome does not seem to correlate with radioulnar convergence in some case series,[10,11] stabilization of the ulnar stump seems to relieve symptom severity. Indications for stabilizing the ulnar stump, optimal surgical technique, and origin of postoperative pain are still debated.

ULNAR STUMP STABILIZATION WITH TENDON TRANSFERS

Various muscle and tendon units, including strips of flexor carpi ulnaris (FCU), extensor carpi ulnaris (ECU), and pronator quadratus, have been used to

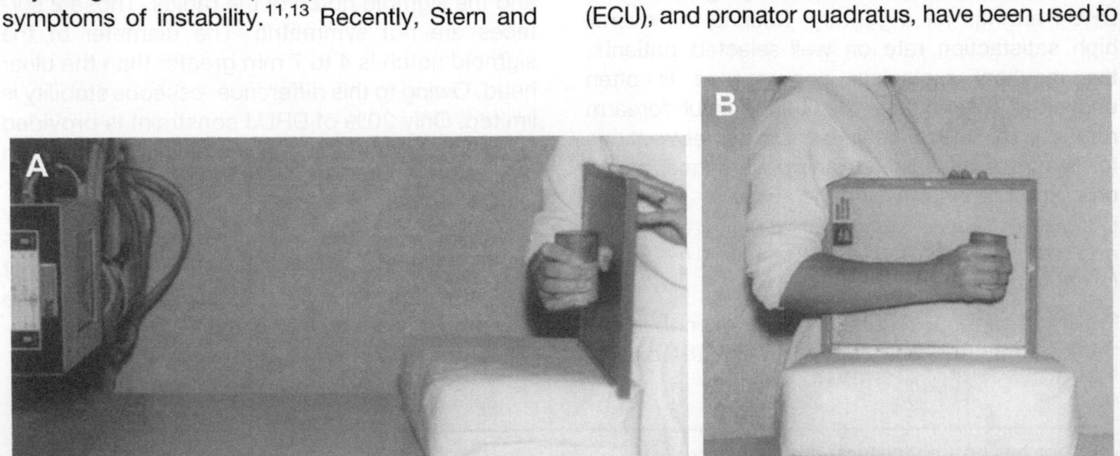

Fig. 1. (*A*) The positioning of the patient with respect to the x-ray beam is shown. (*B*) Patient is holding 2.2 kg with the forearm in neutral position. (*From* Lees VC, Scheker LR. The radiological demonstration of dynamic ulnar impingement. J Hand Surg 1997;22:449; with permission.)

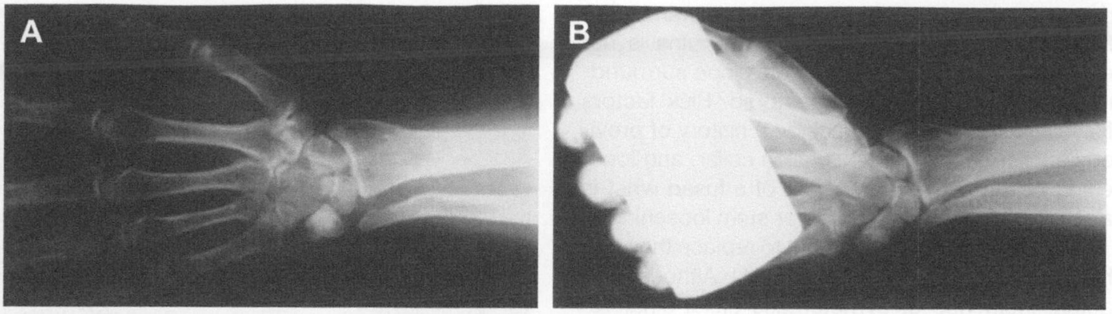

Fig. 2. (*A*) Radiograph of the wrist of a 48-year-old woman who underwent matched hemiresection arthroplasty 1 year before presentation. (*B*) Anteroposterior view of the wrist showing impingement. (*From* Lees VC, Scheker LR. The radiological demonstration of dynamic ulnar impingement. J Hand Surg 1997;22:450; with permission.)

stabilize the ulnar stump.[20–23] Breen and Jupiter[20] reported on 3 patients who underwent FCU and ECU stabilization, reporting increased forearm rotation with no increase in grip strength in all 3. Kleinman and Greenberg[21] stabilized 6 cases using ECU and pronator quadratus and reported complete pain relief with increased forearm motion and grip strength. Syed and colleagues[23] reported on 14 patients stabilized with a strip of FCU tendon. Although radiographic signs of convergence between radius and ulna continued, clinical outcomes were not affected by the presence of this contact.

Based on a small group of patients with no patient-rated outcomes, all 3 studies reported pain relief and improved function, even with ongoing radioulnar convergence. Whether the applied surgical technique, the cause of the DRUJ instability, or the age of the patient was responsible for this positive outcome is unclear.

ULNAR HEAD REPLACEMENT

The first ulnar head implant was designed as a single-piece silicone head.[24] Despite its earlier encouraging results, implant migration, breakage, and silicone synovitis became significant issues, leading to abandonment of the material for this use.[25] Later, Herbert[26] designed a modular implant that consisted of a metallic stem and ceramic head that allowed rotation of the head (**Fig. 3**). Using this implant, van Schoonhoven and colleagues[27] reported complete pain relief in 23 patients at 27 months. Later, the same group in a multicenter trial reported longer-term results of 23 patients 11 years after the index procedure. Their results showed improved patient satisfaction, grip strength, forearm rotation, and pain. One patient developed an infection requiring hardware removal, and 3 had radiographic changes at the articular surface of the radius without stem loosening. Later, Willis and colleagues[28] and Kakar and colleagues,[29] in 2 separate publications, reported outcomes on 19 and 47 patients at 32 and 56 months after the surgery, respectively. Both groups showed significant improvements in Mayo scores, although the improvement in grip strength, pain, and forearm rotation were not as substantial. Two patients in the series by Willis and colleagues[28] and 8 patients in the series by Kakar and colleagues[29] needed a revision. In a review of 22 implants in 20 patients at 54 months, Yen Shipley and colleagues[30] reported that pain and Mayo scores improved regardless of the cause. They revised 3 implants in this series.

Ulnar head implants not only aim to restore DRUJ and ulnar stability but also help support the ulnar side of the wrist, theoretically preventing ulnar translation of the carpus. Studies on cadavers using dynamic loading models demonstrated restoration of load transmission across the wrist and forearm when the ulnar head was replaced with an implant after its resection.[31] Among many variables, resistance to torque improves significantly after implant arthroplasty. However, it is important to keep in mind that successful restoration of painless forearm rotation

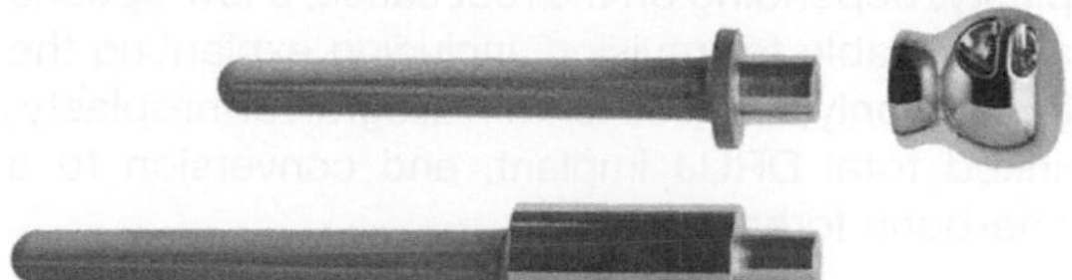

Fig. 3. Modular implant head arthroplasty. The head and stem are manufactured in different sizes, but a universal coupling allows for interchanges of different-sized components. (*From* Berger RA. Ulnar head resection related instability. Hand Clin 2013;29:105; with permission.)

depends on the link between the radius and ulna. Restoring the previous length of the ulna is not enough unless the soft tissue envelope surrounding the ulnar head is well restored. Risk factors for failure of the implant include a history of previous surgery, use of an extension collar, and loosening of the stem.[29] Presence of a fused wrist is also a recognized risk factor for stem loosening.[32]

Indications to use an implant to replace the ulnar head originate from a painful DRUJ. Although the actual incidence of symptomatic distal ulnar resections is debated, many authors recommend performing implant arthroplasty as the primary procedure at the time of ulnar head resection. Contraindications for the ulnar head prosthesis are active infection, active inflammatory arthropathy, trauma leading to inadequate soft tissue support or limited tendon excursion caused by scarring, and neurologic conditions resulting in lack of motor control. The presence of DRUJ instability with a native ulnar head is a relative contraindication for this procedure, because such a deformity will not correct itself, especially if the root cause is ligamentous/capsular insufficiency. Angular malalignment of the sigmoid notch may also present as a pattern of instability and is a relative contraindication for this procedure.

Implant subsidence, loosening, and instability with pain are potential complications that must be addressed (**Fig. 4**). If residual instability is present at the time of surgery or afterward, it may be from soft tissue insufficiency, sigmoid notch insufficiency, or malalignment. In the case of sigmoid notch insufficiency, deepening the notch with a notchplasty may not work and may create further instability and subsidence, necessitating conversion to a fully constrained DRUJ arthroplasty. Additionally, when residual instability is related to inadequate ligamentous and capsular support, using strips of FCU and ECU tendons to provide further stability or conversion to a fully constrained DRUJ arthroplasty may be required. Minor implant loosening can be monitored safely once infection and metal allergy are ruled out.

In the case of a failed ulnar head implant arthroplasty, depending on the root cause, a few options are available for revision, including explanting the implant only, Achilles tendon allograft arthroplasty, linked total DRUJ implant, and conversion to a one-bone forearm.

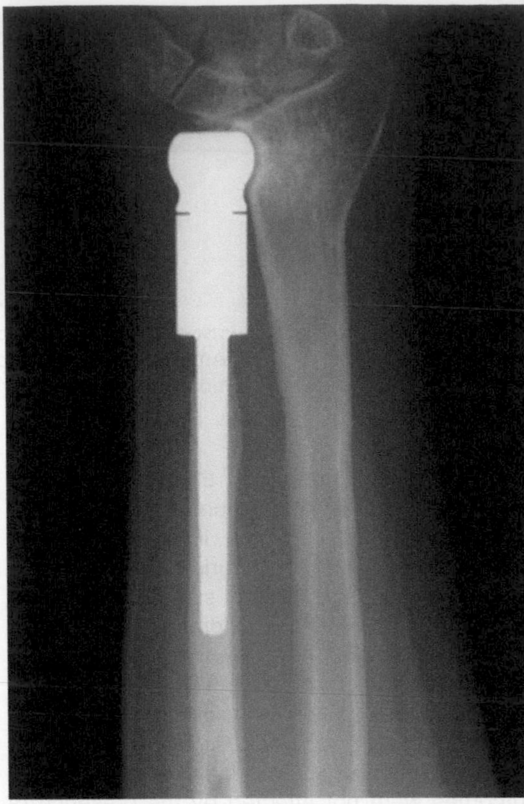

Fig. 4. Posteroanterior radiograph of a wrist 4 years after conversion of a Sauve-Kapandji procedure to an ulnar head implant arthroplasty. Note the subsidence of the implant into the radius, undermining the support for the lunate fossa. (*From* Berger RA. Ulnar head resection related instability. Hand Clin 2013;29:110; with permission).

DISTAL RADIOULNAR JOINT CONSTRAINED ARTHROPLASTY

The shortcomings of ulnar head replacement include reliance on the integrity of soft tissues and painful erosion of the sigmoid notch. To circumvent these problems along with painful DRUJ, Scheker[4] designed an implant aimed at restoring the DRUJ motion in multiple planes, including pronation/supination and radial migration (**Fig. 5**). Indications for this implant are rheumatoid, degenerative, or posttraumatic arthritis of the DRUJ, either as a primary replacement option or after Darrach, Sauvé-Kapandji, or matched resection procedures. In addition, a history of large tumor resections and congenital anomalies, including Madelung deformity, are indications for using this implant.[33] This device can be used on patients with up to 14 cm of the ulna remaining.

Savvidou and colleagues[34] reported on the results of 35 arthroplasties at an average of 5 years, showing significant improvements in active forearm rotation, grip strength (from 48% to 90% of the contralateral side), pain at rest and activity (from 5.11 to 1.02) with a final DASH score of 16. Eleven patients in this report had complications, such as ECU tendonitis, ectopic bone formation,

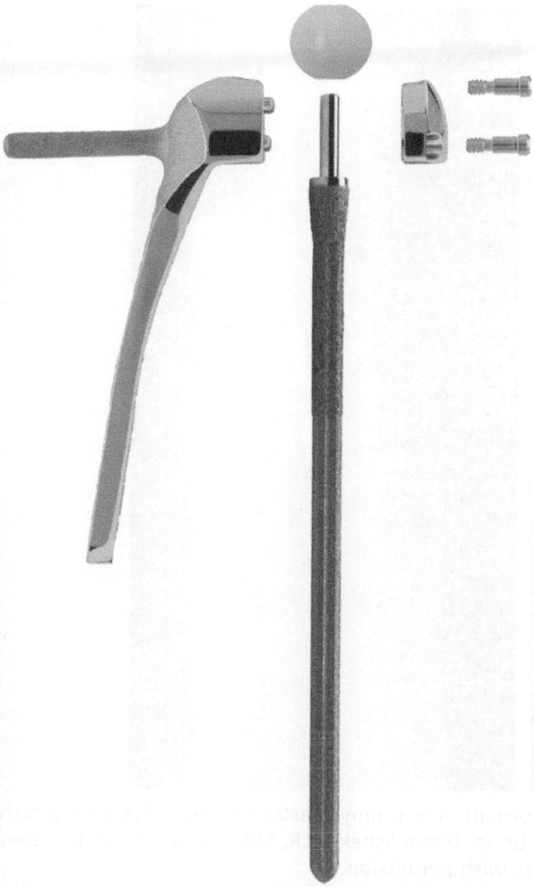

Fig. 5. Self-stabilizing Scheker total distal radioulnar joint has a radius plate with a distal socket, an ulnar stem with an ultrahigh-molecular-weight polyethylene ball, and a ball cover to complete the assembly. The advantage is that it does not require any ligaments from the original joint. (*From* Scheker LR, Martineau DW. Distal radioulnar joint constrained arthroplasty. Hand Clin 2013;29:114; with permission.)

and screw loosening requiring revision. The same group recently published their experience with 17 patients with rheumatoid arthritis with a mean follow-up of 39 months.[35] They reported significant improvements in pain (VAS, 7.3–2.2) and active ROM (forearm pronation and supination improved 39% and 27%, respectively), with a final DASH score of 24. Eight patients (42%) eventually underwent radiocarpal fusions without progression of radioulnar translocation. Two patients underwent revision surgeries because of ulnar stem loosening and ECU tendonitis. Zimmerman and Jupiter[36] reported on 6 cases with this design at 2.4 years after surgery. Their results confirmed improvement in pain, active ROM, and grip strength after the surgery. One patient had ECU tendinitis requiring a revision procedure.

Although results published by Scheker[4] have yet to be reproduced by others, constrained DRUJ arthroplasty clearly provides a unique reconstructive option. Complications include ECU tendinitis, stem loosening, ectopic bone formation, and infection (**Fig. 6**).

ACHILLES ALLOGRAFT INTERPOSITION ARTHROPLASTY

The technique described by Sotereanos and colleagues[37] has the advantages of providing biological reconstruction using an allograft tendon without compromising local tendon and muscle units. Its simple application prevents contact between the radius and ulna and provides stability in pronation and supination. A detailed description of the surgical technique can be found in another publication by Greenberg and Soteranos.[38] Long-term results of this procedure in 26 patients at an average of 79 months showed significant improvements in pain scores (from 8.1 to 1.3), Mayo wrist scores (from 42 to 85), and forearm rotation (average, 28°–41° in pronation and supination).[39] One patient had a radial shaft fracture and 2 had ulnar shaft scalloping. All 3 patients, however, remained asymptomatic. Authors recommend the procedure for a resected ulnar head of up to one-third of its entire length. Patients who underwent a previous Sauve-Kapandji procedure can have the same arthroplasty without the need to interfere with DRUJ fusion. Unfortunately, no other author has yet reproduced or validated the results achieved by Sotereanos and colleagues.[37] Although the procedure may not restore the original anatomy and biomechanics of the forearm, it seems effective enough to relieve pain and instability and can be considered either as a primary procedure or in patients who are not candidates for arthroplasty or other procedures.

ONE-BONE FOREARM

One-bone forearm is usually considered the last option in the management of painful radioulnar convergence. Forearm rotation is sacrificed, whereas radiocarpal and ulnohumeral joint motions are preserved. No clear consensus exists on its indications, but it has been applied in the treatment of open fractures with bone loss, infection, tumor, and congenital differences.[40–42] Peterson and colleagues[40] reported on 19 patients at a mean follow-up of 42 months, noting a 32% nonunion rate after the first surgery. This rate has improved to 28% after revision. One-third of those patients had a fair to poor outcome. Later, Allende

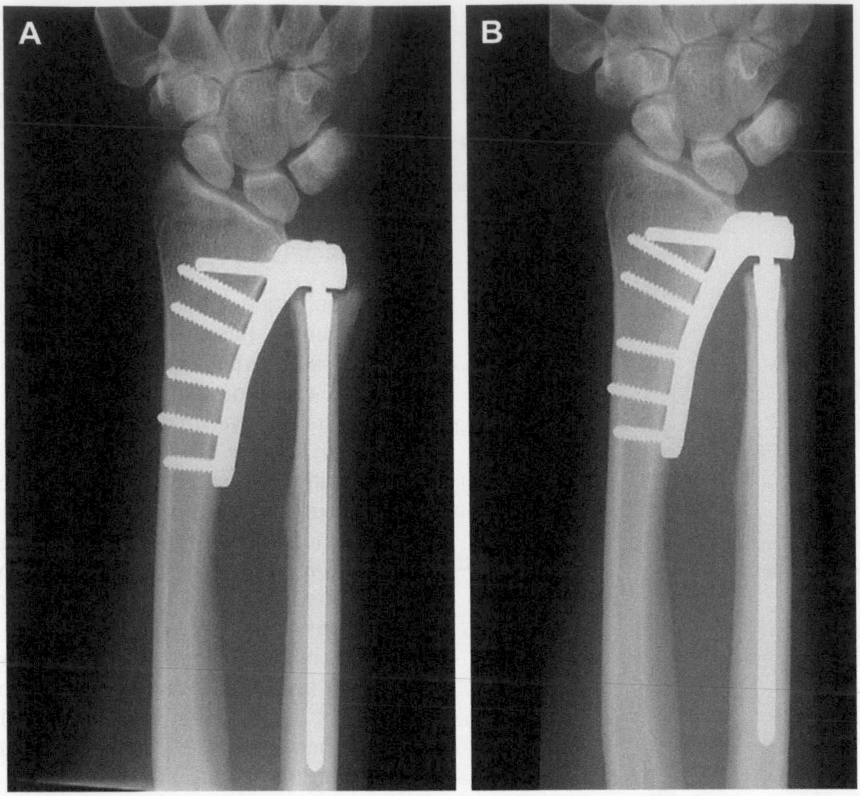

Fig. 6. (*A*) Radiograph of a patient with an ectopic bone formation resulting in extensor carpi ulnaris tendinitis. (*B*) Postoperative radiograph after removal of the ectopic bone. (*From* Scheker LR, Martineau DW. Distal radio-ulnar joint constrained arthroplasty. Hand Clin 2013;29:120; with permission.)

and Allende[41] reported on 7 cases at a mean follow-up of 9.7 years. All patients remained pain-free with 86% of the contralateral grip strength. Finally, Jacoby and colleagues[42] reported on 10 patients at an average follow-up of 6 years. They reported 3 nonunions and 7 revision surgeries. Final DASH and pain scores remained high (77 and 7, respectively). Based on these and other case series, conversion to one-bone forearm seems to have the highest complication rates and to result in substantial loss of function.

SUMMARY

Careful analysis of the literature seems to teach the following lessons:

- Removal of the ulnar head permanently changes forearm dynamics, rotation, and stability of the DRUJ.
- Not every patient with a resected distal ulna will have satisfactory outcome; young ages, and moderate to high activity levels, are associated with poorer outcomes, resulting in pain and limited motion.
- No direct correlation exists between radioulnar convergence, pain, objective, and subjective outcomes, but stabilization of the ulnar stump seems to alleviate pain and improve forearm rotation and functional outcomes.
- Procedures designed to prevent radioulnar convergence include biological methods (AAIA, tendon strip stabilization), implant arthroplasties, and salvage options (one-bone forearm).
- Comparison among various treatment methods is not possible because of the heterogeneous groups of patients, retrospective nature of the studies, and lack of uniform reporting methods.
- Innovators of the AAIA and implant arthroplasties report good and excellent outcomes, but those results have not been reproduced by others and should be able to stand the test of time before becoming common practice.

REFERENCES

1. Werner FW, Palmer AK, Fortino MD, et al. Force transmission through the distal ulna: effect of ulnar

variance, lunate fossa angulation, and radial and palmar tilt of the distal radius. J Hand Surg Am 1992;17(3):423–8.
2. Sauerbier M, Berger RA, Fujita M, et al. Radioulnar convergence after distal ulnar resection: mechanical performance of two commonly used soft tissue stabilizing procedures. Acta Orthop Scand 2003; 74(4):420–8.
3. Sauerbier M, Fujita M, Hahn ME, et al. The dynamic radioulnar convergence of the Darrach procedure and the ulnar head hemiresection interposition arthroplasty: a biomechanical study. J Hand Surg Br 2002;27(4):307–16.
4. Scheker LR. Implant arthroplasty for the distal radioulnar joint. J Hand Surg Am 2008;33(9):1639–44.
5. Lees VC, Scheker LR. The radiological demonstration of dynamic ulnar impingement. J Hand Surg 1997;22:448–50.
6. Buck-Gramcko D. On the priorities of publication of some operative procedures on the distal end of the ulna. J Hand Surg Br 1990;15(4):416–20.
7. Moore EM. Three cases illustrating luxation of the ulna in connection with Colles' fracture. Med Rec 1880;17:305–8.
8. Darrach W. Anterior dislocation of the head of the ulna. Ann Surg 1912;56:802–3.
9. Bell MJ, Hill RJ, McMurtry RY. Ulnar impingement syndrome. J Bone Joint Surg Br 1985;67(1):126–9.
10. McKee MD, Richards RR. Dynamic radio-ulnar convergence after the Darrach procedure. J Bone Joint Surg Br 1996;78(3):413–8.
11. Grawe B, Heincelman C, Stern P. Functional results of the Darrach procedure: a long-term outcome study. J Hand Surg Am 2012;37(12):2475–80.e1–e2.
12. Dingman PV. Resection of the distal end of the ulna (Darrach operation); an end result study of twenty four cases. J Bone Joint Surg Am 1952;34 A(4): 893–900.
13. Tulipan DJ, Eaton RG, Eberhart RE. The Darrach procedure defended: technique redefined and long-term follow-up. J Hand Surg Am 1991;16(3): 438–44.
14. Shearman CP. The long-term outcome following Darrach's procedure for complications of fractures of the distal radius. Injury 1988;19(5):318–20.
15. af Ekenstam F, Engkvist O, Wadin K. Results from resection of the distal end of the ulna after fractures of the lower end of the radius. Scand J Plast Reconstr Surg 1982;16(2):177–81.
16. Kessler I, Hecht O. Present application of the Darrach procedure. Clin Orthop Relat Res 1970; 72:254–60.
17. Bieber EJ, Linscheid RL, Dobyns JH, et al. Failed distal ulna resections. J Hand Surg Am 1988;13(2):193–200.
18. Field J, Majkowski RJ, Leslie IJ. Poor results of Darrach's procedure after wrist injuries. J Bone Joint Surg Br 1993;75(1):53–7.
19. Hartz CR, Beckenbaugh RD. Long-term results of resection of the distal ulna for post-traumatic conditions. J Trauma 1979;19(4):219–26.
20. Breen TF, Jupiter JB. Extensor carpi ulnaris and flexor carpi ulnaris tenodesis of the unstable distal ulna. J Hand Surg Am 1989;14(4):612–7.
21. Kleinman WB, Greenberg JA. Salvage of the failed Darrach procedure. J Hand Surg Am 1995;20(6): 951–8.
22. Tsai TM, Shimizu H, Adkins P. A modified extensor carpi ulnaris tenodesis with the Darrach procedure. J Hand Surg Am 1993;18(4):697–702.
23. Syed AA, Lam WL, Agarwal M, et al. Stabilization of the ulna stump after Darrach's procedure at the wrist. Int Orthop 2003;27(4):235–9.
24. Swanson AB. Implant arthroplasty for disabilities of the distal radioulnar joint. Use of a silicone rubber capping implant following resection of the ulnar head. Orthop Clin North Am 1973;4(2):373–82.
25. Sagerman SD, Seiler JG, Fleming LL, et al. Silicone rubber distal ulnar replacement arthroplasty. J Hand Surg Br 1992;17(6):689–93.
26. van Schoonhoven J, Fernandez DL, Bowers WH, et al. Salvage of failed resection arthroplasties of the distal radioulnar joint using a new ulnar head prosthesis. J Hand Surg Am 2000;25(3):438–46.
27. van Schoonhoven J, Muhldorfer-Fodor M, Fernandez DL, et al. Salvage of failed resection arthroplasties of the distal radioulnar joint using an ulnar head prosthesis: long-term results. J Hand Surg Am 2012;37(7):1372–80.
28. Willis AA, Berger RA, Cooney WP 3rd. Arthroplasty of the distal radioulnar joint using a new ulnar head endoprosthesis: preliminary report. J Hand Surg Am 2007;32(2):177–89.
29. Kakar S, Swann RP, Perry KI, et al. Functional and radiographic outcomes following distal ulna implant arthroplasty. J Hand Surg Am 2012;37(7): 1364–71.
30. Yen Shipley N, Dion GR, Bowers WH. Ulnar head implant arthroplasty: an intermediate term review of 1 surgeon's experience. Tech Hand Up Extrem Surg 2009;13(3):160–4.
31. Sauerbier M, Hahn ME, Fujita M, et al. Analysis of dynamic distal radioulnar convergence after ulnar head resection and endoprosthesis implantation. J Hand Surg Am 2002;27(3):425–34.
32. Berger RA. Implant arthroplasty for treatment of ulnar head resection-related instability. Hand Clin 2013;29(1):103–11.
33. Coffey MJ, Scheker LR, Thirkannad SM. Total distal radioulnar joint arthroplasty in adults with symptomatic Madelung's deformity. Hand(N Y) 2009;4(4): 427–31.
34. Savvidou C, Murphy E, Mailhot E, et al. Semiconstrained distal radioulnar joint prosthesis. J Wrist Surg 2013;2(1):41–8.

35. Galvis EJ, Pessa J, Scheker LR. Total joint arthroplasty of the distal radioulnar joint for rheumatoid arthritis. J Hand Surg Am 2014;39(9):1699–704.
36. Zimmerman RM, Jupiter JB. Outcomes of a self-constrained distal radioulnar joint arthroplasty: a case series of six patients. Hand(N Y) 2011;6(4):460–5.
37. Sotereanos DG, Gobel F, Vardakas DG, et al. An allograft salvage technique for failure of the Darrach procedure: a report of four cases. J Hand Surg Br 2002;27(4):317–21.
38. Greenberg JA, Sotereanos D. Achilles allograft interposition for failed Darrach distal ulna resections. Tech Hand Up Extrem Surg 2008;12(2):121–5.
39. Sotereanos DG, Papatheodorou LK, Williams BG. Tendon allograft interposition for failed distal ulnar resection: 2- to 14-year follow-up. J Hand Surg Am 2014;39(3):443–8.e1.
40. Peterson CA 2nd, Maki S, Wood MB. Clinical results of the one-bone forearm. J Hand Surg Am 1995;20(4):609–18.
41. Allende C, Allende BT. Posttraumatic one-bone forearm reconstruction. A report of seven cases. J Bone Joint Surg Am 2004;86-A(2):364–9.
42. Jacoby SM, Bachoura A, Diprinzio EV, et al. Complications following one-bone forearm surgery for posttraumatic forearm and distal radioulnar joint instability. J Hand Surg Am 2013;38(5):976–82.e1.

The Management of Complications of Small Joint Arthrodesis and Arthroplasty

Ellen S. Satteson, MD[a,b], Matthew A. Langford, MD[a], Zhongyu Li, MD, PhD[a,*]

KEYWORDS

- Arthroplasty • Arthrodesis • Fusion • Nonunion • Distal interphalangeal joint
- Proximal interphalangeal joint • Metacarpophalangeal joint • Carpometacarpal phalangeal joint

KEY POINTS

- Arthrodesis and arthroplasty are often performed to treat pain, stiffness, deformity, and instability related to arthritis and traumatic injury of the small joints of the hand.
- Arthrodesis is more frequently used at the distal interphalangeal and thumb metacarpophalangeal (MP) joints; arthroplasty is more frequently used at the proximal interphalangeal, MP of the fingers, and thumb carpometacarpal joints when possible.
- Postoperative infections after both arthrodesis and arthroplasty are usually managed with oral antibiotics when superficial, but deep infection or osteomyelitis may require hardware removal.
- Common complications following arthrodesis include nonunion, malunion, dorsal skin necrosis, and prominent hardware.
- Arthrodesis revision techniques include fixation with Kirschner wires, tension bands, 90-90 interosseous wires, plates, and screws with or without bone grafting.
- Small joint arthroplasty most often requires silicone implants or nonconstrained arthroplasty (cemented or uncemented surface replacement); common complications following arthroplasty include implant failure, synovitis, recurrent deformities or instability, prosthetic loosening, stiffness, deformity, squeaking, and pain.

COMPLICATIONS AFTER SMALL JOINT ARTHRODESIS

Distal Interphalangeal Joint

A nonunion rate ranging from 3% to 15% is reported for distal interphalangeal (DIP) arthrodesis, with Kirschner wires (K wire), 90-90 interosseous wires, and compression screw techniques.[1–4] **Table 1** shows the reported time to union and nonunion rates with the specific technique used. The thumb interphalangeal (IP) joint was more often included in the DIP category, but some studies did include it in the evaluation of proximal interphalangeal (PIP) arthrodesis instead.

Disclosures: None (Dr Z. Li and Dr E.S. Satteson); The views expressed in this presentation are those of this author and do not necessarily reflect the official policy or position of the Department of the Navy, the Department of Defense, or the US Government. This author is a military service member (or employee of the US Government). This work was prepared as part of this author's official duties (Dr M.A. Langford).

[a] Department of Orthopedic Surgery, Wake Forest School of Medicine, Medical Center Boulevard, Winston-Salem, NC 27157, USA; [b] Department of Plastic Surgery, Wake Forest School of Medicine, Medical Center Boulevard, Winston-Salem, NC 27157, USA
* Corresponding author.
E-mail address: zli@wakehealth.edu

Hand Clin 31 (2015) 243–266
http://dx.doi.org/10.1016/j.hcl.2015.01.002
0749-0712/15/$ – see front matter

Table 1
DIP joint arthrodesis: nonunion rates

Authors	Technique	Number of Joints	Average Time to Union (mo)	Nonunion (%) (n)	Infected Nonunion (%) (n)	Outcomes of Infected Nonunions (n)	Aseptic Nonunion (%) (n)	Outcomes of Aseptic Nonunion (%)	Revision Techniques (n)
Brutus et al,[3] 2006	Compression screw (Mini-Acutrak)	27	2.5	15 (4)	7 (2)	Declined revision (2)	7 (2)	Painless fibrous union (1) Fusion with revision	Crossed K wire (1)
Kocak et al,[2] 2011	Herbert screw (Zimmer, Warsaw, IN)	64	2.8	5 (3)	2[a] (1)	Fusion with immobilization	3 (2)	Fusion with revision (2)	Interosseous and K wire (2) Bone grafting and screw (1)
Matsumoto et al,[4] 2013	Compression screw (Reverse Fix Nail [Tact Medical, Tokyo, Japan])	89	2.5	2 (3)	0	Not applicable	2 (3)	Painless fibrous union (1) Fusion with revision (2)	Bone grafting with longitudinal K wire (1) Bone grafting without screw removal (1)
Stern & Fulton,[1] 1992	K wire	111	2.3[b]	12 (13)	2 (2)	Painless fibrous union (1) Painful nonunion with amputation (1)	10 (11)	Painless fibrous union (11) Fusion with revision (6)	Dorsal bone grafting with longitudinal K wire or interosseous wire (6)
Stern & Fulton,[1] 1992	Interosseous wire	43	2.3[b]	12 (5)	2 (1)	Painless fibrous union (1)	10 (4)	Declined revision (1)	
Stern & Fulton,[1] 1992	Herbert screw (Zimmer, Warsaw, IN)	27	2.3[b]	11 (3)	0	Not applicable	11 (3)		

[a] Infection occurred with secondary revision procedure on previously aseptic nonunion.
[b] Average time to union was reported for all techniques in the study combined but not individually.
Data from Refs.[1–4]

Successful union is usually assessed both radiographically and clinically, with trabecular bridging representing radiographic union and stability with limited pain on examination indicating clinical union. Common reasons for nonunion include poor or inadequate bone stock, under resection of subchondral bone, premature pin removal, and infection.[2] Further surgical intervention is not typically indicated for an asymptomatic DIP nonunion. In the presence of persistent pain, however, revision arthrodesis may be necessary.

Management of complications

Infected nonunion Simple soft tissue infections may be managed with a course of antibiotics. Contrarily, implant removal with immobilization and antibiotics is indicated with deep infections associated with hardware, concern for osteomyelitis, or failure to improve with antibiotic therapy. A formal revision procedure is often needed to achieve subsequent fusion. Some patients, however, may develop auto-fusion or painless fibrous union without further surgery (**Fig. 1**).

When infection results in a symptomatic nonunion, revision arthrodesis may be indicated once the infection is cleared. **Table 1** includes a literature review of the rates of infected nonunion and the ultimate outcomes with immobilization and/or revision. Several revision techniques have been described, including crossed or transverse K wires, screws, and interosseous wires with or without bone grafting.[1–4] The authors prefer headless screws or buried K wires for revision arthrodesis.

Aseptic nonunion In contrast to septic nonunion, hardware removal is not always required. Keeping hardware allows for prolonged attempts at delayed union, which is not possible when infection necessitates hardware removal. Furthermore, the presence of hardware may provide enough stabilization to prevent pain and symptoms in the case of fibrous union.

Regardless of these differences, similar revision techniques can be used using a cortical screw, headless screw, or buried K wires based on the size of the bone and surgeon preference. If poor

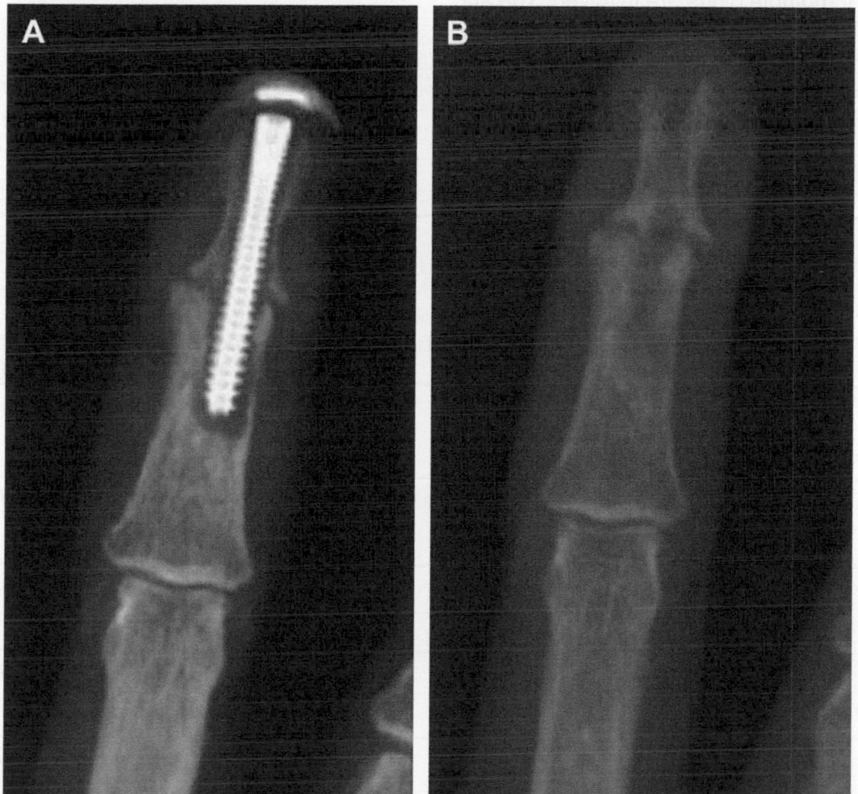

Fig. 1. Infected nonunion of DIP fusion. A 43-year-old woman underwent arthrodesis of her right long finger DIP joint with an Acutrak (Acumed, Hillsboro, OR, USA) 30-mm mini screw for a chronic mallet finger deformity related to rheumatoid arthritis (*A*). She developed a painful, infected nonunion with radiographic signs of osteomyelitis at 6 months after surgery (*B*). DIP auto-fusion occurred after hardware removal and appropriate antibiotic therapy without further revision. (*From* Koman LA, editor. Wake Forest University orthopaedic workbook. Winston-Salem (NC): Wake Forest University Orthopaedic Press; 2014; with permission.)

or inadequate bone stock is the likely underlying cause of nonunion, augmentation of the revision with bone graft should be considered.

Other complications Other common complications include soft tissue infection, nail deformity, and prominent hardware, which are typically managed with oral antibiotics or hardware removal (**Table 2**).

Proximal Interphalangeal Joint

Similar to the DIP joint, arthrodesis of the PIP carries a nonunion rate of 0% to 15%.[5–12] The average time to union, rates of nonunion based on technique, and revision procedures used are detailed in **Table 3**.

Management of complications

Nonunion A stable fixation is paramount for a successful revision. Bone grafting is often necessary to avoid overshortening of the digit. Bone graft can be obtained from the distal radius, olecranon, or iliac crest if multiple digits are involved. The authors have found 90-90 interosseous wires, tension banding, and plating to be useful salvage options when revision arthrodesis is indicated. The use of 90-90 interosseous wires requires the placement of 2 orthogonal loops of a 26-gauge surgical steel wire through 2 pairs of parallel holes drilled using a 0.035-in K wire (**Fig. 2**).

Other complications Additional complications that are commonly described with PIP arthrodesis include superficial or deep infection, dorsal skin necrosis, and prominent hardware; these complications are usually managed with antibiotics, local wound care, and/or hardware removal, respectively.[13] Malunion may also occur and require revision if symptomatic. Reported rates of these complications are listed in **Table 4**.

Thumb Metacarpophalangeal Joint

Although arthritis of the thumb metacarpophalangeal (MP) joint is less common than the carpometacarpal (CMC) joint, arthrodesis may be indicated in cases of arthritis, trauma, instability, or hyperextension deformity secondary to CMC arthritis. Fusion can be achieved using K wires, tension bands, screws, plates, or intramedullary interlocking devices.[13–19]

Management of complications

Nonunion Nonunion rates range from 0% to 20% (**Table 5**). Symptomatic nonunions require revision. Suggested techniques include tension banding or plating with bone grafting (**Fig. 3**).[14,16,17]

Table 2
DIP joint arthrodesis: other complication rates

Authors	Technique	Number of Joints	Superficial Infection	Deep Infection or Osteomyelitis	Skin Necrosis (%) (n)	Prominent Hardware (%) (n)	Malunion (%) (n)
Brutus, et al,[3] 2006	Compression screw (Mini-Acutrak)	27	4 (1)	11 (3)	4 (1)	11 (3)	None reported
Kocak, et al,[2] 2011	Herbert screw	64	0	2[a] (1)	None reported	8 (5)	None reported
Matsumoto, et al,[4] 2013	Compression screw (Reverse Fix Nail)	79	0	0	0	1 (1)	0
Stern & Fulton,[1] 1992	K wire	111	1 (1)	5 (5)	3 (3)	0	4 (4)
Stern & Fulton,[1] 1992	Interosseous wire	43	2 (1)	7 (3)	2 (1)	0	2 (1)
Stern & Fulton,[1] 1992	Herbert screw	27	4 (1)	4 (1)	15 (4)	7 (2)	4 (1)

[a] Infection occurred with secondary revision procedure on previously aseptic nonunion.
Data from Refs.[1–4]

Table 3
PIP joint arthrodesis: nonunion rates

Authors	Technique	Number of Joints	Average Time to Union (mo)	Nonunion (%) (n)	Infected Nonunion (%) (n)	Outcomes of Infected Nonunions (n)	Aseptic Nonunion (%) (n)	Outcomes of Aseptic Nonunion (%)	Revision Techniques (n)
Ayres et al,[5] 1998	Herbert screw	51	Not reported[a]	2 (1)	0	Not applicable	2 (1)	Fusion with revision	Miniplate fixation with bone grafting
Büchler & Aiken,[6] 1988	Corticocancellous bone graft and plate	25	Range of 1.5–3.0	8 (2)	4 (1)	Fusion with revision (1)	4 (1)	Fusion with revision (1)	Cancellous bone graft with plate (1) Without plate (1)
Høgh & Jensen,[7] 1982	K wire and cerclage	43[b]	2	7 (3)	1 (2)	Amputation (1)	6 (14)	Painless fibrous union (4) Revision (1) Amputation (1)	Not reported
Leibovic & Strickland,[8] 1994	K wire	99	2.5	21 (21)	1[c] (1)	Amputation (1)	21 (21)	Painless fibrous union (6) Fusion with revision (8)	Plate (7) Tension band (3)
Leibovic & Strickland,[8] 1994	Tension band	66	2.8	5 (3)	0	Not applicable	3 (2)	Nonunion with revision (5) No revision attempted (5)	Herbert screw (2) K wire (1)
Leibovic & Strickland,[8] 1994	Herbert screw	35	2.3	0	0	Not applicable	0	Not applicable	
Leibovic & Strickland,[8] 1994	Plate	4	3	50 (2)	0	Not applicable	50 (2)	Painless fibrous union	
Stern et al,[9] 1993	Tension band	290[d]		3 (9)	0	Not applicable	3 (9)	Painless fibrous union (3) Fusion with revision (5) Elected for amputation (1)	Not reported
Stahl & Rozen,[10] 2001	Tension band	72[e]	1.9 (trauma) 3.3 (arthritis)	0	0	Not applicable	0	Not applicable	Not applicable
Uhl & Schneider,[11] 1992	Tension band	75[f]	3	1 (1)	0	Not applicable	1 (1)	Painless fibrous union (1)	Not applicable

[a] Union rate of 98% at 6 weeks.
[b] Includes 23 PIP, 7 thumb IP, 4 thumb MP, and 9 DIP joints.
[c] Osteomyelitis occurred during secondary fusion attempt for primary nonunion.
[d] Includes 213 PIP, 60 thumb MP, and 17 finger MP joints.
[e] Includes 41 PIP, 20 thumb IP, 9 thumb MP, and 2 small finger MP joints.
[f] Includes 32 PIP, 8 thumb IP, and 35 thumb MP joint.
Data from Refs.[5–11]

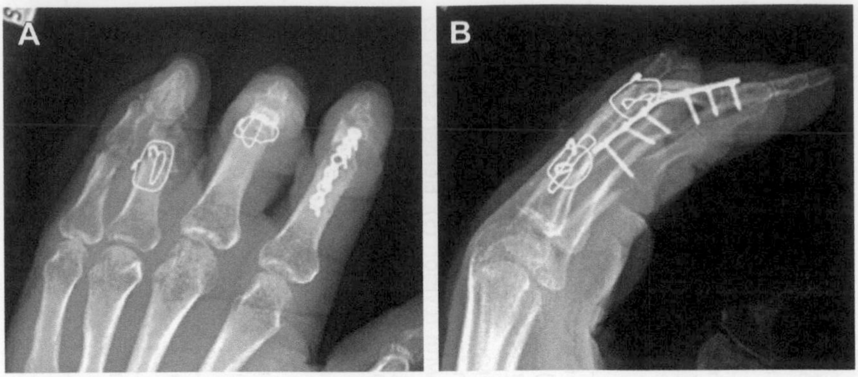

Fig. 2. PIP 90-90 interosseous wiring and plating. (*A, B*) Tension banding of the left long and ring PIP joints with plating of the index PIP related to an extensive table saw injury in a right-hand-dominant, 49-year-old male woodworker. (*From* Koman LA, editor. Wake Forest University orthopaedic workbook. Winston-Salem (NC): Wake Forest University Orthopaedic Press; 2014; with permission.)

Table 4
PIP joint arthrodesis: other complication rates

Authors	Technique	Number of Joints	Malunion (%) (n)	Superficial Infection (%) (n)	Deep Infection or Osteomyelitis (%) (n)	Prominent Hardware (%) (n)
Ayres et al,[5] 1998	Herbert screw	51	None reported[a]	None reported	None reported	4
Büchler & Aiken,[6] 1988	Corticocancellous bone graft and plate	25	0	None reported	4 (1)	None reported
Høgh & Jensen,[7] 1982	K wire and cerclage	43[b]	None reported	None reported	3 (7)	None reported
Leibovic & Strickland,[8] 1994	K wire	99	4 (4)	2 (2)	1[c] (1)	0
Leibovic & Strickland,[8] 1994	Tension band	66	0	0	0	9 (6)
Leibovic & Strickland,[8] 1994	Herbert screw	35	0	3 (1)	0	3 (1)
Leibovic & Strickland,[8] 1994	Plate	4	0	0	0	0
Stern et al,[9] 1993	Tension band	290[d]	1 (3)	3 (10)	0	9 (25)
Stahl & Rozen,[10] 2001	Tension band	72[e]	0	3 (2)	0	7 (5)
Uhl & Schneider,[11] 1992	Tension band	75[f]	0	1 (1)	0	23 (17)

[a] Union rate of 98% at 6 weeks.
[b] Includes 23 PIP, 7 thumb IP, 4 thumb MP and 9 DIP joints.
[c] Osteomyelitis occurred during secondary fusion attempt for primary nonunion.
[d] Includes 213 PIP, 60 thumb MP, and 17 finger MP joints.
[e] Includes 41 PIP, 20 thumb IP, 9 thumb MP, and 2 small finger MP joints.
[f] Includes 32 PIP, 8 thumb IP, and 35 thumb MP joint.
Data from Refs.[5–11]

Table 5
Thumb MP joint arthrodesis: complication rates

Authors	Technique	Number of Joints	Average Time to Union (mo)	Nonunion (%) (n)	Outcomes of Nonunions (n)	Revision Techniques (n)	Malunion (%) (n)	Superficial Infection (%) (n)	Deep Infection or Osteomyelitis (%) (n)	Prominent Hardware (%) (n)
Bicknell et al,[13] 2007	K wire (10 with bone graft)	48	2.6	0	Not applicable	Not applicable	0	4 (2)	0	2 (1)
Huffman & Rayan,[14]	K wire with bone graft	42	1.7	5 (2)	Painless fibrous union (1) Lost to follow-up (1)	Not applicable	None reported	12 (5)	0	5 (2)
Messer et al,[15]	Cannulated screw	18	2.5	0	Not applicable	Not applicable	None reported	6 (1)	0	6 (1)
Rasmussen et al,[18]	Plate	51	Not reported	2 (1)	Fusion with revision (1)	Repeat plating with bone graft (1)	0	0	0	6 (3)
Schmidt et al,[17]	Cannulated screw and threaded washer	26	2.5	4 (1)	Fusion with revision (1)	Tension banding (1)	0	0	0	0
Stanley et al,[16]	K wire	42	Not reported	12 (5)	Fusion with revision (1) Painless fibrous union with revision (4)	Not reported	None reported	0	0	0
Vanderzanden et al,[19] 2014	Intramedullary interlocking device	17	2	0	Not applicable	Not applicable	0	0	0	0

Data from Refs.[13–19]

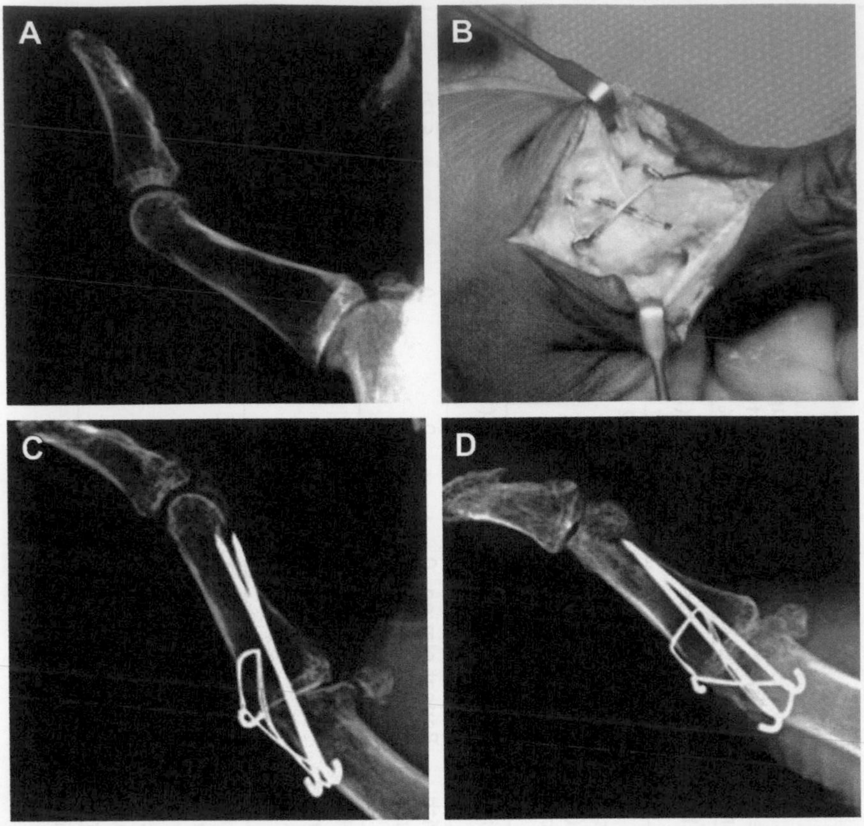

Fig. 3. Tension band arthrodesis of thumb MP. Thumb MP fusion performed in a right-hand-dominant, 57-year-old man who developed right MP instability with hyperextension following a stroke. (*A*) Preoperative hyperextensibility. (*B*) Tension band positioning. (*C, D*) Radiographs 2 months postoperatively. (*From* Koman LA, editor. Wake Forest University orthopaedic workbook. Winston-Salem (NC): Wake Forest University Orthopaedic Press; 2014; with permission.)

Other complications In addition to the other expected postoperative complications of surgical site infection, malunion, and prominent hardware (see **Table 5**), Stanley and colleagues[16] also reported postoperative extensor pollicis longus (EPL) rupture in 2 out of 42 MP fusions performed using a K-wire technique that involved placement of a longitudinal wire. Evaluation of these cases led them to recommend the avoidance of longitudinal K-wire placement when possible and use of a radiograph to confirm that the tip of the wire sits distal to the CMC joint. For patients with IP stiffness following MP arthrodesis, in one cited case, Rasmussen and colleagues[18] report tenolysis as a successful means of improving motion.

Thumb Carpometacarpal Joint

The thumb CMC joint is commonly affected by osteoarthritis, resulting in pain that may not respond to nonoperative therapies.[20] Although tendon interposition and synthetic arthroplasty techniques are commonly used, arthrodesis is a valuable option reserved for patients younger than 50 years or individuals prioritizing grip strength, such as manual laborers.[21] Several studies comparing arthrodesis with arthroplasty have reported higher rates of complications with CMC arthrodesis, making knowledge of the appropriate management of these complications of great importance to those performing the procedure.[20,22]

Management of complications

Nonunion The literature suggests that achieving fusion at the thumb CMC joint may be more challenging than other small joints of the hand, with nonunion rates ranging from 0% to 58%.[20–24] Although several primary arthrodesis techniques have been reported, including K wire, tension banding, plating with a locking plate, staples, and compression screws (**Fig. 4**),[20–24] revision arthrodesis is less frequently described (**Table 6**).[20,23] Locking plate is the authors' choice for CMC arthrodesis as it provides strong fixation. Conversion to a trapeziectomy with ligament

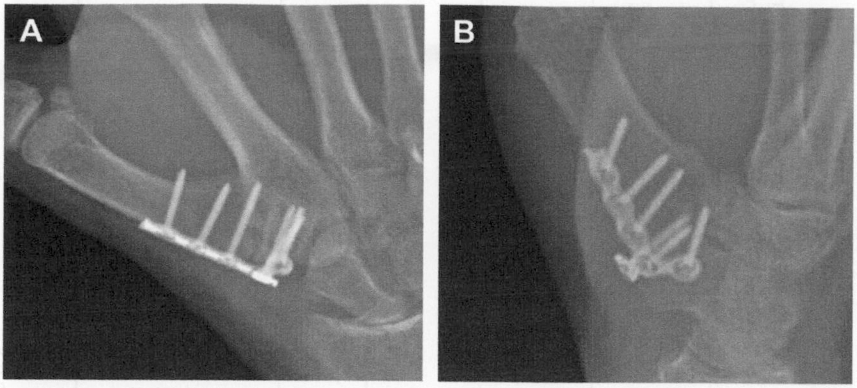

Fig. 4. CMC plating. (*A, B*) Arthrodesis of the CMC joint with a plate and screws for posttraumatic arthritis in a right-hand-dominant, 53-year-old, male butcher with a history of a Darrach procedure as a teenager. (*From* Koman LA, editor. Wake Forest University orthopaedic workbook. Winston-Salem (NC): Wake Forest University Orthopaedic Press; 2014; with permission.)

reconstruction and tendon interposition (LRTI) also provides a satisfactory result in those patients with nonunion or persistent pain.[21,23]

Other complications A review of the literature suggests that superficial infection, radial nerve neuritis, and prominent hardware are the most common complications (see **Table 6**). Other less frequently cited complications include increased peritrapezial arthritis compared with the nonoperative side,[20,21,24] complex regional pain syndrome,[21] extensor tendonitis,[23] and intraoperative fracture.[21] The authors and others (Kevin Chung, MD, personal communication, 2014) have also encountered flexor pollicis longus (FPL) ruptures related to migration of a screw that required a palmaris longus (PL) graft or tendon transfer from the flexor digitorum superficialis (FDS) of the ring finger (**Fig. 5**).

COMPLICATIONS AFTER SMALL JOINT ARTHROPLASTY

In contrast to arthrodesis, arthroplasty of any sort is generally regarded as a useful option for providing pain relief while maintaining motion when performed in appropriately selected patients. However, like arthrodesis, arthroplasty is not without risk.

Proximal Interphalangeal Joint

Arthroplasty of the PIP comes in multiple forms, with silicone implants, the most popular current form, having been around since the 1960s when they were initially popularized by Swanson. Two broad categories of implants are currently in clinical use: silicone joint replacement and nonconstrained resurfacing. Nonconstrained arthroplasty uses several materials, including various metal types on polymer (both cemented and uncemented) and pyrocarbon.[25]

Silicone arthroplasty

When arthroplasty is performed, silicone is still the standard technique owing to its consistent long-term results, providing good pain relief while maintaining adequate function. Even with its high praise in the literature, revision rates range from 2% to 16%.[26–30] A review of 70 articles has identified breakage, continued pain, infection, implant loosening, decreased range of motion, bony block, instability, and synovitis as the primary indications for revision (**Table 7**).[26–29]

Several investigators have looked at complication rates related to different surgical approaches, including dorsal, palmar, lateral, or a combination. Drake and Segalman[31] reviewed the literature and found no significant differences based on approach. Herren and Simmen[32] report that the volar approach is associated with a smaller number of complications, although there was not a statistically significant difference. They did suggest that the volar approach may be beneficial if collateral ligament integrity was crucial. The volar approach might reduce extensor lag, but joint exposure could be challenging. For revision arthroplasty, the authors prefer to use the same incision as used for the primary surgery if possible.

Nonconstrained arthroplasty

Pyrolytic carbon as well as cemented and uncemented surface replacement arthroplasty (SRA) with metal (cobalt-chrome or titanium) and ultra-high molecular weight polyethylene require adequate soft tissue support to prevent subluxation and dislocation. Preoperative malalignment is a relative contraindication for reconstruction.

Table 6
Thumb CMC joint arthrodesis: complication rates

Authors	Technique (n)	Number of Joints	Average Time to Union (mo)	Nonunion (%) (n)	Outcomes of Nonunions (n)	Revision Techniques (n)	Radial Sensory Neuritis (%) (n)	Superficial Infection (%) (n)	Deep Infection or Osteomyelitis (%) (n)	Prominent Hardware (%) (n)
Forseth & Stern,[23] 2003	Plate	26	Not reported	8 (2)	Fusion with revision (1) Interposition arthroplasty (1)	Plate (1)	8 (2)	4 (1)	0	23 (6)
Fulton & Stern,[24] 2001	K wire with bone graft	59		7 (4)	Fusion with revision (1) Painless fibrous union (3)	Plate with bone graft (1)	0	7 (4)	0	3 (2)
Hartigan, et al,[20] 2001	K wire (40) Minicondylar plate (16) Tension band (2)	58	Not reported	16 (9)	Fusion with revision (3) Painless fibrous union (6)	Plate with bone graft (3)	2 (1)	3 (2)	2 (1)	3 (2)
Mureau, et al,[22] 2001[a]	K wire +/– bone graft	32	2.1	7 (2)	Painless fibrous union (5) Painful nonunion (2)	Revision (1)[b] K wire removal (1)	2 (7)	3 (1)	0	9 (3)
Rizzo, et al,[21] 2009[c]	K wires (101) Tension band +/– K wires (11) Staples (8) Plate (3) Screw (2) None (1)	126	Not reported	13 (17)	Fusion with revision (6) Interposition arthroplasty (3) Painless fibrous union (8)	Bone grafting (fixation technique not specified)	6 (5)	8[d] (11)	0	2 (3)

[a] Fourteen of the 32 arthrodeses included bone graft. Three of the 7 nonunions occurred in these patients.
[b] Outcome results following secondary procedures (unspecified revision technique and K wire removal) were not reported.
[c] Ninety of the 126 arthrodeses were augmented with supplemental bone graft. Eleven of the 17 nonunions occurred in bone grafted joints.
[d] Included pin migration, loosening, and infection.
Data from Refs.[20–24]

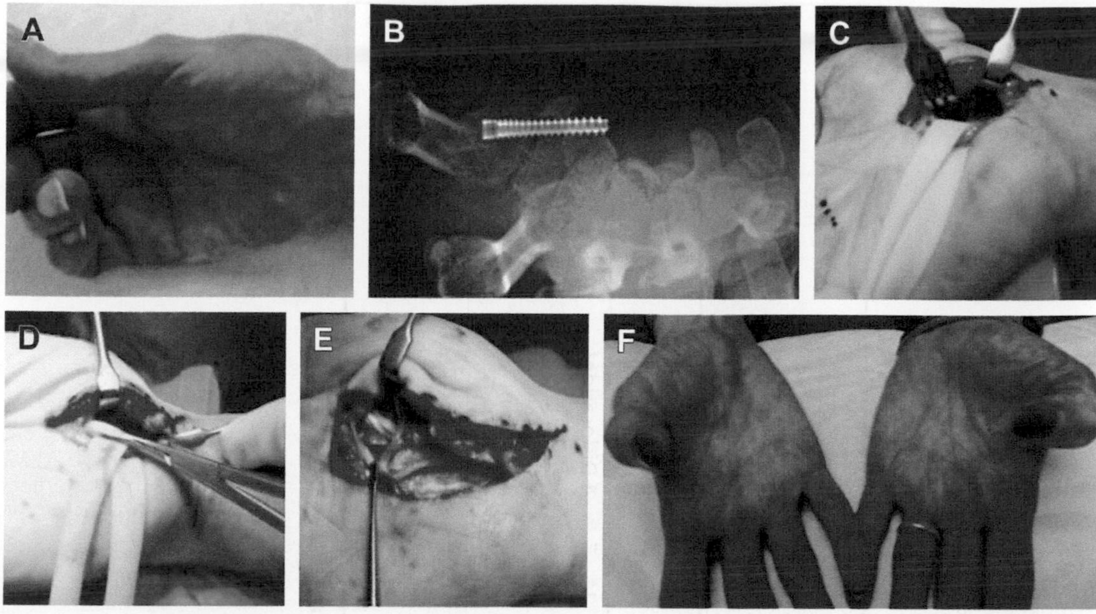

Fig. 5. Tendon transfer for FPL rupture following thumb CMC fusion with headless screw. A 59-year-old woman presented with a right FPL rupture 15 years after CMC arthrodesis with a headless screw. (*A*) Preoperative inability to flex the thumb IP joint. (*B*) Radiograph showing migration of the headless screw into the carpal tunnel. (*C*) Visibly prominent screw with absence of FPL tendon in its usual anatomic location. (*D*) The distal end of the transected FPL. (*E*) Transfer of the ring FDS to the distal FPL. (*F*) Postoperative thumb flexion compared with the unaffected contralateral side. (*From* Koman LA, editor. Wake Forest University orthopaedic workbook. Winston-Salem (NC): Wake Forest University Orthopaedic Press; 2014; with permission.)

Although inadequate collateral ligaments are considered to be an absolute contraindication, joint stabilization with external fixation for 6 to 8 weeks could be considered if joint instability occurs after bone resection.[33]

Nonconstrained implants were designed to counteract some of the problems of silicone implants; however, the complication rates for nonconstrained implants are not insignificant. These complications include instability, loosening, stiffness, deformity, squeaking, pain, and infection. Reoperation rates range from 6% to 58%.[34–38] A review by Pritsch and Rizzo[34] found that the most common cause of revision was extensor mechanism dysfunction, accounting for two-thirds of the revisions. Surgical approach also had a statistically significant impact with the Chamay, the central slip reflection approaches having the highest complication rates at 87%; 61% of cases using an extensor split approach presented with extensor dysfunction, whereas the lateral approach had the lowest complication rate at 33%. The 3 complications that were listed as most common for these approaches included adhesions, incompetence, and imbalance resulting in swan neck deformity. Reoperations for lateral instability were significantly more common in patients with inflammatory conditions, preexisting volar plate contractures, and pyrolytic carbon implants. In another study, Jennings and Livingstone[39] found that 39% of the uncemented components loosened at 3 years compared with 4% in the cemented group. A major drawback that has led to abandonment of the use of cemented prosthetics in the hand is the inability to remove the implant should revision be needed (**Table 8**).

Management of complications

Extensor mechanism problems tend to be the most frequently seen complications following PIP arthroplasty.[34] Adhesions may require tenolysis. In the event of extensor disruption, however, a reconstruction or revision to arthrodesis must be considered as direct repair is often not possible. Revision of the implant is often required when there is instability, loosening or a periprosthetic fracture.[29,34,40] The average number of reoperations for failed arthroplasty is 1.6 per digit.[34] If there is adequate bone stock and soft tissue support, a revision to a new nonconstrained implant is possible with or without concomitant bone grafting. When soft tissue support is inadequate, options include transition to, or replacement of, a silicone implant. Salvage measures include resection arthroplasty, arthrodesis, and amputation.

Table 7
PIP joint silicone arthroplasty: complications

Author	Implant	Number of Joints (n)	Pain (n)	Particulate Synovitis/ Silicone Lymphadenopathy (n)	Bone Changes (n)	Implant Fracture (n)	Implant Loosening (n)	Infection (n)	Removal (n)
Foliart,[26] 1995	Swanson	2463	Not reported	4 Synovitis/none reported	29	39	6 Dislocation 8 Instability 1 Subluxation	21	52[a]
Takigawa et al,[27] 2004	Swanson	70	16 (Grade 1, 2, or 3 pain)	0/0	8 Radiolucency 32 Hinge bone formation 11 Heterotopic bone 46 Sclerosis	11	4 Dislocation/ instability/ subluxation 18 Implant deformation	1	9[b] (Revisions)
Herren et al,[29] 2014	Silicone	34[c]	14	Not reported	Not reported	18	8 Deviation (3 of which also had implant fracture)	Not reported	4 (Revisions)

[a] Twenty-one implant fracture, 9 continued pain, 5 infection, 4 particulate synovitis, 4 loosening, 9 miscellaneous.
[b] Three Swanson revisions, 2 metal-polyethylene revisions, 1 biometric revision, 1 fusion, 1 disarticulation.
[c] Nine were for decreased active range of motion with or without pain.
Data from Refs.[26,27,29]

Table 8
PIP joint nonconstrained arthroplasty: complications

Author	Implant	Number of Joints (n)	Tendon Adhesions (n)	Extensor Mechanism Failure (n)	Collateral Ligament Failure (n)	Loosening (n)	Bony Changes (n)	Dislocation/ Malalignment (n)	Infection (n)	Revision (n)
Pritsch & Rizzo,[34] 2011[a]	Pyrolytic carbon and SRA	203 Pyrolytic carbon 91 SRA	34/6/5 Extensor 2/1/0 Flexor	9/8/3	10/6/2	17/9/2	4/0/0	13/6/2 Swan neck 4/0/0 Malalignment	0/1/1	76[b]
Wijk et al,[37] 2010	Pyrolytic carbon	53	1	None reported	None reported	1	None reported	2	1	7[c]
Jennings & Livingstone,[39] 2008	SRA	43[d]	1	None reported	None reported	2 Cemented 16 Uncemented	15 Stress shielding 9 Radiolucency	5 Swan neck 1 Angulation	None reported	11 (Loosening in 10, pain in 1)

[a] First revision/second revision/third revision.
[b] Forty-five joints single reoperation, 19 joints had 2 reoperation, 11 joints had 3 reoperations, 1 joint had 4 reoperations. Average 1.6 reoperations per joint.
[c] Additional 2 revisions caused by pain.
[d] Eighty-six components: 45 cemented, 41 uncemented.
Data from Refs.[34,37,39]

Arthrodesis is not without its own complications in this setting though. Jones and colleagues[40] showed that in 13 fingers undergoing fusion after arthroplasty, only 8 achieved union without additional surgery. Four fingers achieved union with repeat operations, and 1 went on to nonunion.

Vascularized toe joint transfer is a viable option for experienced surgeons after failed arthroplasty, although patient selection is paramount. A revision rate of 29% is comparable with the 33% seen with pyrolytic carbon arthroplasty but still higher than those after silicone arthroplasty.[41] With a natural joint, vascularized toe joint transfer is less susceptible to resorption and failure once healed, but poor range of motion is a concern.

Metacarpophalangeal Joint

Silicone arthroplasty

Silicone arthroplasty for the MP joint remains the standard in significantly deformed joints.[42,43] As with the PIP joint, soft tissue restraints are not required in the hinged silicone implants, but complications are still associated with their use. Implant fracture rate varies among the different types of silicone implants available. Tägil and colleagues[44] found a higher implant fracture rate in silicone implants with more flexion or range of motion. With time, the implant survival decreased, whereas the revision rate increased. Another study examined 1336 MP joint silicone arthroplasties and found a fracture rate of 42% at 10 years with a revision rate of 17%. At 17 years, the fracture rate was 66% with a revision rate of 37%.[45] The investigators found that previous thumb CMC replacement, thumb MP joint fusion, and manipulation under anesthesia (MUA) of the arthroplasty were associated with a significantly higher rate of revision. Previous PIP joint replacement placed the MP joint arthroplasty at a statistically significant higher chance of fracture. Improvements in fracture and implant survival rates were seen with crossed intrinsic transfer, realignment of the wrist, and soft tissue balancing. The overall reported revision rate was 5.7% (**Table 9**).

Nonconstrained arthroplasty

Similar to the PIP joint, nonconstrained implants come in pyrolytic carbon and metal-plastic varieties. Successful surgery depends on adequate bone stock and sufficient adjacent soft tissues for stability.[42] These criteria tend to make this type of implant more suitable for osteoarthritic and degenerative joint pathologies, though early rheumatoid arthritis with little deformity is not a contraindication when used in conjunction with synovectomy and extensor centralization. Cook and colleagues[46] evaluated 151 pyrolytic carbon MP implants with 8 years of follow-up, showing an overall revision rate of 12%. Implant survivorship analysis showed a 2.1% annual failure rate with a calculated 16-year survivorship of 70.3%. Revisions were required for subluxation, dislocation, flexion contracture, stiffness, loosening, tendon rupture, and implant fracture (**Table 10**).[46,47]

Management of complications

As with the PIP joint, management of postoperative complications depends on which problem has arisen. A thorough knowledge of the options and the ability to be creative are required for any surgeon performing small joint arthroplasty. For the MP joint, the primary treatment of a failed arthroplasty is revision arthroplasty.[48] Although it is occasionally possible to revise a failed nonconstrained arthroplasty to another nonconstrained implant, the more common revision approach is replacement with a silicone implant. Salvage, when revision arthroplasty fails, ranges from arthrodesis to resection arthroplasty without reimplantation to amputation.

Joint stiffness may require manipulation, tenolysis, or tissue rebalancing. If the implant has fractured, a revision of the implant is typically required in nonconstrained implants; however, in silicone implants, this is not always the case. It is theorized that even though a silicone implant is fractured and no longer functioning as intended, it is still able to act as an interposition, thus, alleviating pain. Periprosthetic fractures can be treated with closed reduction and casting, open reduction with cerclage, or even revision arthroplasty.

Thumb Carpometacarpal Joint

Thumb CMC joint osteoarthritis is exceedingly common. According to Becker and colleagues,[49] rates may be as high as 100% in women older than 91 years and 93% in men older than 81 years. Surgery rates, however, do not reach these prevalence rates, with only 3 of 2321 patients with available CMC radiographs having evidence of surgery at this joint. Nevertheless, CMC arthroplasty is a procedure commonly performed by the hand surgeon with a variety of surgical options available. Trapeziectomy alone is the original, well-described arthroplasty technique that some investigators still recommend.[50–52] Additional surgical procedures have been developed as a response to patient complaints of substantial weakness and pain that was thought to be caused by subsidence of the thumb metacarpal.[53,54]

Implant arthroplasty

The reported implant arthroplasties include silicone trapezial replacement; metal-plastic

Table 9
MP joint silicone arthroplasty: complications

Author	Implant	Number of Joints (n)	Pain (n)	Particulate Synovitis/ Silicone Lymphadenopathy (n)	Bony Changes (n)	Implant Fracture (n)	Implant Loosening (n)	Infection (n)	Revision (n)
Foliart,[26] 1995	Swanson	13,031	Not reported	6/13	424	312	43 Dislocation 27 Instability 29 Subluxation	64	87[a] (Removal)
Goldfarb & Stern,[43] 2003	Silicone	208	152 (Occasional to constant)	None reported	416 of 416 Phalanges/ metacarpals[b]	130 Broken 45 Severely deformed	Overall average 2.2-mm implant subsidence	Not reported	14
Trail et al,[45] 2004[c]	Silicone	1336	Not reported	4	2 (spur)	39	9 Deformity 4 Dislocation 2 Loosening	2	76

[a] Forty-five implant fracture, 25 infection, 8 loosening/instability, 6 particulate synovitis, 3 m scellaneous.
[b] A total of 296 with sclerotic rim, 76 with radiolucent zone, 76 with cysts: proximal phalanx more likely to have more severe changes (*P*<.05), osseous resorption (radiolucency or cysts) associated with metacarpal shortening (*P*<.05).
[c] Numbers provided after total number of joints are only the numbers causing revision, not incidence; additional 14 revisions caused by stiffness.
Data from Refs.[26,43,45]

Table 10
MP joint nonconstrained arthroplasty: complications

Author	Implant	Number of Joints (n)	Tendon Adhesions (n)	Extensor Mechanism Failure (n)	Collateral Ligament Failure (n)	Loosening (n)	Bony Changes (n)	Dislocation/ Malalignment (n)	Infection (n)	Revision (n)
Cook et al,[46] 1999	Pyrolytic carbon	151	None reported	None reported	None reported	See revision explanation	50/53 with sclerotic rim 34/53 with subsidence 12/53 with radiolucency	See revision explanation	None reported	18[a]
Parker et al,[47] 2007	Pyrolytic carbon	142 (12 Revisions from silicone)	2	1	None reported	53 Axial subsidence 4 Stem angulation	101 Radiolucent line 30 Erosions	4 Dislocation/ subluxation	None reported	10[b]

[a] Four revisions to another pyrolytic carbon with bone cement or graft: 1 for stiffness, 1 for stiffness and loosening, and 2 for flexion contracture. Fourteen revisions to other implants: 10 Swanson replacements for subluxation, flexion contracture, stiffness, and dislocation; 2 replaced with carbon implants for loosening and dislocation; 1 Sutter silicone implant for pain, loosening, stiffness; 1 cemented metal and plastic for implant fracture.

[b] Six soft tissue rebalancing, 1 closed MUA, 2 extensor tenolysis (1 also had soft tissue rebalancing), 1 extensor mechanism repair, 1 ray amputation for pain.

Data from Cook SD, Beckenbaugh RD, Redondo J, et al. Long-term follow-up of pyrolytic carbon metacarpophalangeal implants. J Bone Joint Surg Am 1999;81(5):635–48; and Parker WL, Rizzo M, Moran SL, et al. Preliminary results of nonconstrained pyrolytic carbon arthroplasty for metacarpophalangeal joint arthritis. J Hand Surg Am 2007;32(10):1496–505.

Table 11
Thumb CMC joint arthroplasty: complications

Author	Implant	Number of Joints (n)	Loosening (n)	Dislocation (n)	Heterotopic Bone (n)	Fracture (n)	Subsidence (n)	Revisions (n)	Revisions (Procedure)
Pellegrini & Burton,[58] 1986	Silicone	32	Not applicable	35% Subluxation	None reported	None reported	50% Implant height loss	25%	Soft tissue interposition
Badia & Sambandam,[60] 2006	Braun-Cutter	26	1 (Posttraumatic)	None reported	None reported	None reported	None reported	1	Implant revision
Nicholas & Calderwood,[61] 1992	Caffinière	20	1	1	None reported	None reported	1	None at time of publishing	Not applicable
Chakrabarti et al,[62] 1997	Caffinière	93	21	1	None reported	2 (cup)	None reported	11 (12 Surgeries)	5 Implant revision 6 Implant excision 1 Neuroma excision
van Cappelle et al,[63] 1999	Caffinière	77	27 (44%)	3	None reported	None reported	None reported	16 (18 Surgeries)	7 Fusion/excision 2 Secondary salvage 11 Implant revisions
Wachtl et al,[64] 1998	Caffinière and Ledoux	88 43 Caffinière 45 Ledoux	23[a,b] 9 Caffinière 14 Ledoux	5 1 Caffinière 4 Ledoux	None reported	None reported	Yes (no details)	27 10 Caffinière 17 Ledoux	Not addressed 9 Loose/1 dislocate 14 Loose/4 dislocate
Adams et al,[65] 2009	Orthosphere (Wright Medical Technology, Memphis, TN)	50	Not applicable	0 7 Subluxations	1	15	47	4 (1 HO, 1 subluxation, 2 pain)	1 HO excision 3 Soft tissue interposition

[a] Number involved in revisions.
[b] Total loosening not given: Caffinière group: 24% of stems, 28% of cups; Ledoux group: 5% of stems, 46% of cups.
Data from Refs.[58,60–65]

implants; hemiarthroplasty; ceramic balls; and a polycaprolactone-based polyurethaneurea interposition, the Artelon spacer (Artimplant, Vastra Frölunda, Sweden).[55] Silicone replacements first became popular in the 1970s but later fell out of favor because of instability, wear, wear debris, problems with cold flow, and foreign body synovitis.[56–59] The most prevalent metal-plastic implant with extensive follow-up, is the de le Caffinière prosthesis, although there are other implants in this group available.[60] Unfortunately, these implants are fraught with a high complication rate and catastrophic failure after a short-term symptom relieve. The complications associated with these prostheses are aseptic loosening, subsidence, heterotopic bone, dislocation, and trapezial fracture, with up to a 31% revision rate (**Table 11**).[58,60–66]

Management of complications

Management options of complications following implant arthroplasty of the thumb CMC joint are limited from an implant standpoint. When adequate bone stock still remains, revision of the loose components is possible.[67,68] When there is inadequate bone stock, revision options become similar to those for suspension arthroplasty (**Fig. 6**). Salvage of failed implant arthroplasty does not have high success rates. Conolly and Rath[68] showed that revision of soft tissue stabilization after silicone arthroplasty carried a 47% fair and poor outcome satisfaction rate.

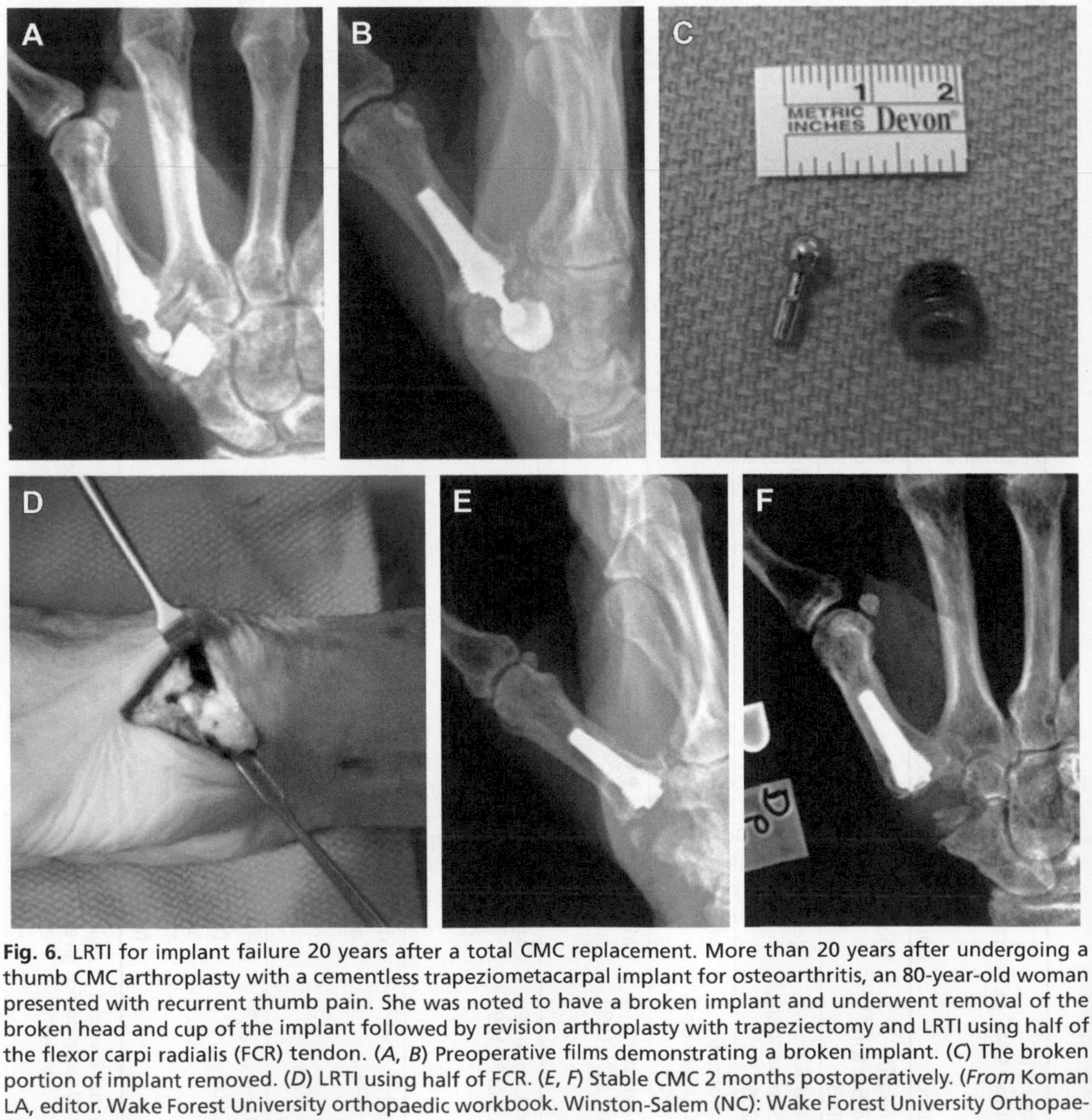

Fig. 6. LRTI for implant failure 20 years after a total CMC replacement. More than 20 years after undergoing a thumb CMC arthroplasty with a cementless trapeziometacarpal implant for osteoarthritis, an 80-year-old woman presented with recurrent thumb pain. She was noted to have a broken implant and underwent removal of the broken head and cup of the implant followed by revision arthroplasty with trapeziectomy and LRTI using half of the flexor carpi radialis (FCR) tendon. (*A, B*) Preoperative films demonstrating a broken implant. (*C*) The broken portion of implant removed. (*D*) LRTI using half of FCR. (*E, F*) Stable CMC 2 months postoperatively. (*From* Koman LA, editor. Wake Forest University orthopaedic workbook. Winston-Salem (NC): Wake Forest University Orthopaedic Press; 2014; with permission.)

Table 12
Thumb CMC joint suspension arthroplasty: complications

Author	Technique	Number of Joints (n)	Tendon Rupture/ Adhesions (n)	Scar Tenderness/ Infection (n)	Pain (n)	Sensory Change (n)	Lacerated Palmar Cutaneous Median Nerve (n)	Neuroma (n)	Instability (n)	CRPS (n)	Revisions (n)
Wajon et al,[70] 2009	T	134	None reported	2	1	7	2	1	1	2	Not reported
	T & LRTI	168	15	4	2	5	3	1	1	7	Not reported
	T & LR	15	None reported	None reported	None reported	None reported	None reported	None reported	None reported	None reported	Not reported
	T & TI	59	6	1	None reported	4	3	None reported	None reported	None reported	None reported
Cooney et al,[72] 2006	T & interposition arthroplasty	606	None reported	None reported	17	None reported	None reported	2 (After revision)	Second most common reason for revision	None reported	17[a]
Megerle et al,[73] 2011	LRTI	343	1	None reported		1	None reported	None reported	None reported	None reported	19[b] (7 Rerevisions)

Abbreviations: CRPS, chronic regional pain syndrome; T, trapeziectomy.
[a] Ten LRTI revisions, 5 interposition arthroplasties, 2 silicone arthroplasties.
[b] Twelve primary revisions were 6 repeat arthroplasty, 2 thumb MC to index MC fusion, 2 complete wrist denervation, 1 neurolysis sensory branch radial nerve, 1 FCR tenolysis.
Data from Refs.[70,72,73]

Suspension arthroplasty

Common suspension arthroplasty techniques include simple distraction arthroplasty, trapeziectomy with interposition, and trapeziectomy with LRTI. Ligament reconstruction can be performed with flexor carpi radialis (FCR), extensor carpi radialis longus (ECRL), abductor pollicis longus (APL), or a Mini Tightrope (Arthrex, Naples, FL).[69] Interposition can also be done in several ways. The use of split or whole FCR, PL, APL, or ECRL have been described.

Numerous studies have reported similar overall outcomes after thumb CMC suspension arthroplasty, regardless of the technique used.[70,71] In general, 80% to 90% of patients are satisfied postoperatively.[55] In 2 large reviews, revision rates of 2.3% to 4.7% were reported after a total of 997 CMC arthroplasties (**Table 12**).[72,73]

Management of complications

Thumb metacarpal subsidence after thumb CMC suspension arthroplasty is common, but revision is not necessary if the patient is asymptomatic. Common indications for revision are persistent pain and instability. If pain persists after an LRTI procedure, a thorough workup to exclude infection and scaphotrapezial (ST) arthritis is warranted. Resection of the proximal portion of the trapezoid may eliminate pain if ST arthritis is the source. Dislocation of the anchovy resulting in pain and instability also occurs occasionally. Thumb metacarpal and scaphoid impingement requires a revision ligament reconstruction.

Several techniques for ligament reconstruction have been described. The Thompson procedure uses a slip of APL for suspension if a partial FCR is intact. If the FCR is compromised, then the

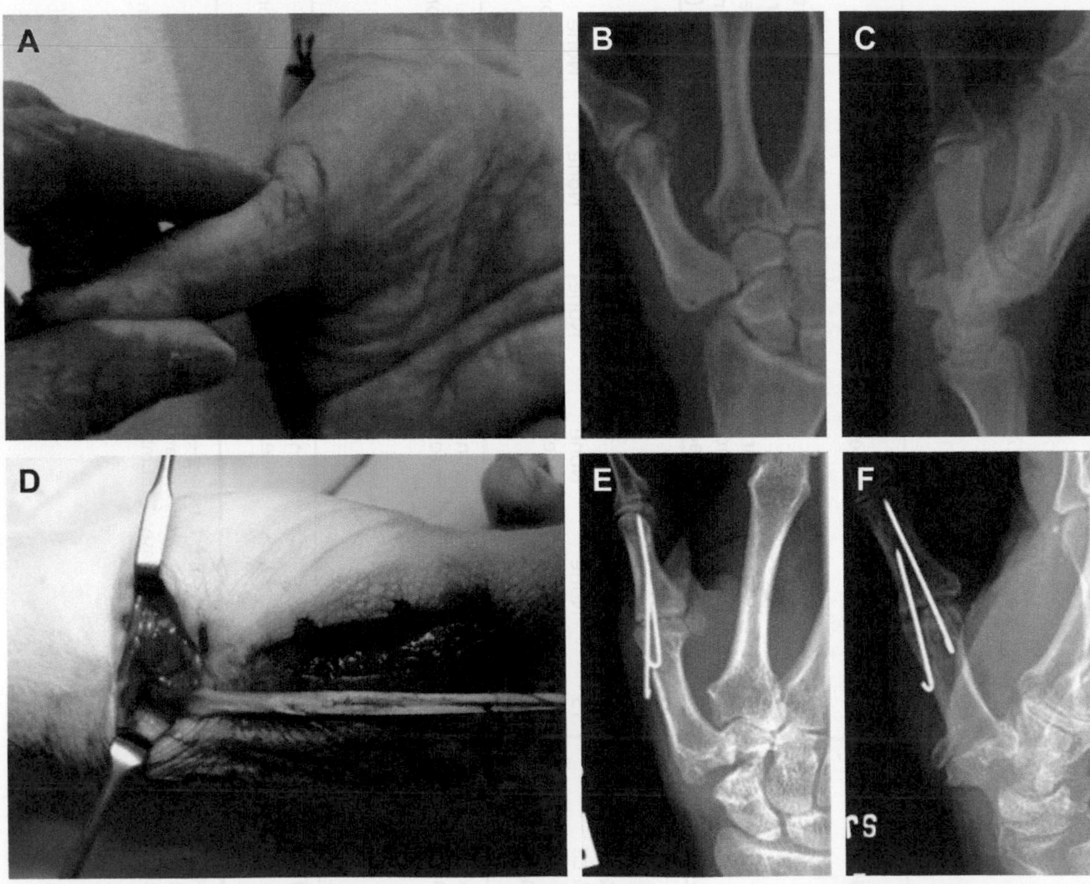

Fig. 7. Revision LRTI using ECRL. A 54-year-old woman failed LRTI using the FCR tendon at an outside institution. She underwent revision LRTI with ECRL as well as MP fusion. (*A*) Clinical CMC instability with MP hyperextension. (*B, C*) Failure of initial LRTI with collapse and instability of the CMC joint and hyperextension of the MP. (*D*) ECRL after proximal transection and distal pull through for interposition. (*E, F*) Stable CMC with maintenance of interposition height 6 months postoperatively. (*From* Koman LA, editor. Wake Forest University orthopaedic workbook. Winston-Salem (NC): Wake Forest University Orthopaedic Press; 2014; with permission.)

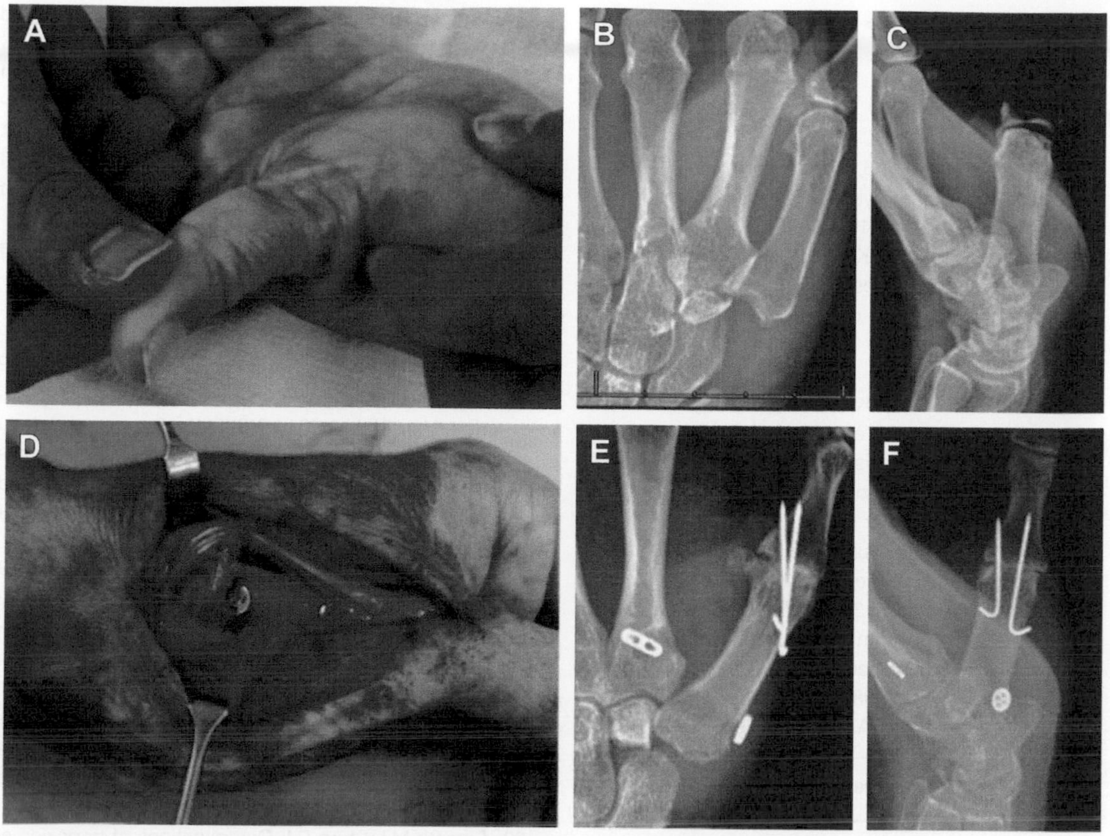

Fig. 8. Mini Tightrope for revision LRTI. A 48-year old woman underwent left LRTI using FCR for CMC arthritis with joint instability. She subsequently developed persistent pain and instability and underwent revision LRTI using a Mini Tightrope and tendon allograft as well as MP arthrodesis for an associated hyperextension deformity. She also underwent contralateral LRTI with FCR, which also required revision with a Mini Tightrope. (*A*) Clinical CMC instability following initial LRTI. (*B, C*) Radiographs following initial LRTI. (*D*) Intraoperative positioning of Tightrope. (*E, F*) Postoperative radiographs with stable CMC and fused MP 5 months following revision. (*From* Koman LA, editor. Wake Forest University orthopaedic workbook. Winston-Salem (NC): Wake Forest University Orthopaedic Press; 2014; with permission.)

ECRL can be used for suspension purposes (**Fig. 7**). The radial half of the ECRL tendon is divided proximal to the extensor retinaculum, passed underneath the EPL tendon, and pulled through a bone tunnel made over the base of the thumb metacarpal where it is then weaved to itself with the thumb distracted distally. If ECRL transfer is not available, a free tendon graft with a Mini Tightrope may be considered (**Fig. 8**). Thumb metacarpal-to-index metacarpal fusion as well as costochondral or bone graft fusion may provide rigid stability of the CMC joint to alleviate pain. An additional relatively new option is trapezial replacement with a titanium prosthesis.

Revision of a failed CMC suspension arthroplasty can be challenging. It is important to remember that although most patients do very well, those who do not may require significant additional work before their satisfaction level reaches that of the majority. Psychosocial factors, such as worker's compensation, legal status, and secondary gain, may also complicate the outcome of the surgery. In a review of 15 patients, Renfree and Dell[74] found that in patients requiring revision, an average of 3 additional procedures were required before the patients were satisfied with their results.

SUMMARY

Even though small joint arthrodesis and arthroplasty are commonly performed by most hand surgeons, their associated complications remain a frequent challenge. Although the literature is often sparse in its offerings of management options for these complications, careful evaluation of patients' outcome goals and the likely underlying cause of the specific complication can help guide treatment options to maintain a satisfactory outcome.

REFERENCES

1. Stern PJ, Fulton DB. Distal interphalangeal joint arthrodesis: an analysis of complications. J Hand Surg Am 1992;17(6):1139–45.
2. Kocak E, Carruthers KH, Kobus RJ. Distal interphalangeal joint arthrodesis with the Herbert headless compression screw: outcomes and complications in 64 consecutively treated joints. Hand (N Y) 2011;6(1):56–9.
3. Brutus JP, Palmer AK, Mosher JF, et al. Use of a headless compressive screw for distal interphalangeal joint arthrodesis in digits: clinical outcome and review of complications. J Hand Surg Am 2006;31(1):85–9.
4. Matsumoto T, Nakamura I, Miura A, et al. Distal interphalangeal joint arthrodesis with the reverse fix nail. J Hand Surg Am 2013;38(7):1301–6.
5. Ayres JR, Goldstrohm GL, Miller GJ, et al. Proximal interphalangeal joint arthrodesis with Herbert screw. J Hand Surg Am 1998;13(4):600–3.
6. Büchler U, Aiken MA. Arthrodesis of the proximal interphalangeal joint by solid bone grafting and plate fixation in extensive injuries to the dorsal aspect of the finger. J Hand Surg Am 1988;13(4): 589–94.
7. Høgh J, Jensen PO. Compression-arthrodesis of finger joints using Kirschner wires and cerclage. Hand 1982;14(2):149–52.
8. Leibovic SJ, Strickland JW. Arthrodesis of the proximal interphalangeal joint of the finger: comparison of the use of the Herbert screw with other fixation methods. J Hand Surg Am 1994;19(2):181–8.
9. Stern PJ, Gates NT, Jones TB. Tension band arthrodesis of small joints in the hand. J Hand Surg Am 1993;18(2):194–7.
10. Stahl S, Rozen N. Tension-band arthrodesis of the small joints of the hand. Orthopedics 2001;24(10): 981–3.
11. Uhl RL, Schneider LH. Tension band arthrodesis of finger joints: a retrospective review of 76 consecutive cases. J Hand Surg Am 1992;17(3):518–22.
12. Lister G. Intraosseous wiring of the digital skeleton. J Hand Surg Am 1978;3(5):427–35.
13. Bicknell RT, MacDermid J, Roth JH. Assessment of thumb metacarpophalangeal joint arthrodesis using a single longitudinal K-wire. J Hand Surg Am 2007; 32(5):677–84.
14. Messer TM, Nagle DJ, Martinez AG. Thumb metacarpophalangeal joint arthrodesis using the AO 3.0-mm cannulated screw: surgical technique. J Hand Surg Am 2002;27(5):910–2.
15. Schmidt CC, Zimmer SM, Boles SD. Arthrodesis of the thumb metacarpophalangeal joint using cannulated screw and threaded washer. J Hand Surg Am 2004;29(6):1044–50.
16. Stanley JK, Smith EJ, Muirhead AG. Arthrodesis of the metacarpo-phalangeal joint of the thumb: a review of 42 cases. J Hand Surg Br 1989;14(3):291–3.
17. Huffman R, Rayan GM. Thumb metacarpophalangeal arthrodesis with local bone grafting. Hand Surg 2011;16(1):55–61.
18. Rasmussen C, Roos S, Boecstyns M. Low-profile plate fixation in arthrodesis of the first metacarpophalangeal joint. J Hand Surg Eur Vol 2011;36(6): 509–13.
19. Vanderzanden JC, Adams BD, Guan JJ. MCP arthrodesis using an intramedullary interlocking device. Hand (N Y) 2014;9(2):209–13.
20. Hartigan BJ, Stern PJ, Kiefhaber TR. Thumb carpometacarpal osteoarthritis: arthrodesis compared with ligament reconstruction and tendon interposition. J Bone Joint Surg Am 2001;83-A(10):1470–8.
21. Rizzo M, Moran SL, Shin AY. Long-term outcomes of trapeziometacarpal arthrodesis in the management of trapeziometacarpal arthritis. J Hand Surg Am 2009;34(1):20–6.
22. Mureau MA, Rademaker RP, Verhaar JA, et al. Tendon interposition arthroplasty versus arthrodesis for the treatment of trapeziometacarpal arthritis: a retrospective comparative follow-up study. J Hand Surg Am 2001;26(5):869–76.
23. Forseth MJ, Stern PJ. Complications of trapeziometacarpal arthrodesis using plate and screw fixation. J Hand Surg Am 2003;28(2):342–5.
24. Fulton DB, Stern PJ. Trapeziometacarpal arthrodesis in primary osteoarthritis: a minimum two-year follow-up study. J Hand Surg Am 2001;26(1):109–14.
25. Sweets TM, Stern PJ. Proximal interphalangeal joint prosthetic arthroplasty. J Hand Surg Am 2010; 35(7):1190–3.
26. Foliart DE. Swanson silicone finger joint implants: a review of the literature regarding long-term complications. J Hand Surg Am 1995;20(3):445–9.
27. Takigawa S, Meletiou S, Sauerbier M, et al. Long-term assessment of Swanson implant arthroplasty in the proximal interphalangeal joint of the hand. J Hand Surg Am 2004;29(5):785–95.
28. Merle M, Villani F, Lallemand B, et al. Proximal interphalangeal joint arthroplasty with silicone implants (NeuFlex) by a lateral approach: a series of 51 cases. J Hand Surg Eur Vol 2012; 37(1):50–5.
29. Herren DB, Keuchel T, Marks M, et al. Revision arthroplasty for failed silicone proximal interphalangeal joint arthroplasty: indications and 8-year results. J Hand Surg Am 2014;39(3):462–6.
30. Lin HH, Wyrick JD, Stern PJ. Proximal interphalangeal joint silicone replacement arthroplasty: clinical results using an anterior approach. J Hand Surg Am 1995;20(1):123–32.

31. Drake ML, Segalman KA. Complications of small joint arthroplasty. Hand Clin 2010;26(2):205–12.
32. Herren DB, Simmen BR. Palmar approach in flexible implant arthroplasty of the proximal interphalangeal joint. Clin Orthop Relat Res 2000;(371):131–5.
33. Sears ED, Chung KC. Arthroplasty procedures in the hand. In: Chung KC, Evans GR, editors. Chung: hand and upper extremity reconstruction. 1st edition. Edinburgh (United Kingdom): Saunders/Elsevier; 2009. p. 180.
34. Pritsch T, Rizzo M. Reoperations following proximal interphalangeal joint nonconstrained arthroplasties. J Hand Surg Am 2011;36(9):1460–6.
35. Bravo CJ, Rizzo M, Hormel KB, et al. Pyrolytic carbon proximal interphalangeal joint arthroplasty: results with minimum two-year follow-up evaluation. J Hand Surg Am 2007;32(1):1–11.
36. Luther C, Germann G, Sauerbier M. Proximal interphalangeal joint replacement with surface replacement arthroplasty (SR-PIP): functional results and complications. Hand (N Y) 2010;5(3):233–40.
37. Wijk U, Wollmark M, Kopylov P, et al. Outcomes of proximal interphalangeal joint pyrocarbon implants. J Hand Surg Am 2010;35(1):38–43.
38. Chung KC, Ram AN, Shauver MJ. Outcomes of pyrolytic carbon arthroplasty for the proximal interphalangeal joint. Plast Reconstr Surg 2009;123(5): 1521–32.
39. Jennings CD, Livingstone DP. Surface replacement arthroplasty of the proximal interphalangeal joint using the PIP-SRA implant: results, complications and revisions. J Hand Surg Am 2008;33(9):1565.e1–11.
40. Jones DB Jr, Ackerman DB, Sammer DM, et al. Arthrodesis as a salvage for failed proximal interphalangeal joint arthroplasty. J Hand Surg Am 2011;36(2):259–64.
41. Squitieri L, Chung KC. A systematic review of outcomes and complications of vascularized toe joint transfer, silicone arthroplasty, and PyroCarbon arthroplasty for posttraumatic joint reconstruction of the finger. Plast Reconstr Surg 2008;121(5):1697–707.
42. Rizzo M. Metacarpophalangeal joint arthritis. J Hand Surg Am 2011;36(2):345–53.
43. Goldfarb CA, Stern PJ. Metacarpophalangeal joint arthroplasty in rheumatoid arthritis. A long-term assessment. J Bone Joint Surg Am 2003;85-A(10): 1869–78.
44. Tägil M, Geijer M, Malcus P, et al. Correlation between range of motion and implant fracture: a 5 year follow-up of 72 joints in 18 patients in a randomized study comparing Swanson and Avanta/Sutter MCP silicone prosthesis. J Hand Surg Eur Vol 2009;34:743–7.
45. Trail IA, Martin JA, Nuttall D, et al. Seventeen-year survivorship analysis of Silastic metacarpophalangeal joint replacement. J Bone Joint Surg Br 2004; 86(7):1002–6.
46. Cook SD, Beckenbaugh RD, Redondo J, et al. Long-term follow-up of pyrolytic carbon metacarpophalangeal implants. J Bone Joint Surg Am 1999;81(5): 635–48.
47. Parker WL, Rizzo M, Moran SL, et al. Preliminary results of nonconstrained pyrolytic carbon arthroplasty for metacarpophalangeal joint arthritis. J Hand Surg Am 2007;32(10):1496–505.
48. Burgess SD, Kono M, Stern PJ. Results of revision metacarpophalangeal joint surgery in rheumatoid patients following previous silicone arthroplasty. J Hand Surg Am 2007;32(10):1506–12.
49. Becker SJ, Briet JP, Hageman MG, et al. Death, taxes, and trapeziometacarpal arthrosis. Clin Orthop Relat Res 2013;471(12):3738–44.
50. Gervis WH. Excision of the trapezium for osteoarthritis of the trapezio-metacarpal joint. J Bone Joint Surg Br 1949;31B(4):537–9.
51. Gervis WH, Wells T. A review of excision of the trapezium for osteoarthritis of the trapezio-metacarpal joint after twenty-five years. J Bone Joint Surg Br 1973;55(1):56–7.
52. Mahoney JD, Meals RA. Trapeziectomy. Hand Clin 2006;22(2):165–9.
53. Murley AH. Excision of the trapezium in osteoarthritis of the first carpo-metacarpal joint. J Bone Joint Surg Br 1960;42B(3):502–7.
54. Iyer KM. The results of excision of the trapezium. Hand 1981;13(3):246–50.
55. Forthman CL. Management of advanced trapezio-metacarpal arthrosis. J Hand Surg Am 2009;34(2): 331–4.
56. Swanson AB. Disabling arthritis at the base of the thumb: treatment by resection of the trapezium and flexible (silicone) implant arthroplasty. J Bone Joint Surg Am 1972;54(3):456–71.
57. Peimer CA. Long-term complications of trapeziometacarpal silicone arthroplasty. Clin Orthop Relat Res 1987;(220):86–98.
58. Pellegrini VD Jr, Burton RI. Surgical management of basal joint arthritis of the thumb. Part 1. Long-term results of silicone implant arthroplasty. J Hand Surg Am 1986;11(3):309–24.
59. Bozentka DJ. Implant arthroplasty of the carpometacarpal joint of the thumb. Hand Clin 2010;26(3): 327–37.
60. Badia A, Sambandam SN. Total Joint arthroplasty in the treatment of advanced stages of thumb carpometacarpal joint osteoarthritis. J Hand Surg Am 2006;31(10):1605–14.
61. Nicholas RM, Calderwood JW. De la Caffinière arthroplasty for basal thumb joint osteoarthritis. J Bone Joint Surg Br 1992;74(2):309–12.
62. Chakrabarti AJ, Robinson AH, Gallagher P. De la Caffinière thumb carpometacarpal replacements. 93 cases at 6 to 16 years follow-up. J Hand Surg Br 1997;22(6):695–8.

63. van Cappelle HG, Elzenga P, van Horn JR. Long-term results and loosening analysis of de la Caffinière replacements of the trapeziometacarpal joint. J Hand Surg Am 1999;24(3):476–82.
64. Wachtl SW, Guggenheim PR, Sennwald GR. Cemented and non-cemented replacements of the trapeziometacarpal joint. J Bone Joint Surg Br 1998; 80(1):121–5.
65. Adams BD, Pomerance J, Nguyen A, et al. Early outcome of spherical ceramic trapezial-metacarpal arthroplasty. J Hand Surg Am 2009;34(2):213–8.
66. Cooney WP, Linscheid RL, Askew LJ. Total arthroplasty of the thumb trapeziometacarpal joint. Clin Orthop Relat Res 1987;(220):35–45.
67. Sondergaard L, Konradsen L, Rechnagel K. Long-term follow-up of cemented Caffinière prosthesis for trapezio-metacarpal arthroplasty. J Hand Surg Br 1991;16(4):428–30.
68. Conolly WB, Rath S. Revision procedures for complications of surgery for osteoarthritis of the carpometacarpal joint of the thumb. J Hand Surg Br 1993;18(4):533–9.
69. Braun BM, Li Z, Wiesler ER. Dissatisfaction after trapezial-metacarpal arthroplasty. J Hand Surg Am 2014;39(5):973–5.
70. Wajon A, Carr E, Edmunds I, et al. Surgery for thumb (trapeziometacarpal joint) osteoarthritis. Cochrane Database Syst Rev 2009;(4):CD004631.
71. Vermeulen GM, Slijper H, Feitz R, et al. Surgical management of primary thumb carpometacarpal osteoarthritis: a systematic review. J Hand Surg Am 2011;36(1):157–69.
72. Cooney WP, Leddy TP, Larson DR. Revision of thumb trapeziometacarpal arthroplasty. J Hand Surg Am 2006;31(2):219–27.
73. Megerle K, Grouls S, Germann G, et al. Revision surgery after trapeziometacarpal arthroplasty. Arch Orthop Trauma Surg 2011;131(2):205–10.
74. Renfree KJ, Dell PC. Functional outcome following salvage of failed trapeziometacarpal joint arthroplasty. J Hand Surg Br 2002;27(1):96–100.

Management of Complications of Ligament Injuries of the Wrist

Sreenadh Gella, MBBS, MS (Orth), FRCS (T&O), Jennifer L. Giuffre, MD, FRCSC, Tod A. Clark, MD, MSc, FRCSC*

KEYWORDS

• Complications • Scapholunate ligament • Lunotriquetral ligament • Carpal instability • SLAC

KEY POINTS

- Early accurate diagnosis of intrinsic carpal ligament injuries (scapholunate [SL], lunotriquetral [LT]) provides for best outcomes.
- Delayed diagnosis of SL and LT injuries has been shown to lead to arthritis within 10 years of injury if not treated.
- Conservative management of SL and LT injuries is inadequate with poor outcomes; operative intervention is indicated to manage pain, dysfunction, and delay the natural history of disease.
- Despite improvements in our knowledge of these injuries, and a variety of surgical techniques, no single treatment has proven superior; treatment should be individualized.
- Complications of treatment and general surgical risks are common and must be minimized by careful selection of surgical technique and prevention.

Intrinsic ligament injuries are common and often underdiagnosed in the wrist. Both scapholunate (SL) and lunotriquetral (LT) injuries are routinely missed acutely. Complex combined injuries are much less common, but also often unrecognized. The complex biokinematics of wrist motion are affected by these injuries and complications are common. In this article, we review the available literature surrounding the prevention and treatment of complications resulting from injury to the SL and LT ligaments.

SCAPHOLUNATE LIGAMENT

Avoiding complications in SL ligament injuries is best done by making an accurate early diagnosis. The acute "wrist sprain" should be considered an SL tear or scaphoid fracture until proven otherwise. Close examination of the SL interval in patients with more obvious carpal injuries is crucial because SL tears can be associated with carpal and distal radius fractures.[1,2] Diagnosis relies on an accurate history, clinical suspicion, and appropriate radiographs (**Fig. 1**). Often clenched fist images, contralateral wrist x-rays and even cineradiography are included for thorough assessment.[3] MRI has recently been found to have low sensitivity but high specificity in detection.[4] Additionally, MR arthrography can improve detection rates.[5] These studies can be even more difficult to interpret when patient presentation is delayed and symptoms are mild.

Failure to identify an SL injury acutely can result in progression to SL advanced collapse (SLAC).[6] Although an isolated SL injury alters the forces across the radioscaphoid joint, it is not until the secondary stabilizers, including the scaphotrapezoid–trapezial joint, the volar radiocarpal ligaments, and the dorsal intercarpal ligament, are injured that the wrist is prone to pancarpal disease

Section of Orthopedic and Plastic Surgery, Panam Clinic, University of Manitoba, 75 Poseidon Bay, Winnipeg, Manitoba R3M 3E4, Canada
* Corresponding author.
E-mail address: tclark@panamclinic.com

Hand Clin 31 (2015) 267–275
http://dx.doi.org/10.1016/j.hcl.2015.01.003

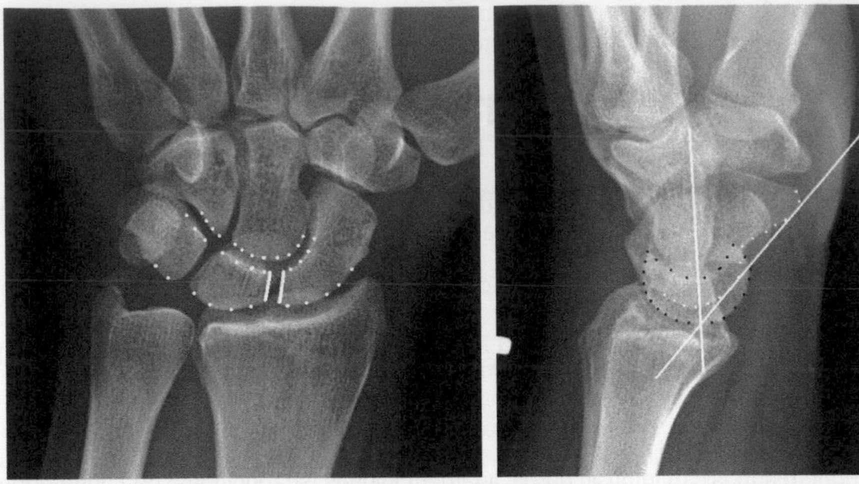

Fig. 1. Wrist posteroanterior (*left*) and lateral (*right*) radiographs. Posteroanterior smooth carpal alignment (*dotted lines*) of Gilula's lines and scapholunate (SL) interval (normal, <4 mm). The lateral–SL angle is normally 30° to 60°.

owing to altered biomechanics of the wrist.[7–10] Although the natural history and timeline of this degenerative progression is variable, most agree that changes occur within 10 years and severe changes are present by 15 to 20 years after the ligament tear.[11,12] Nonoperative treatment has never been shown to alter the natural history and, as a result, surgical management of these injuries is accepted. The management and complications of SL injuries before arthritis are described, followed by a discussion of SL injuries in the presence of arthritis.

Casting

Results from casting alone in the management of acute SL injuries have been poor. Tang and coworkers[13] followed 20 patients for 1 year after a concomitant distal radius and SL injury treated with casting and found uniformly poor results. SL distances did not change (3.4 mm initial and 3.8 mm at 1 year) and 8 of the 20 patients required operative intervention at 1 year.[13] The literature does not document results of casting isolated SL tears, but the general consensus is that treatment of complete SL tears, if diagnosed early, should be operative. Unfortunately, there is no consensus on the appropriate treatment options.

Closed Reduction and Pinning

Given the difficulty in assessing the SL interval, even on good quality plain films, it is not surprising that intraoperative fluoroscopic views are often less than optimal. The technical challenges inherent in a closed reduction and pinning have resulted in some suggestion of concomitant wrist arthroscopy. Whipple treated 40 patients with this technique and reported 83% success in acute (<3 month) minimally displaced (<3 mm) injuries.[14] Patients not fitting these criteria had poor results at 1 year both radiographically and symptomatically.[14] Similarly, Darlis and associates[15] followed 11 patients for approximately 3 years after arthroscopic pinning and debridement. At the time of surgery, these patients were greater than 3 months from injury and had suboptimal results. Complications included the requirement of further surgery (fusions, capsulodesis) in 3 patients and persistent SL widening on radiographs at final follow-up. Overall, closed reduction and percutaneous pinning is technically challenging and does not afford the ability to heal the SL ligament itself. If anatomic positioning of the SL interval can be achieved, long-term maintenance of the joint interval is likely reliant on stability based on fibrous tissue rather than a functional SL ligament.

Arthroscopy Alone

Debridement procedures have been attempted to improve pain, although reports are limited. Lee and colleagues[16] followed a group of 14 patients (16 wrists) with partial intrinsic ligament tears (6 SL and 10 LT) treated with arthroscopic debridement and thermal shrinkage for 4 years. These patients noted statistically significant improvement in both pain scores and grip strength without signs of carpal collapse or widening of the affected joint interval. It is important to note this group had no static or dynamic radiographic instability but rather arthroscopic identification of only grade 1 and 2 tearing (**Table 1**). A similar pediatric population with arthroscopic debridement of grade 2 SL tears had generally successful results at 30 months of follow-up.[17]

Table 1
Geissler's arthroscopic classification

Grade	Radio Carpal View, SL Ligament	Midcarpal View, SL Space
1	Attenuation/ hemorrhage	Nil abnormal
2	Attenuation/ hemorrhage	Space less than probe width
3	Incongruency	Arthroscopic probe can be passed
4	Incongruency—gap	Arthroscope of 2.7 mm can be passed

Abbreviation: SL, scapholunate.
Adapted from Geissler WB. Arthroscopic management of scapholunate instability. Chir Main 2006;25(Suppl 1):S187–96.

Long-term follow-up (>20 years) of these groups is crucial to determine whether the secondary scapho-trapezoid–trapezial and extrinsic ligament restraints withstand the increasing forces demanded of them with incomplete intrinsic stability. Early complications with this treatment are rare and pain seems to be improved, but whether this management offers SLAC prevention is not yet known.

Thermal Shrinkage

In an attempt to tighten the SL ligament and capsule, electrocautery has been used to heat and tighten collagen tissue based on similar treatment for shoulder instability. Again, this should be considered only in low-grade tears. Darlis and colleagues[18] demonstrated short-term (19 month) success for motion (78% contralateral), pain control, and Mayo wrist scores. This group also cautioned that the results were very early and need be limited to early SL disease. Shih and Lee[19] followed 19 patients for 21 months and noted 79% success. Four patients developed recurrent instability. Based on available data, there is no recommendation for this treatment in grade 3 or 4 SL tears (see **Table 1**). Complications of this treatment, aside from failure, can include thermal injuries to the wrist bone cartilages. This damage can be minimized by ensuring arthroscopic fluid enters and exits the joint rapidly through both inflow and outflow portals.

Open Reduction Internal Fixation

In more significant acute SL injuries (Geissler grade 3 or 4), identifying and reducing the torn ligament has become popular. This procedure affords an anatomic reduction of the SL interval and dorsal portion of the ligament via transosseous sutures or suture anchor fixation generally combined with intercarpal immobilization by pin fixation. Major complications, although rare, include arthrofibrosis, infection, and complex regional pain. Careful identification of the superficial radial nerve through the dorsal incision while pinning the SL and scaphocapitate intervals prevents injury to the nerve. Rosati and associates[20] demonstrated 88% success with this technique at 3 years. Complications included loss of reduction (8%) and late failure (4%). A similar study noted the development of lunate avascular necrosis in 1 patient and a 17% overall failure rate.[21–23] Minimizing anchor failure requires appropriate anchor sizing, suture type, suture size, and knot fixation to avoid pullout. The best data regarding anchor types and outcomes arise from the shoulder literature; however, this involves a dynamic motor component (rotator cuff), so whether this relates well to the static ligament of the wrist is unknown.

Capsulodesis

SL instability has been treated for decades by attempting to limit scaphoid flexion and thereby correct the increased SL angle associated with SL instability. Blatt[24] originally used the dorsal capsule to anchor the scaphoid to the distal radius. Many modifications have been made to date with a goal of not crossing the radiocarpal joint. Complications most notably are motion loss (flexion), weakness, and late failure. Baxamusa and Williams[25] noted all these problems after having excellent early results. During the course of only a 30-month follow-up, Wyrick and associates[26] noted persistent pain in all patients, reduced grip strength, and progressive stiffness. Deshmukh and colleagues[27] demonstrated poor or fair results in 52% of their patients during follow-up. Gajendran and colleagues[28] had 58% good and excellent results at 7 year follow-up; however, they noted progressive radiologic deterioration in 42%. Although complications are common with capsulodesis, there are no large studies comparing this treatment with the others. Given the longer follow-up available for this treatment, it is certainly possible other treatment modalities will perform similarly in the long term. We think capsulodesis is an excellent adjunct to open reduction and internal fixation of acute injuries, but worry about its use as an isolated treatment for chronic SL instability given the data to date.

Tenodesis

In chronic cases of SL insufficiency with reducible carpal collapse, multiple tenodesis procedures exist using the flexor carpi radialis to reduce the scaphoid. Brunelli's original procedure did cross the radiocarpal joint and limited wrist flexion.[29] Garcia-Elias and colleagues,[30] and Van Den Abbeele and associates,[31] and others have modified this procedure to spare the radiocarpal joint. Moran compared the results of tenodesis and capsulodesis for chronic SL insufficiency and found at 3 years no differences in wrist motion (63% and 64% contralateral, respectively) or grip strength (87% and 91%).[32] There was 1 complete failure that required fusion. Talwalkar and associates[33] reported a series of 167 tenodesis procedures and demonstrated at a 4-year follow-up, 79% satisfaction, grip strength deterioration by an average of 20%, and range of motion loss by an average of 31%. Ongoing symptoms warranted partial or total wrist fusion in only 4 patients with 1 notable complex regional pain syndrome. These results have been confirmed in other smaller series.[34,35] In treatment of chronic SL instability, all patients must be aware that the improvements in pain scores are related to decreasing range of motion of the wrist. As such, mild arthrofibrosis should be considered a goal rather than a complication (**Fig. 2**).

Ligament Reconstruction

Free tendon grafts to reconstruct the central SL ligament have recently been popularized by Lee and colleagues.[36] Long-term data does not exist; however, it has been noted that maintenance of the normal SL angle and SL interval was improved in cadaveric models.[36] Complications inherent to this technique include potential risk to the radial artery and superficial radial nerve with a radial snuff box incision. Additionally, the exact positioning of the SL intraosseous bone tunnels is needed to ensure the axis of rotation is correct and tendon cutout through the bone tunnel does not occur. The authors caution that in general many techniques work well in the early follow-up period; however long-term studies are required to evaluate the longevity of the technique.

Chronic Scapholunate Ligament Injury: The Scapholunate Advanced Collapse Wrist

The classification system used in the SLAC wrist is an excellent method by which to assess the complications of an SL ligament injury (**Fig. 3**). Moderate intraobserver reliability was found with this system.[37] In stage 1, injuries that increase joint forces result in radial styloid–scaphoid arthrosis. These injuries progress to involving the entire radioscaphoid articulation in stage 2 disease and to finally include the lunocapitate articulation in stage 3. As a result, it is important to intervene as early in the process as possible to mitigate more profound arthritic changes.

Many excellent recent papers exist that review the stages of SL injuries.[38–41] Garcia-Elias, Wolfe, and others have described a progression of injury from the occult partial tear requiring limited treatment if any to more advanced disease requiring ligament reconstruction or salvage procedures. These are shown in **Table 2** such that a review of complications can follow. It is important to note that the classification of SL tears requires the use of clinical timelines (acute, chronic), imaging (plain films, possibly fluoroscopy), and arthroscopic assessment in some cases. Geissler's arthroscopic classification has been recognized as a basis for assisting in clinical decision making (see **Table 1**).[42]

Scapholunate advanced collapse, grade 1

Arthrosis of the radiostylo–scaphoid articulation alone has classically been managed with radial styloidectomy either open or arthroscopic.[43] This aims to treat the source of pain without addressing the etiology (SL instability). The radioscaphocapitate ligament is of critical importance. Overly

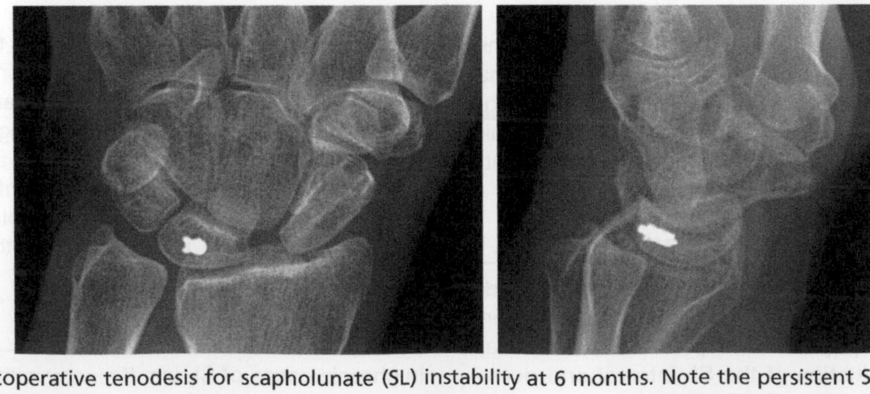

Fig. 2. Postoperative tenodesis for scapholunate (SL) instability at 6 months. Note the persistent SL gap despite correction of SL angle.

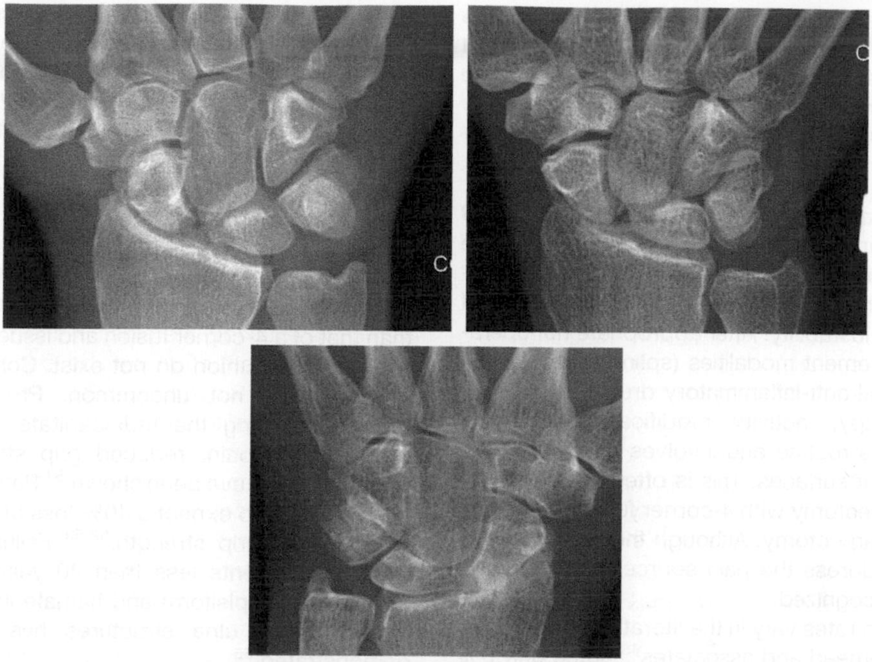

Fig. 3. Scapholunate advanced collapse (SLAC). (*Top left*) Stage 1 styloscaphoid arthritis. (*Top right*) Stage 2 entire scaphoid fossa involved. (*Bottom*) Capitolunate joint arthrosis.

aggressive resection of the styloid can result in ulnar translocation of the carpus resulting from destabilization of the origin of the radioscaphocapitate ligament.[44] This result can be minimized by ensuring resection of the styloid is limited to 4 to 7 mm. Ulnar translocation is a significant complication and must be avoided, because treatment requires radiolunate arthrodesis. Arthroscopic

Table 2
Stages of scapholunate instability

	I. Occult	II. Dynamic	III. SL Dissociation	IV. DISI	V. SLAC
Injured ligaments	Partial SLIL	Incompetent or complete SLIL; partial volar extrinsics	Complete SLIL, volar or dorsal extrinsics	Complete SLIL, volar extrinsics, secondary changes in RL, ST, DIC ligaments	As in stage IV
X-rays	Normal	Usually normal	SL gap ≥3 mm; RS angle ≥60°	SL angle ≥70°, SL gap ≥3 mm, RL ≥15°, CL ≥15°	I. Styloid DJD II. RS DJD III. CL DJD IV. Pancarpal DJD
Stress x-rays	Normal, abnormal fluoroscopy	Abnormal	Grossly abnormal	Unnecessary	Unnecessary
Treatment	Pinning or capsulodesis	SLIL repair with capsulodesis	SLIL repair with capsulodesis vs triligament reconstruction	Reducible: triligament reconstruction Fixed: intercarpal arthrodesis	Intercarpal arthrodesis or PRC

Abbreviations: CL, capitolunate; DIC, dorsal intercarpal; DISI, dorsal intercalated segment instability; DJD, degenerative joint disease; PRC, proximal row carpectomy; RL, radiolunate; RS, radioscaphoid; SL, schapolunate; SLAC, scapholunate advanced collapse; SLIL, scapholunate interosseous ligament; ST, scaphotrapezoid.

From Kitay A, Wolfe SW. Scapholunate instability: current concepts in diagnosis and management. J Hand Surg Am 2012;37(10):2184; with permission.

resection requires careful portal placement at the 1, 2 and 3, 4 portal sites to protect the superficial radial nerve. It is not uncommon to combine the styloidectomy with one of the tenodesis or other procedures, as discussed, in an attempt to prevent further SLAC progression.

Scapholunate advanced collapse, grades 2 and 3

More advanced arthritic changes involving the entire radioscaphoid joint and possibly the midcarpal joint are the end result or complication of chronic SL instability. After appropriate nonoperative management modalities (splinting, injections, nonsteroidal anti-inflammatory drugs, analgesics, physiotherapy, activity modification), surgical treatment is routine and involves excision of the arthritic joint surfaces. This is often in the form of a scaphoidectomy with 4-corner fusion or a proximal row carpectomy. Although these procedures certainly address the pain source, complications are well-recognized.

Nonunion rates vary in the literature for 4-corner fusion. Ashmead and associates[45] noted only 3% nonunion in a 4-year follow-up of 100 patients, whereas others[46] have noted 8.5% nonunion using similar fixation techniques. The type of fixation may influence the union rates. The literature has shown nonunion rates with circular plates to be as high as 25% nonunion, whereas other series have shown union rates of 100%.[47–49] Regardless of fixation mode, it is imperative to debride fusion surfaces to healthy bleeding cancellous bone and provide strict wrist immobilization until fusion. Using these principles, nonunion rates continue to be very low. Bone graft obtained from Lister tubercle can be used primarily or for the treatment of nonunion if needed (**Fig. 4**).

Other notable complications, such as dorsal impingement between the capitate and radius, prominent dorsal hardware (staples, plates), or malreductions of the radiolunate joint,[50] can be prevented with careful operative technique. The lunate must be reduced to neutral when fusing the midcarpal joint; otherwise, the final range of motion will favor extension owing to the dorsally tilted lunate and dorsal impingement. The authors temporarily pin the radiolunate joint to maintain the lunate in appropriate neutral alignment and find this an advantageous maneuver.

Proximal row carpectomy is relatively simple and useful in lower demand patients with advanced SLAC wrist. Immobilization time is less than that of a 4-corner fusion and issues regarding hardware and union do not exist. Complications, however, are not uncommon. Progression of arthritis involving the radiocapitate joint, unexplained wrist pain, reduced grip strength, and loss of motion have been shown.[51] Patients should be counseled to expect a 40% loss of motion and 20% loss of grip strength.[52,53] Failure rates increase in patients less than 40 years of age.[54] Although rare, pisiform and hamate impingement against distal ulna structures has also been demonstrated.[55]

Despite the more technically demanding nature of the 4-corner fusion and the possible issues reported with it, we use this treatment routinely in all laborers and most patients under 50 years of age to maintain wrist height (purported to retain strength). Careful recessing of dorsal hardware under the dorsal lip of the lunate and close intraoperative assessment for dorsal impingement should be performed before capsular closure.

Complications and the management of total wrist arthrodesis are the focus of the article by Chung elsewhere in this issue.

LUNOTRIQUETRAL INJURY

In comparison with SL injuries, LT pathology is less common and less well understood. As a result, reported series are small and no definitive treatment

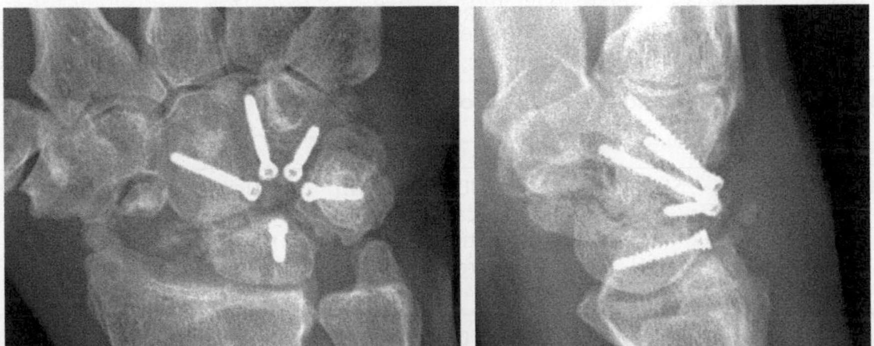

Fig. 4. Postoperative midcarpal fusion for scapholunate advanced collapse wrist at 4 months. Note the hardware prominence and delayed union despite bone grafting.

regime exists.[56] Reagan and associates[57] described the injury in 1984 and noted that outcomes are based on timing of diagnosis. In addition to acute trauma, Shin[58] noted that LT injuries can be attritional, resulting from ulnar positive variance and advancing age. Classic complications of nonoperative treatment include chronic ulnar-sided wrist pain, carpal collapse (volar intercalated segment instability), wrist stiffness, weak grip, ulnar neuropathy, and progressive arthrosis.[58,59]

Carpal collapse or progressive wrist pain are indications to further investigate the wrist with wrist arthroscopy, arthrograms, or cineradiography to confirm diagnosis. Diagnosis can be difficult because no gap exists at the LT joint despite tearing of this ligament.

Acute injuries can be managed with ligament repair; however, given that the diagnosis is difficult to make in the acute setting, this has been a very rare treatment. Knoll and colleagues[60] did not demonstrate any significant complications with this management aside from 1 pin site infection.

Arthroscopy with or Without Thermal Shrinkage

Similar results to the SL complex have been found in early grade LT tears. In the absence of complications, Weiss and co-workers[61] demonstrated 100% success with debridement alone and others have found similar findings combining thermal treatment of the ligament.[16] Moskal and associates[62] combined arthroscopy with an open capsulodesis and noted success despite a 20% incidence of neuritis and extensor carpi ulnaris tendinitis.

Lunotriquetral Arthrodesis

Results of LT arthrodesis are quite variable, mostly as a result of nonunion. Although good clinical results have been obtained, nonunion rates have varied from 0% to 57%.[63–65] Choice of fixation method may be an important factor in achieving fusion. With staple fixation, nonunion rates were reported to be 50% in 1 study, whereas with screw fixation, nonunion rates have been shown to be 9% to 46%. K-wire fixation has been generally abandoned, having an unacceptable 80% nonunion rate in 1 study.[66,67] Shin and colleagues[68] performed LT arthrodesis in 22 patients. The authors stated that, with arthrodesis, the probability of remaining free of complications at 5 years was less than 1%. Of those patients who underwent a LT arthrodesis, 40.9% developed nonunion and 22.7% developed ulnocarpal impaction. The probability of not requiring further surgery at 5 years was 21.8% in arthrodesis.[68] Compression fixation between the lunate and triquetrum and ulna shortening in cases of ulnar positive variance can minimize these adverse events. Mirza and co-workers[69] demonstrated success in a group of LT tears with ulnar shortening osteotomy alone. Ulna shortening theoretically tightens the ulnar carpal complex while reducing loading on the lunate and LT interval.

Lunotriquetral Reconstruction

In the absence of arthrosis, ligament reconstruction using a slip of extensor carpi ulnaris showed encouraging results.[70] With careful operative technique, complication rates have been lower at 5-year follow-up than either the fusion or repair cohorts in 1 study.[68] Inherent risks of surgery are injury to the dorsal sensory ulnar nerve and extensor tendons, and complications from pisotriquetral pain as seen in 11% of cases in 1 series.[71]

SUMMARY

Both SL and LT ligament injuries are difficult to diagnose acutely. Treating the acute injury yields better outcomes. When left untreated, an undefined percentage of patients progresses to carpal collapse and altered wrist biomechanics. Treatment options available strive to control pain and prevent arthrosis. Although generally beneficial, these surgical options have significant associated risks and complications. During the consent process, patients should be informed of the potential loss of motion and hand strength, residual pain, procedure failure, requirement for subsequent surgery, and general surgical risks. Unfortunately, the literature contains data derived from case series. Larger, comparative studies are required for stronger evidence-based recommendations.

REFERENCES

1. Bjelland JC, Bush JC. Secondary rotational subluxation of the carpal navicular associated with a Smith's type fracture. Ariz Med 1977;31(4):267–8.
2. Rosenthal DI, Schwartz M, Phillips WC, et al. Fracture of the radius with instability of the wrist. AJR Am J Roentgenol 1983;141(1):113–6.
3. Pliefke J, Stengel D, Rademacher G, et al. Diagnostic accuracy of plain radiographs and cineradiography in diagnosing traumatic scapholunate dissociation. Skeletal Radiol 2008;37(2):139–45.
4. Mayer S, Hahn P, Bruckner T, et al. Diagnostic value of preoperatively performed MRI regarding lesions of the scapholunate ligament in clinical routine. Handchir Mikrochir Plast Chir 2013;45(1):26–32.
5. Pahwa S, Srivastava DN, Sharma R, et al. Comparison of conventional MRI and MR arthrography in the

evaluation of wrist ligament tears: a preliminary experience. Indian J Radiol Imaging 2014;24(3):259–67.
6. Watson HK, Ballet FL. The SLAC wrist: scapholunate advanced collapse pattern of degenerative arthritis. J Hand Surg Am 1984;9(3):358–65.
7. Blevens AD, Light TR, Jablonsky WS, et al. Radiocarpal articular contact characteristics with scaphoid instability. J Hand Surg Am 1989;14:781–90.
8. Burgress RC. The effect of rotatory subluxation of the scaphoid on the radio-scaphoid contact. J Hand Surg Am 1987;12:771–4.
9. Short WH, Werner FW, Green JK, et al. Biomechanical evaluation of the ligamentous stabilizers of the scaphoid and lunate. J Hand Surg Am 2002;27:991–1002.
10. Short WH, Werner FW, Green JK, et al. Biomechanical evaluation of the ligamentous stabilizers of the scaphoid and lunate: part II. J Hand Surg Am 2005;30:24–34.
11. Watson HK, Ryu J. Evolution of arthritis of the wrist. Clin Orthop Relat Res 1986;(202):57–67.
12. Talwalkar SC, Hayton MJ, Stanley JK. Wrist osteoarthritis. Scand J Surg 2008;97(4):305–9.
13. Tang JB, Shi D, Gu YQ, et al. Can cast immobilization successfully treat scapholunate dissociation associated with distal radius fractures? J Hand Surg Am 1996;21(4):583–90.
14. Whipple TL. The role of arthroscopy in the treatment of scapholunate instability. Hand Clin 1995;11(1):37–40.
15. Darlis NA, Kaufmann RA, Giannoulis F, et al. Arthroscopic debridement and closed pinning for chronic dynamic scapholunate instability. J Hand Surg Am 2006;31(3):418–24.
16. Lee JI, Nha KW, Lee GY, et al. Long-term outcomes of arthroscopic debridement and thermal shrinkage for isolated partial intercarpal ligament tears. Orthopedics 2012;35(8):e1204–9.
17. Earp BE, Waters PM, Wyzykowski RJ. Arthroscopic treatment of partial scapholunate ligament tears in children with chronic wrist pain. J Bone Joint Surg Am 2006;88(11):2448–55.
18. Darlis NA, Weiser RW, Sotereanos DG. Partial scapholunate ligament injuries treated with arthroscopic debridement and thermal shrinkage. J Hand Surg Am 2005;30(5):908–14.
19. Shih JT, Lee HM. Monopolar radiofrequency electrothermal shrinkage of the scapholunate ligament. Arthroscopy 2006;22(5):553–7.
20. Rosati M, Parchi P, Cacianti M, et al. Treatment of acute scapholunate ligament injuries with bone anchor. Musculoskelet Surg 2010;94(1):25–32.
21. Bickert B, Sauerbier M, Germann G. Scapholunate ligament repair using the Mitek bone anchor. J Hand Surg Br 2000;25(2):188–92.
22. Burkhart SS. Suture anchor insertion angle and the deadman theory. Arthroscopy 2009;25(12):1365 [author reply: 1365–6].
23. Clevenger TA, Beebe MJ, Strauss EJ, et al. The effect of insertion angle on the pullout strength of threaded suture anchors: a validation of the deadman theory. Arthroscopy 2014;30(8):900–5.
24. Blatt G. Capsulodesis in reconstructive hand surgery. Dorsal capsulodesis for the unstable scaphoid and volar capsulodesis following excision of the distal ulna. Hand Clin 1987;3(1):81–102.
25. Baxamusa TH, Williams CS. Capsulodesis of the wrist for scapholunate dissociation. Tech Hand Up Extrem Surg 2005;9(1):35–41.
26. Wyrick JD, Youse BD, Kiefhaber TR. Scapholunate ligament repair and capsulodesis for the treatment of static scapholunate dissociation. J Hand Surg Br 1998;23(6):776–80.
27. Deshmukh SC, Givissis P, Belloso D, et al. Blatt's capsulodesis for chronic scapholunate dissociation. J Hand Surg Br 1999;24:215–20.
28. Gajendran VK, Peterson B, Slater RR Jr, et al. Long-term outcomes of dorsal intercarpal ligament capsulodesis for chronic scapholunate dissociation. J Hand Surg Am 2007;32(9):1323–33.
29. Brunelli GA, Brunelli GR. A new surgical technique for carpal instability with scapho-lunar dislocation (Eleven cases). Ann Chir Main Memb Super 1995;14(4–5):207–13.
30. Garcia-Elias M, Lluch AL, Stanley JK. Three ligament tenodesis for the treatment of scapholunate dissociation: indications and surgical technique. J Hand Surg Am 2006;31(1):125–34.
31. Van den Abbeele KL, Loh YC, Stanley JK, et al. Early results of a modified Brunelli procedure for scapholunate instability. J Hand Surg Br 1998;23(2):258–61.
32. Moran SL, Ford KS, Wulf CA, et al. Outcomes of dorsal capsulodesis and tenodesis for treatment of scapholunate instability. J Hand Surg Am 2006;31(9):1438–46.
33. Talwalkar SC, Edwards AT, Hayton MJ, et al. Results of tri-ligament tenodesis: a modified Brunelli procedure in the management of scapholunate instability. J Hand Surg Br 2006;31(1):110–7.
34. Chabas JF, Gay A, Valenti D, et al. Results of the modified Brunelli tenodesis for treatment of scapholunate instability: a retrospective study of 19 patients. J Hand Surg Am 2008;33(9):1469–77.
35. De Smet L, Van Hoonacker P. Treatment of chronic static scapholunate dissociation with the modified Brunelli technique: preliminary results. Acta Orthop Belg 2007;73(2):188–91.
36. Lee SK, Zlotolow DA, Sapienza A, et al. Biomechanical comparison of 3 methods of scapholunate ligament reconstruction. J Hand Surg Am 2014;39(4):643–50.
37. Vishwanathan K, Hearnden A, Talwalker S, et al. Reproducibility of radiographic classification of scapholunate advanced collapse (SLAC) and scaphoid nonunion advanced collapse (SNAC) wrist. J Hand Surg Eur Vol 2013;38(7):780–7.

38. Pappou IP, Basel J, Deal DN. Scapholunate ligament injuries: a review of current concepts. Hand (N Y) 2013;8(2):146–56.
39. Manuel J, Moran SL. The diagnosis and treatment of scapholunate instability. Orthop Clin North Am 2007; 38(2):261–77.
40. Chim H, Moran SL. Wrist essentials. The diagnosis and management of scapholunate ligament injuries. Plast Reconstr Surg 2014;134(2):312e–22e.
41. Kitay A, Wolfe SW. Scapholunate instability: current concepts in diagnosis and management. J Hand Surg Am 2012;37(10):2175–96.
42. Geissler WB. Arthroscopic management of scapholunate instability. Chir Main 2006;25(Suppl 1): S187–96.
43. Birman MV, Danoff JR, Rosenwasser MP. Arthroscopic wrist debridement and radial styloidectomy for late-stage scapholunate advanced collapse wrist (SS-49). Arthroscopy 2012;28(6):e26–7.
44. Slutsky DJ, Nagle DJ. Techniques in wrist and hand arthroscopy. Chapter 24. 1st edition. London: Churchill Livingston; 2007. p. 201.
45. Ashmead D 4th, Watson HK, Damon C, et al. Scapholunate advanced collapse wrist salvage. J Hand Surg Am 1994;19(5):741–50.
46. Krakauer JD, Bishop AT, Cooney WP. Surgical treatment of scapholunate advanced collapse. J Hand Surg Am 1994;19(5):751–9.
47. Bedford B, Yang SS. High fusion rates with circular plate fixation for four-corner arthrodesis of the wrist. Clin Orthop Relat Res 2010;468(1):163–8.
48. Merrell GA, McDermott EM, Weiss AP. Four-corner arthrodesis using a circular plate and distal radius bone grafting: a consecutive case series. J Hand Surg Am 2008;33(5):635–42.
49. Khan SK, Ali SM, McKee A, et al. Outcomes of four-corner arthrodesis using the Hubcap circular plate. Hand Surg 2013;18(2):215–20.
50. Shin AY. Four-corner arthrodesis. J Am Soc Surg Hand 2001;1:93–111.
51. Baumeister S, Germann G, Dragu A, et al. Functional results after proximal row carpectomy (PRC) in patients with SNAC-/SLAC-wrist stage II. Handchir Mikrochir Plast Chir 2005;37(2):106–12 [in German].
52. Kremer T, Sauerbier M, Trankle M, et al. Functional results after proximal row carpectomy to salvage a wrist. Scand J Plast Reconstr Surg Hand Surg 2008;42(6):308–12.
53. Stern PJ, Agabegi SS, Kiefhaber TR, et al. Proximal row carpectomy. J Bone Joint Surg Am 2005; 87(Suppl 1(Pt 2)):166–74.
54. Wall LB, Didonna ML, Kiefhaber TR, et al. Proximal row carpectomy: minimum 20-year follow-up. J Hand Surg Am 2013;38(8):1498–504.
55. Kluge S, Schindele S, Herren D. Two cases of pisiform bone impingement syndrome after proximal row carpectomy. Arch Orthop Trauma Surg 2014; 134(7):1017–22.
56. Mitsuyasu H, Patterson RM, Shah MA, et al. The role of the dorsal inter- carpal ligament in dynamic and static scapholunate instability. J Hand Surg Am 2004;29:279–88.
57. Reagan DS, Linscheid RL, Dobyns JH. Lunotriquetral sprains. J Hand Surg Am 1984;9:502–14.
58. Shin AY, Battaglia MJ, Bishop AT, et al. Lunotriquetral instability: diagnosis and treatment. J Am Acad Orthop Surg 2000;8:170–9.
59. Ritt M, Linscheid RL, Cooney WP, et al. The lunotriquetral joint: kinematic effects of sequential ligament sectioning, ligament repair, and arthrodesis. J Hand Surg Am 1998;23:432–45.
60. Knoll VD, Allan C, Trumble TE. Trans-scaphoid perilunate fracture dislocations: results of screw fixation of the scaphoid and lunotriquetral repair with a dorsal approach. J Hand Surg Am 2005;30(6):1145–52.
61. Weiss AP, Sachar K, Glowacki KA. Arthroscopic debridement alone for intercarpal ligament tears. J Hand Surg Am 1997;22(2):344–9.
62. Moskal MJ, Savoie FH 3rd, Field LD. Arthroscopic capsulodesis of the lunotriquetral joint. Clin Sports Med 2001;20(1):141–53, ix–x.
63. Kirschenbaum D, Coyle MP, Leddy JP. Chronic lunotriquetral instability: diagnosis and treatment. J Hand Surg Am 1993;18(6):1107–12.
64. Guidera PM, Watson HK, Dwyer TA, et al. Lunotriquetral arthrodesis using cancellous bone graft. J Hand Surg Am 2001;26(3):422–7.
65. Sennwald GR, Fischer M, Mondi P. Lunotriquetral arthrodesis. A controversial procedure. J Hand Surg Br 1995;20(6):755–60.
66. Vandesande W, De Smet L, Van Ransbeeck H. Lunotriquetral arthrodesis, a procedure with a high failure rate. Acta Orthop Belg 2001;67(4):361–7.
67. Nelson DL, Manske PR, Pruitt DL, et al. Lunotriquetral arthrodesis. J Hand Surg Am 1993;18:1113–20.
68. Shin AY, Weinstein LP, Berger RA, et al. Treatment of isolated injuries of the lunotriquetral ligament. A comparison of arthrodesis, ligament reconstruction, and ligament repair. J Bone Joint Surg Br 2001;83:1023–8.
69. Mirza A, Mirza JB, Shin AY, et al. Isolated lunotriquetral ligament tears treated with ulnar shortening osteotomy. J Hand Surg Am 2013;38(8):1492–7.
70. De Smet L, Janssens I, van de Sande W. Chronic lunotriquetral ligament injuries: arthrodesis or capsulodesis. Acta Chir Belg 2005;105(1):79–81.
71. Shahane SA, Trail IA, Takwale VJ, et al. Tenodesis of the extensor carpi ulnaris for chronic, post-traumatic lunotriquetral instability. J Bone Joint Surg Br 2005; 87:1512–5.

Management of Complications of Wrist Arthroplasty and Wrist Fusion

Michael P. Gaspar, MD[a], Patrick M. Kane, MD[a],
Eon K. Shin, MD[a,b,*]

KEYWORDS

• Wrist complications • Arthroplasty • Arthrodesis • Fusion • Total partial revision

KEY POINTS

- The wrist joint contains many bony articulations, allowing for many different options of partial (or total) fusion or arthroplasty to treat painful arthritis.
- The high functional demands of the wrist make many of these procedures susceptible to complications and failure.
- Preventative measures and careful patient selection are of utmost importance in avoiding complications.
- Despite vigilant preoperative measures, complications still often occur.
- Although complications sometimes can be managed conservatively, they often require surgical management, which can be extensive in many cases.

INTRODUCTION

Arthrodesis has long been a solution for painful end-stage arthritis, not only of the wrist but also several joints in the body.[1,2] Successful arthrodesis of any joint can offer a stable and pain-free construct, although typically at the expense of mobility and some degree of functionality. This potential sacrifice is of special concern with the wrist, where motion and functionality are more important than the ability to bear weight compared with joints of the lower extremity.

Wrist arthroplasty in its various forms is a newer alternative for treatment of painful arthritis, approximating the motion of a healthy wrist.[3] As implant design and surgical techniques have improved, the indications for wrist arthroplasty have concomitantly expanded. Even with the latest implants and techniques, however, the durability of wrist arthroplasty components is limited. Thus, arthroplasty is typically reserved for older patients or those with fewer physical demands.[4]

Together, wrist arthrodesis and arthroplasty form a spectrum of available treatments for end-stage arthritis about the wrist. Because of the numerous articulations about the wrist, arthroplasty and arthrodesis each has its own specific indications, corresponding to the location of disease.

This article first reviews the different types of fusions and arthroplasties available for the wrist, including a discussion regarding the indications and contraindications for performing each surgery. The article concludes by presenting complications associated with each procedure type, detailing the current methods to address these complications, including preventative measures to avoid such complications and tactics to treat them once they have occurred.

[a] The Philadelphia Hand Center, 834 Chestnut Street, Suite G114, Philadelphia, PA 19107, USA; [b] Department of Orthopedic Surgery, Thomas Jefferson University Hospital, 132 South 10th Street, Philadelphia, PA 19107, USA
* Corresponding author. The Philadelphia Hand Center, 834 Chestnut Street, Suite G114, Philadelphia, PA 19107.
E-mail address: ekshin@handcenters.com

Hand Clin 31 (2015) 277–292
http://dx.doi.org/10.1016/j.hcl.2015.01.004
0749-0712/15/$ – see front matter

hand.theclinics.com

INDICATIONS

Prior to the advent of wrist arthroplasty for treatment of end-stage arthritis, arthrodesis was considered the standard treatment.[5] It is widely considered that the development of wrist arthroplasty techniques have lagged behind other large joint reconstructive procedures, such as the hip, knee, and shoulder, because overall outcomes after wrist arthrodesis with respect to symptom palliation were acceptable.[5–8] Eventually, as interest grew in finding a solution for painful end-stage wrist arthritis that relieved pain and maintained motion, wrist arthroplasty techniques developed and are now considered an alternative to fusion. Because there is significant overlap in the indications for performing either of these 2 procedures, it is often just as judicious to consider the contraindications.

The wrist joint is unique compared with other major joints of the body in that numerous bones and articulations compose the totality of the joint. When compared with other major joints that may present as candidates for arthroplasty, it is not surprising that there are several partial or limited options to consider before performing a total fusion or arthroplasty. Thus, during the initial work-up and planning, it is important to correlate patient complaints with physical examination findings and radiographs to target the areas that need to be addressed.

For patients with posttraumatic arthritis, imaging the contralateral side for comparison and preoperative planning can be helpful.[9] When assessing patients and evaluating radiographs, particular attention should be paid to areas with higher known incidence of pathology, such as the distal radioulnar joint (DRUJ), the scapholunate (SL) interval, the scaphotrapeziotrapezoid (STT) joint, and the triangular fibrocartilage complex (TFCC).[3,9,10]

Although standard wrist radiographs are generally sufficient for evaluation and surgical planning, advanced imaging is often necessary to assess details of specific disease processes. MRI can help distinguish Kienböck disease from ulnar impaction syndrome.[11] CT can also be useful in further delineating degenerative processes when standard radiographs are difficult to interpret. Most degenerative arthritis seen in the wrist is localized about the scaphoid, so a detailed history and physical examination can help elucidate such information.

Once the extent of the disease is revealed and surgical intervention is deemed appropriate, the surgeon must take into consideration the medical, demographic, and even socioeconomic factors that may affect the outcome of surgery, particularly with respect to contraindications.

SURGICAL OPTIONS: ARTHRODESIS

Arthrodesis procedures about the wrist can range from single joint fusion to total wrist fusion, depending on the extent of the disease at the time of surgery and any predicted progression of disease. Because a significant proportion of degenerative disease about the wrist involves the scaphoid or one of its articulations, a majority of these limited wrist fusion options involve the scaphoid.

Radiocarpal Arthrodesis

Both radioscapholunate (RSL) and radiolunate (RL) arthrodeses are typically performed as a treatment of progression of posttraumatic conditions.[12] RSL arthrodesis is often the initial treatment of choice for patients with a history of intra-articular distal radius fractures who progress to significantly painful posttraumatic arthrosis.[13] It can also be a treatment of choice for stabilization of carpal collapse deformities in those with a stable midcarpal joint. Similarly, RL arthrodesis is most commonly used to treat posttraumatic arthrosis at the RL joint, particularly in patients with deformity in the lunate fossa of the radius[14] and in rheumatoid patients to reseat the lunate into the fossa in the radius to correct ulnar subluxation of the wrist. Both RSL and RL arthrodeses can also be used to treat ulnar translocation of the carpus after significant ligamentous disruption. Because both types of limited arthrodesis rely on a stable midcarpal joint for optimal postoperative function, the presence of midcarpal disease or instability is an absolute contraindication for either procedure (**Figs. 1–3**).[12]

Midcarpal Arthrodesis

STT arthrodesis is a mainstay treatment of STT arthritis[12,15] as well as early-stage Kienböck disease prior to the onset of carpal collapse.[15–17] It has also been used for treatment of chronic SL dissociation but with mixed results.[18] Conversely, scaphocapitate arthrodesis is rarely used to treat arthritis but rather to provide a functional result similar to treatment options for STT arthritis, allowing for its use in the reduction of the SL interval and for offloading the lunate in the treatment of Kienböck disease.[19,20] Scaphoid excision with 4-corner fusion can be used in treating SL advanced collapse (SLAC) or scaphoid nonunion advanced collapse (SNAC) (**Figs. 4** and **5**).[21,22]

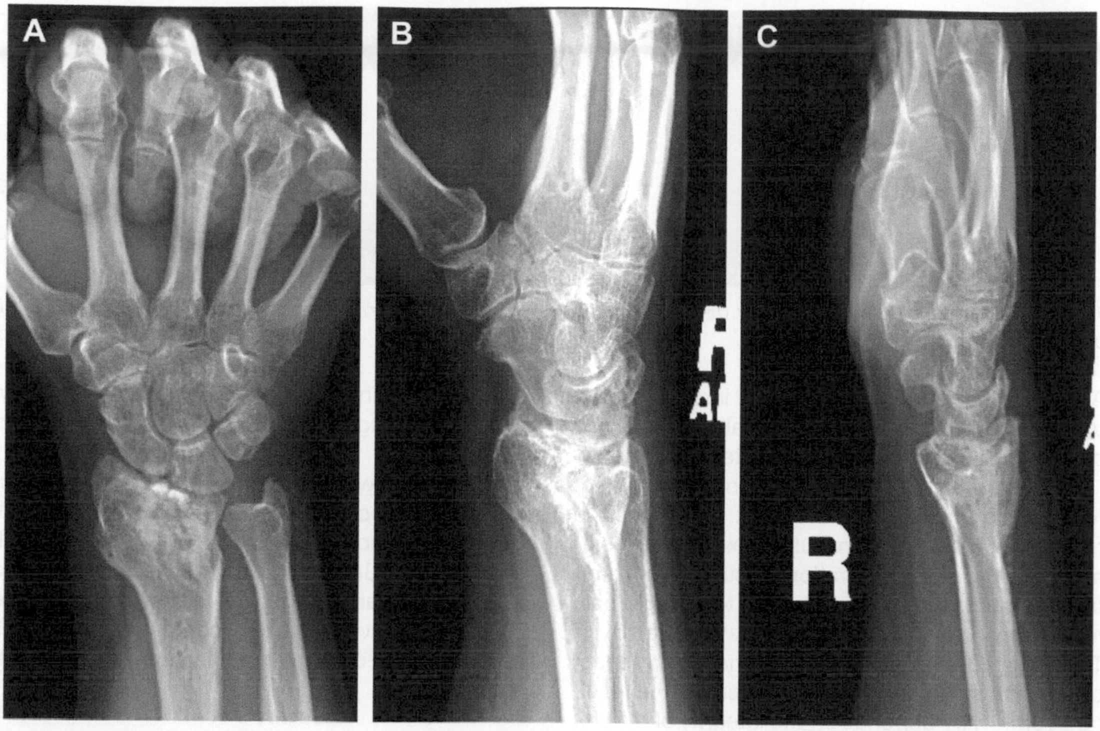

Fig. 1. (*A*) Anteroposterior, (*B*) oblique, and (*C*) lateral views of the right wrist in a patient with significant arthrosis at the radiocarpal joint after a distal radius fracture sustained remotelyas.

Total Wrist Arthrodesis

Finally, total wrist arthrodesis is indicated for primary treatment of pancarpal arthritis, particularly in those patients who are high demand. It can also be used as a salvage procedure for failed limited wrist fusions as well as partial or total wrist arthroplasties (TWAs). Studies have generally shown excellent results with long-term outcomes after wrist arthrodesis (**Fig. 6**).[23,24]

SURGICAL OPTIONS: ARTHROPLASTY

Just as with arthrodesis, there is a range of options with arthroplasty from partial to complete. Again, the partial arthroplasty options provide a more targeted approach depending on the location and extent of the disease, whereas TWA is typically performed to address pancarpal arthritis at the wrist.

Resection Arthroplasty

For disease located at the DRUJ, there are several arthroplasty options, including the Darrach procedure, hemiresection interposition technique (HIT) arthroplasty, the Sauvé-Kapandji procedure, and distal ulna arthroplasty.[25–30] DRUJ pathology can have several etiologies, including degenerative, posttraumatic, inflammatory, and congenital.[29]

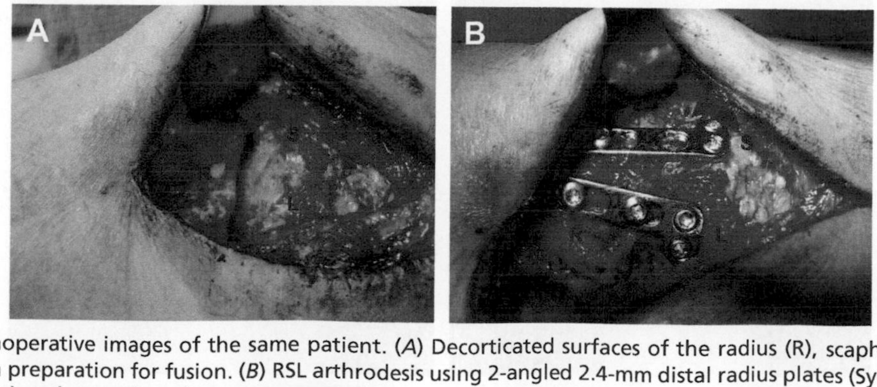

Fig. 2. Intraoperative images of the same patient. (*A*) Decorticated surfaces of the radius (R), scaphoid (S), and lunate (L) in preparation for fusion. (*B*) RSL arthrodesis using 2-angled 2.4-mm distal radius plates (Synthes, Paoli, Pennsylvania) and cancellous iliac crest autograft.

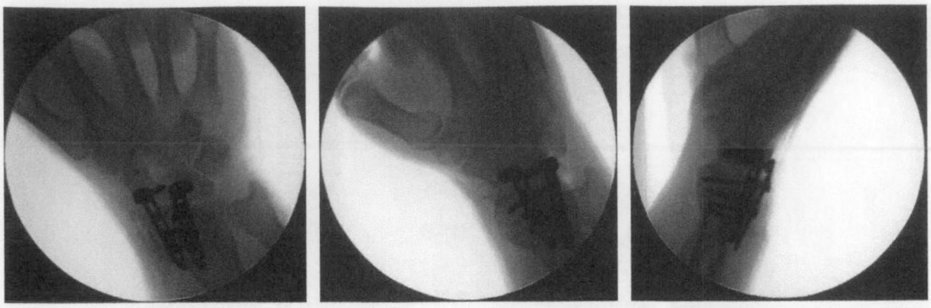

Fig. 3. Postoperative anteroposterior (*left*), oblique (*middle*) and lateral (*right*) fluoroscopic images of the same patient as **Figs. 1** and **2**.

Also, DRUJ dysfunction, forearm instability, and ulnar impaction syndrome often all coexist,[31] so surgical treatment should be selected accordingly.

The Darrach procedure, the oldest form of resection arthroplasty in the wrist, describes the resection of the distal ulna just proximal to the sigmoid notch with preservation of surrounding soft tissue structures.[25,32] The goal is to provide pain relief while maintaining postoperative stability.[25] The HIT involves removal of just the radial aspect of the ulna and insertion of soft tissue in the resultant void.[28] HIT depends on the integrity of the soft tissue stabilizers, in particular the TFCC, and thus should only be performed with an intact TFCC.[28,33] The Sauvé-Kapandji technique involves fusion of the DRUJ and resection of a portion of the ulna just proximal to the sigmoid notch,[26,27] creating a proximal ulnar pseudoarthrosis allowing forearm rotation, eliminating DRUJ pain and instability, and preventing ulnar translation of the carpus (**Fig. 7**).[26,27]

Proximal row carpectomy (PRC) is a resection arthroplasty technique for treatment of radiocarpal disease secondary to SNAC, SLAC, and Kienböck disease.[34,35] Because PRC is essentially used to address the same issues as 4-corner fusion, there have been several studies comparing outcomes of the 2 procedures with variable results (**Figs. 8** and **9**).[22,36,37]

Implant Arthroplasty

Options for implant arthroplasties of the wrist continue to expand as technology improves and as longer-term outcomes are made available from older prostheses. For DRUJ pathology, there

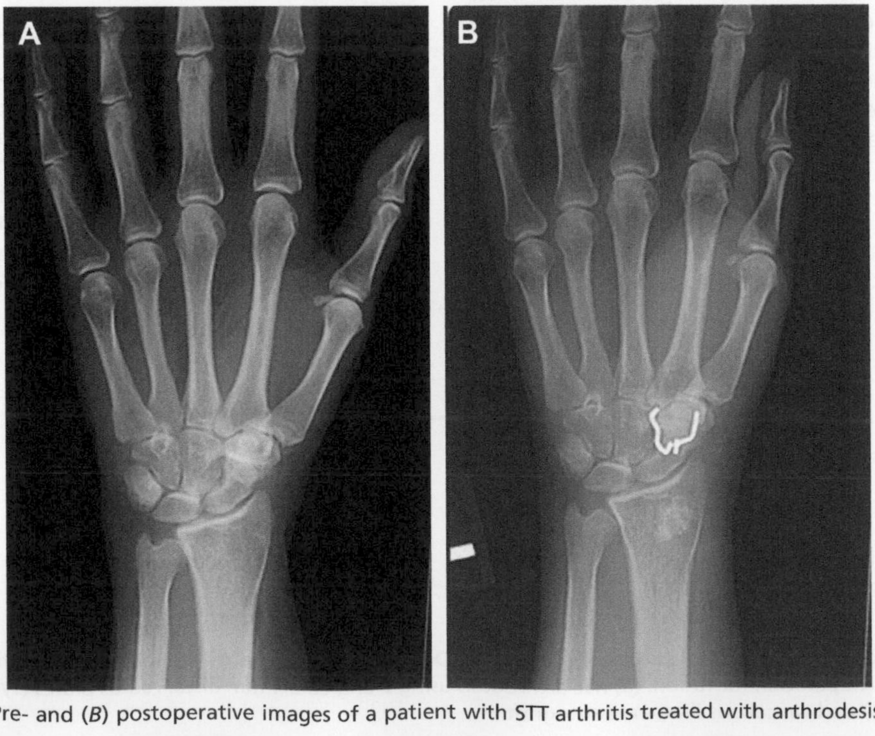

Fig. 4. (*A*) Pre- and (*B*) postoperative images of a patient with STT arthritis treated with arthrodesis.

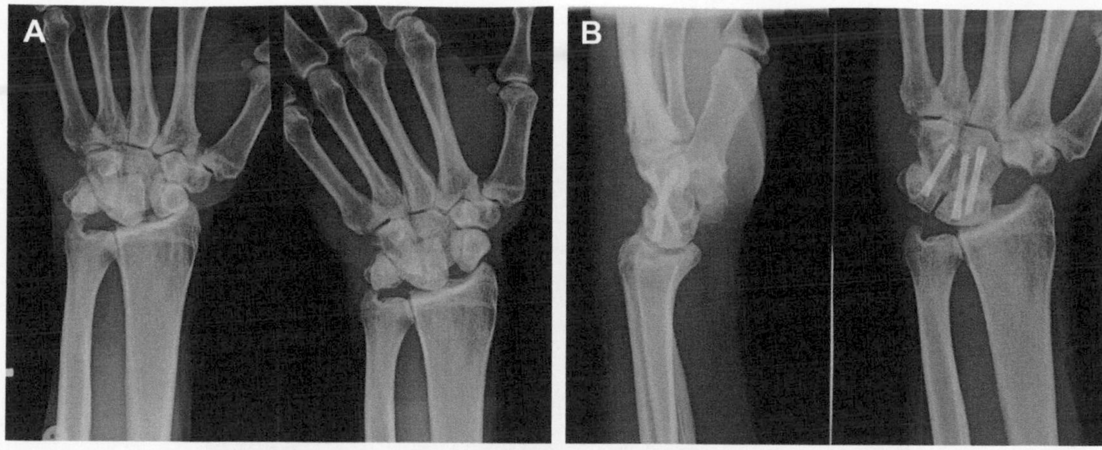

Fig. 5. (*A*) Anteroposterior (*left*) and scaphoid-view (*right*) radiographs of a patient with SLAC wrist. (*B*) Post-operative lateral (*left*) and anteroposterior (*right*) radiographs after treatment with scaphoid excision and 4-corner intercarpal arthrodesis.

are again multiple implant options. Partial ulnar head arthoplasty involves resection of focal areas of diseased ulna and placement of the prosthesis with minimal soft tissue disruption.[38] It is contraindicated after Darrach resection because the entire distal ulna is already excised.

Total ulnar head arthroplasty involves a complete resection of the ulnar head with the insertion of a stemmed implant and is intended to treat instability in addition to pain.[30,40] In cases of complete DRUJ disruption, there are total DRUJ arthroplasty implants available. This procedure completely replaces the DRUJ with an implant that is affixed to both the ulna and the radius with a mobile bearing between them.[30] Both the ulnar head implant and the DRUJ replacement are typically performed for failed resection arthroplasty and represent salvage procedures (**Fig. 10**).

TWA, like arthrodesis, addresses pancarpal arthritis rather than focal areas of disease. The materials used for implants, as well as modes of fixation, have evolved over the years. As a result, the survivorship of these implants has improved. It is important to emphasize, however, that survivorship of even the latest models of implants is highly dependent on patient selection, and their use in patients who exceed their designed capabilities can lead to implant failure, which is often catastrophic.

Decades of trial and error with TWA technology have led to the current total wrist replacement devices that include a proximal component affixed to the distal end of the radius with a stemmed component and a distal component fixed to the distal carpus and metacarpals.[41–43] As in total joint replacements in other large joints, patient selection is of paramount importance. Ideal surgical candidates are those with low-demand lifestyles seeking pain relief without completely giving up motion at the wrist. There are also hemiarthroplasty options in which only a proximal component—inserted into the distal

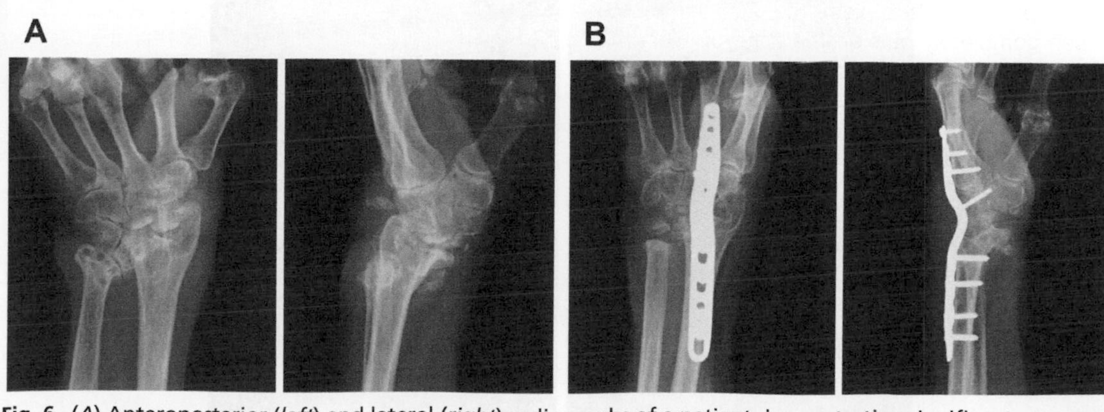

Fig. 6. (*A*) Anteroposterior (*left*) and lateral (*right*) radiographs of a patient demonstrating significant pancarpal and DRUJ arthritis. (*B*) Post-operative anteroposterior (*left*) and lateral (*right*) radiographs after treatment with total wrist fusion using a dorsal plate, and distal ulna resection.

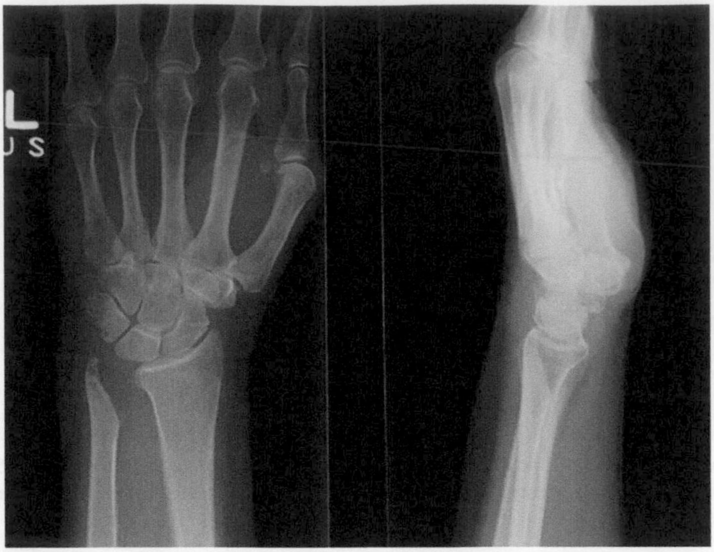

Fig. 7. Post-operative anteroposterior (*left*) and lateral (*right*) radiographs after performing HIT for DRUJ arthritis.

radius—is used, typically performed in conjunction with PRC.[44,45]

Although osteoarthritis (OA) and rheumatoid arthritis (RA) patients compose the majority of total wrist replacement candidates, there are some patients within those groups for whom this surgery is contraindicated. Some patients with OA continue to be physically active and may not be willing to limit their activities to accommodate their new prosthesis. Patients with highly reactive RA and concomitantly poor bone quality may represent poor candidates owing to their high likelihood of failure. Other contraindications include those unable to adhere to postoperative restrictions (such as those with dementia or other mental illness) or those who depend on their upper extremities for ambulation either chronically or acutely (**Fig. 11**).

COMPLICATIONS AND MANAGEMENT: ARTHRODESIS

As with fusion at other joints of the body, complications from wrist arthrodesis are thought largely preventable and highly dependent on patient selection. Nonunion is the most likely complication after wrist fusion, and its occurrence is multifactorial.[46,47] The larger surface area of the wrist articulations relative to other joints in the body is a factor that must be considered for successful fusion. This is usually addressed by meticulous removal of all articular cartilage and direct apposition of the surfaces. A second key factor in the development of union is the stability of the fixation.

For total wrist fusion that addresses degenerative and posttraumatic conditions, dorsal

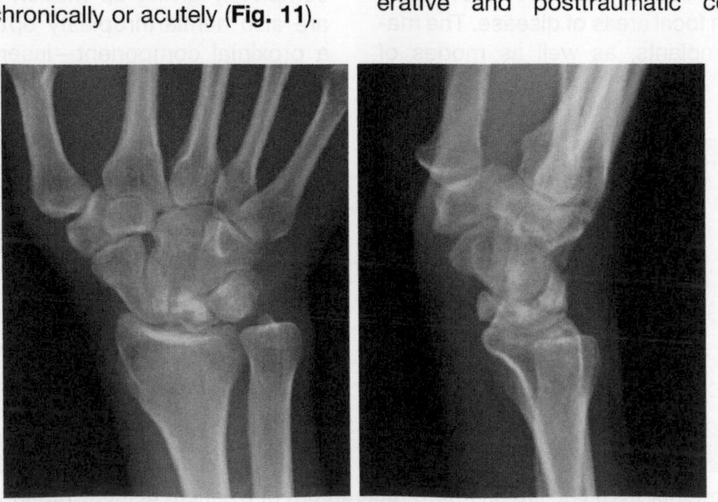

Fig. 8. Advanced Kienböck disease. Note the significant collapse and sclerosis of the lunate seen on the anteroposterior view (*left*).

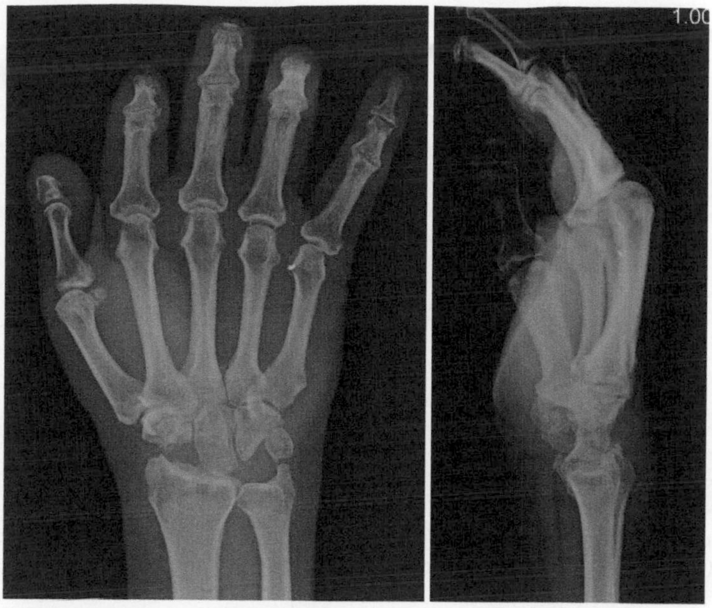

Fig. 9. Postoperative radiographs of the same patient's wrist from Fig. 8, after PRC.

compression plating has provided the most promising results with regard to high union rates and, therefore, is considered the standard.[24,48–52] In cases of inflammatory arthritis, however, there is increased concern for implant failure with plating due to poor bone quality, in addition to concerns with wound healing. Many patients with inflammatory arthropathies can have particularly thin skin on the dorsum of the hand. Thus, the use of Steinmann pins, Kirschner wires, screws, and/or intramedullary rods has been advocated in these patients along with extensive synovectomy and ulnar head excision.[53–56] Similarly, the optimal construct for intercarpal fusions is less definitive, with variable results noted between pin and screw fixation versus circular compression plating.[57–59]

With regard to patient selection, factors that affect bone quality should be evaluated. Patients with severely osteopenic bone and those with a history of smoking have much higher reported rates of nonunion.[47] Similarly, the type and quality of the bone graft that is used should be considered.

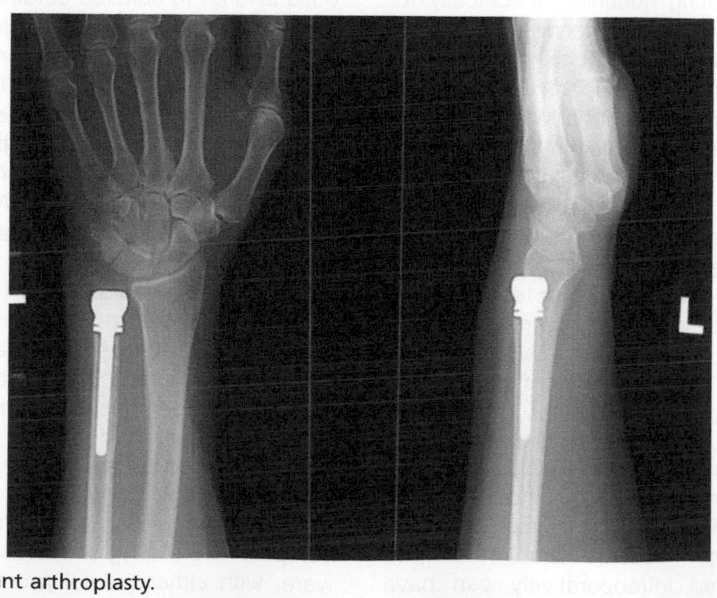

Fig. 10. Ulnar implant arthroplasty.

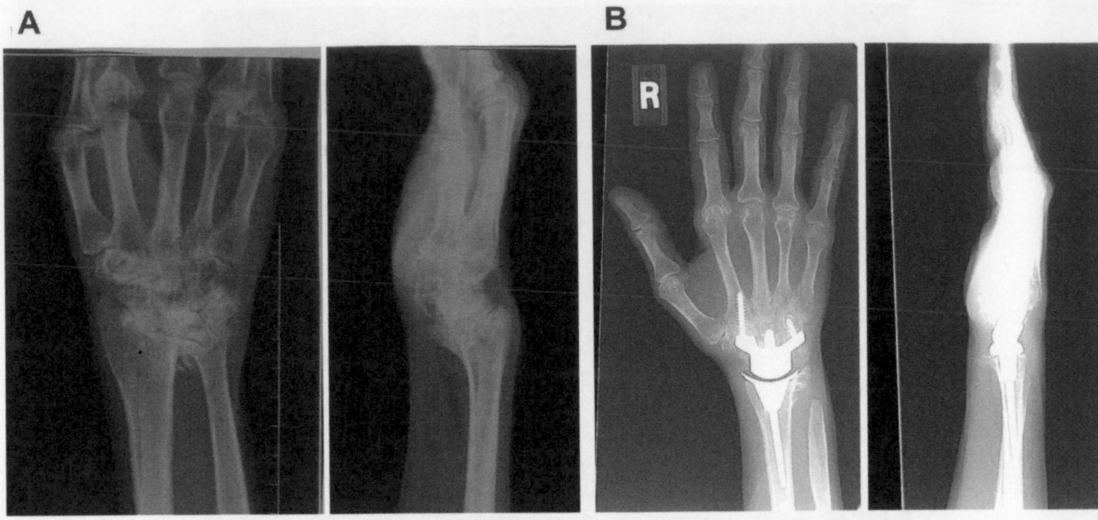

Fig. 11. (*A*) Anteroposterior (*left*) and lateral (*right*) radiographs of a patient demonstrating significant pancarpal and DRUJ arthritis. (*B*) Postoperative anteroposterior (*left*) and lateral (*right*) radiographs after TWA and distal ulna resection.

Although there is no good comparative literature evaluating the different bone graft substrates, anecdotally many surgeons find that the excised carpal bones are too sclerotic for optimal use as autograft and advocate the use of cancellous autograft from iliac crest or distal radius.[60,61] If nonunion still occurs, the mainstay treatment is revision fixation with bone graft (**Fig. 12**).[47]

An alternative or adjunct to revision surgery may be the use of an implantable bone stimulator, which shows promise in animal models[62–64] and variable success in treatment of nonunions at other sites.[65,66] Although data regarding its successful use in treating nonunion specifically for wrist fusion are limited, it has been reported.[67]

Another concerning complication after wrist arthrodesis is infection. Superficial infections occur far more frequently, with a rate of approximately 3%, versus deep infections at approximately 0.5%.[46,48,57] Superficial infections often stem from wound issues, particularly caused by the thin skin that is present on the dorsum of the wrist in many patients.[68] Higher-risk patients include those with preexisting diabetes and those with compromised immune function, acquired through disease or iatrogenic, such as RA patients who take steroids and/or other immune modulators.[69–71]

Deep infections, although far less likely, can often lead to more devastating problems. Significant hematoma formation as a result of the extensive bony preparation required for fusion can serve as a nidus for deep infection.[47] Thus, careful hemostasis performed intraoperatively can have profound effects for prevention of deep infection. Additionally, a well-made postoperative splint and compression dressing can help minimize hematoma formation. Literature on infections in the wrist arthrodesis is somewhat limited, but the most common organisms involved are skin pathogens *Staphylococcus aureus* and *Streptococcus epidermis*.[68] Thus, universally standard precautions, such as aseptic technique and prophylactic antibiotics, are also critical.

When deep infections occur, operative irrigation and débridement with removal of hardware is the treatment of choice, followed by a course of antibiotics tailored to cultures obtained from the site of infection.[68] Typically, an antibiotic regimen of at least 4 weeks in duration is necessary to eradicate the bony infection.[68] Consultation with an infectious disease specialist is always warranted, especially if a patient is immunocompromised or suffers from other medical comorbidities that preclude optimal treatment options.[72] When infection occurs before bony union is present, there is the additional challenge of keeping the wrist stabilized while the infection clears prior to reimplantation of any hardware. Literature is limited regarding this situation, but the best treatment in this case is placement of a temporary external fixator while the patient undergoes appropriate antibiotic therapy to treat the infection.[68,72]

Hardware complications, although not as devastating as nonunion and infection, may still pose a significant challenge. Some studies using dorsal compression plating report symptomatic hardware, with either painful prominence or bursitis

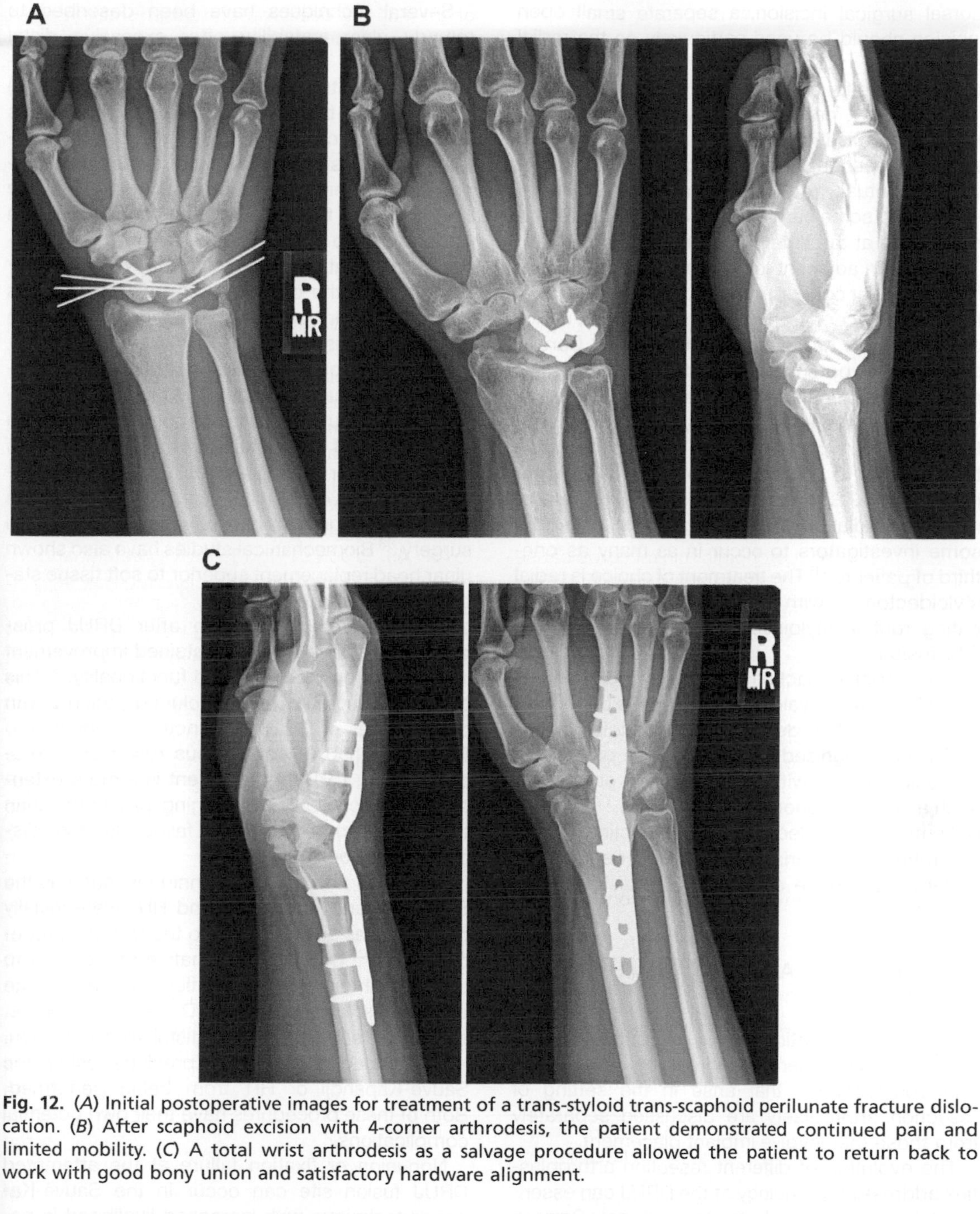

Fig. 12. (*A*) Initial postoperative images for treatment of a trans-styloid trans-scaphoid perilunate fracture dislocation. (*B*) After scaphoid excision with 4-corner arthrodesis, the patient demonstrated continued pain and limited mobility. (*C*) A total wrist arthrodesis as a salvage procedure allowed the patient to return back to work with good bony union and satisfactory hardware alignment.

as high as one-third to two-thirds of patients, frequently requiring hardware removal.[24,49,51] It is recommended that the dorsal plate not be removed prior to clear evidence of bony union, with some guidelines recommending that the plate be maintained at least 6 months and even up to 12 months postoperatively.[47]

Injuries to neurovascular structures may occur, with dorsal sensory branches of the ulnar and radial nerves at highest risk.[46,48,58] Both plating and pin fixation place these structures at risk, and to date there is no study that demonstrates that one method has a lower sensory nerve injury rate than the other. To prevent such injuries from occurring during an open dorsal approach, it is recommended that the sensory branches are kept within the flaps and that excessive retraction is avoided.[47] If pins are placed outside of the dorsal surgical incision, a separate small open incision should be used particularly on the radial side, where the dorsal sensory radial nerve branches are found.

Additionally, carpal tunnel syndrome is a well-known complication after wrist fusion, with some studies presenting rates as high as 10%, half of which eventually require a carpal tunnel release.[48] As a result, some surgeons advocate a carpal tunnel release at the time of the wrist fusion surgery.

Arthritis in adjacent joints is a complication that is of particular concern in limited fusions. After STT fusions, adjacent trapeziometacarpal and radiocarpal arthritis has been reported.[17,73–75] Careful screening of potential limited fusion patients for preexisting adjacent arthrosis is an important preventative measure. Additionally, it is critical that the scaphoid remain anatomically reduced relative to the radius to prevent development of adjacent joint disease. STT fusion also has a high rate of resultant radial styloid impingement, noted by some investigators to occur in as many as one-third of patients.[76] The treatment of choice is radial styloidectomy, with some investigators advocating routine styloidectomy at the time of the STT fusion.[74,75]

Ulnocarpal impaction may also occur and is typically more prevalent when fusion is performed in excessive ulnar deviation.[46] When this complication is recognized in ulnar-positive patients, it is ideally treated with a joint-leveling procedure, such as an ulnar shortening osteotomy.[77] In those patients with inadequate DRUJ function, ulnar-neutral/negative variance, and lower demand requirements, simple excision of the distal ulna is often adequate.[77]

COMPLICATIONS AND MANAGEMENT: ARTHROPLASTY

Potential complications after arthroplasty of the wrist are also numerous and can be devastating. The complications that arise in the setting of resection arthroplasty are discussed separately from those that involve implant placement.

The evolution of different resection arthroplasties addressing pathology at the DRUJ can essentially be traced back to the original Darrach procedure.[25,32] Although outcomes after distal ulna resection are acceptable with regard to pain, motion, and grip strength,[25] they can be associated with several complications. Most notably, instability of the ulnar remnant is observed, which leads to radioulnar impingement. Additionally, loss of the ulnar support of the carpus can lead to carpal collapse or even ulnar translocation of the carpus.

Several techniques have been described to remedy ulnar instability after excessive distal ulna resection. Tenodesis using weaves of a proximally based strip of extensor carpi ulnaris (ECU) and a distally-based strip of flexor carpi ulnaris (FCU) tendon can successfully stabilize a symptomatically unstable ulna[78] and is thought superior to using either ECU or FCU alone.[79,80] The use of Achilles tendon allograft as an interposition graft has also shown success in a small series.[81–84] Additionally, transfer of the pronator quadratus to the dorsum of the ulna for use as an interposition graft has been described with good outcomes.[85,86]

In addition to the soft tissue stabilization procedures, both ulnar head and DRUJ replacement implants can be used as salvage for failed resection arthroplasty of the distal ulna.[40,87–89] Long-term outcomes after ulnar head replacement for treatment of failed distal ulnar resection have shown promise even greater than 10 years after the initial surgery.[88] Biomechanical studies have also shown ulnar head replacement superior to soft tissue stabilization after failed Darrach.[90]

Similarly, 5-year follow-up after DRUJ prosthesis placement showed sustained improvement in patients' reported pain and functionality.[89] This particular study, however, included patients with other causes of DRUJ dysfunction in addition to those who had failed previous resection arthroplasty. Also, DRUJ replacement is a more extensive and technically challenging procedure than the salvage procedures for failed Darrach (discussed previously).[91]

Resection arthroplasty techniques, such as the Sauvé-Kapandji technique and HIT, were initially developed as an alternative to the Darrach procedure.[26–28,33] These are alternative procedures to the Darrach distal ulna resection and not salvage procedures after a failed Darrach procedure, because the results of the distal ulna resection, as described by Darrach, preclude either the Sauvé-Kapandji or HIT from being performed. Both of these procedures have their own potential complications.

Nonunion or fixation failure at the attempted DRUJ fusion site can occur in the Sauvé-Kapandji technique with increased likelihood in patients with poor bone stock or quality, as often seen in patients with RA.[27] A modified version of this technique is termed *shelf arthroplasty* by Masada and colleagues. This procedure removes a portion of the distal ulna, rotates it perpendicular to the long axis of the radius, and fixes it into the sigmoid notch via compression screw. It has been reported with good outcomes after minimum 5-year follow-up.[92]

Both the original and modified Sauvé-Kapandji techniques have the potential complications of radioulnar convergence at the remaining ulnar stump and of reossification at the pseudoarthrosis site. As a preemptive measure to prevent ulnar impingement, it is strongly recommended that the ulna be resected as distally as possible, because the ulnar side of the radius becomes more ridgelike to accommodate the interosseous membrane with proximal movement.[93] This morphology is thought to contribute to the painful symptoms of impingement. Ross and colleagues describe a salvage technique in which the pseudoarthrosis is taken down, an intercalary graft is used to restore ulnar length, and HIT is performed to provide rotation, with successful outcomes in a small set of patients.[94]

Although there is no established regimen for treatment of reossification at the site of the original pseudoarthrosis, one study reported acceptable outcomes with medical management using antiinflammatory steroids in a small number of patients. Simple excision of the reossification site can also be performed.[93]

Implant arthroplasties of the wrist share many of the same complications seen in other joints of the body and can prove challenging to treat. A majority of partial implant arthroplasties of the wrist (partial or total ulnar head replacement and DRUJ total arthroplasty) are still performed as salvage procedures (described previously), but there is an increase in their use as primary treatment of DRUJ pathologies or congenital disorders, such as Madelung deformity and Ehlers-Danlos syndrome.[91] Regardless of their indication for use, the complications that arise are typically the same.

For ulnar head prostheses, the most common reported complication is recurrent instability.[87,88] This is often the result of inadequate soft tissue coverage and can be treated with reinforcement of the soft tissue repair, such as with a retinacular flap.[88] If that is not possible to perform, such as in a multiply operated wrist lacking adequate soft tissue, conversion to a total DRUJ arthroplasty can be considered. One study reports a single case of stem loosening, which was subsequently corrected with revision to a larger diameter stem.[88] This same study reported another case of heterotopic ossification first noted radiographically nearly 4 years postoperatively that was treated conservatively.

Similar results were found in a study looking at DRUJ arthroplasty, with a single patient experiencing heterotopic ossification at the distal ulna, also treated nonoperatively.[91] Implant loosening has not been consistently noted with newer DRUJ implant technologies. There have not been any reports of significant deep infection with DRUJ arthroplasty requiring implant removal, but that may be secondary to the small number of surgeries that are performed (**Fig. 13**).

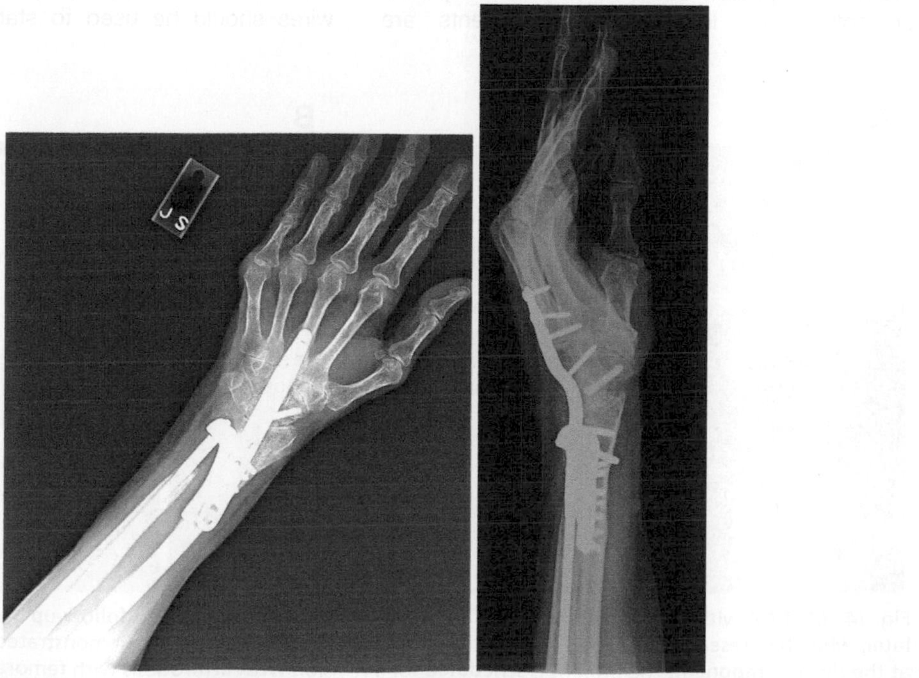

Fig. 13. Anteroposterior (*left*) and lateral (*right*) radiographs after, total wrist arthrodesis and distal ulna arthroplasty using a Scheker implant.

The ultimate choice for salvage of the unstable forearm that has failed the methods described previously is creation of a radioulnar synostosis and a 1-bone forearm.[95,96] In addition to eliminating forearm rotation, the poor overall outcomes of this procedure cause many to consider it a last resort for treatment of painful forearm instability.[95–97]

Despite continuous advances in implant technology and surgical techniques for TWA, complications may occur. Instability and implant loosening are the most common TWA complications but often are preventable. Newer technologies that rely on the distal component fixed to the carpus with concomitant intercarpal fusion have significantly reduced the incidence of loosening compared with older models fixed into the metacarpal shafts.[98,99]

When loosening occurs, it is possible that revision arthroplasty can correct the problem if a patient's bone stock is reasonable. The safest and most generally accepted solution, however, is conversion to a wrist fusion. Positive outcomes have been reported using both iliac crest autograft and femoral head allograft to address bone voids when converting to a fusion. The use of femoral head allograft avoids the morbidity associated with harvesting iliac crest.[100,101] A wrist arthrodesis plate as well as a postoperative splint should be used to ensure bony union prior to activity.[102,103]

Instability can also be predicted by patient selection, because postoperative dislocation is most often a result of excessive joint laxity and/or soft tissue imbalance. RA patients are especially susceptible, because the combination of poor bone stock and attenuated wrist capsule due to synovitis is likely to contribute to a very lax wrist joint.

If instability occurs, surgeons must evaluate technique and component selection. As with loosening, it is possible that revision of one or all of the components may provide the solution, again if there is adequate remaining bone stock. When instability is thought the result of an attenuated wrist capsule, there have been positive outcomes reported with the use of soft tissue allograft to augment the capsule.[4] If an acute trauma has caused instability or dislocation, a trial of immobilization with either casting or a spanning external fixator may be successful.[98] When these techniques do not correct the instability, or if revision is not feasible, conversion to arthrodesis is the most ideal treatment (**Fig. 14**).[103–105]

Intraoperative complications during TWA include fracture and tendon laceration. Proper preparation of the radius prior to implantation of the radial component is vital to avoid fracture. If the intramedullary canal is inadequately prepared or the cortical bone is weakened, then placement of the press-fit radial component may cause fracture.[3,6] Thus, it is recommended to use fluoroscopy judiciously to ensure proper alignment of broaches to the medullary canal.[3,4,106] In addition, it is recommended to prepare the canal so that the trial component can be fully seated with minimal force. If fracture occurs, circumferential cerclage wires should be used to stabilize the fracture,

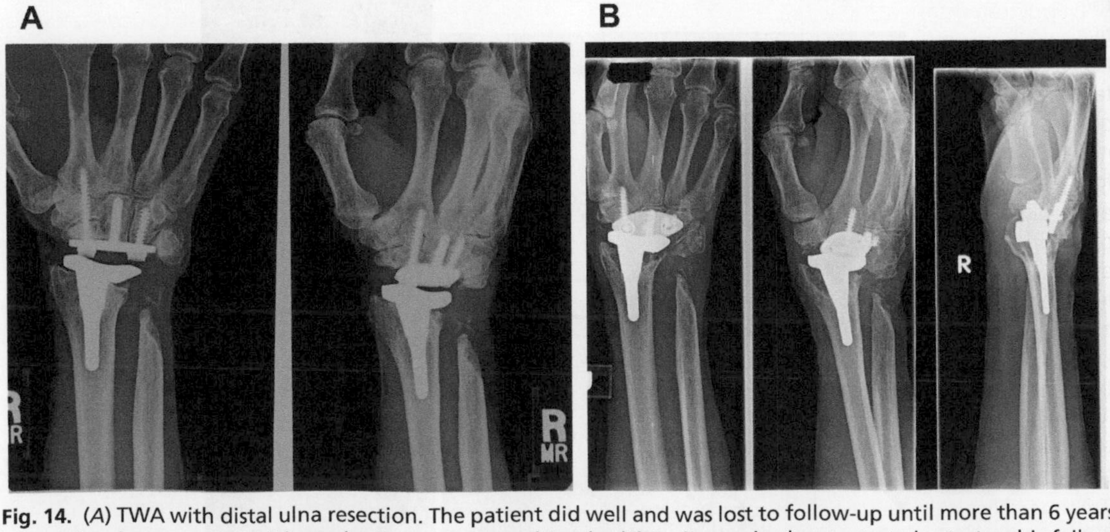

Fig. 14. (*A*) TWA with distal ulna resection. The patient did well and was lost to follow-up until more than 6 years later, when he presented with gradually increasing wrist pain. (*B*) Radiographs demonstrated catastrophic failure at the distal component. The patient is scheduled for a revision wrist arthrodesis with femoral head allograft. It is suspected that gradual polyethylene wear and subsequent osteolysis led to the failure of fixation of the distal component.

and postoperative rehabilitation should be adjusted accordingly by delaying motion until the fracture heals. Unfortunately, these precautions can eventually lead to loss of motion due to capsular stiffness.

Unlike the radial component, the distal carpal component usually has a stem in addition to screws. If fracture occurs distally, bone grafting and longer screws that span the fracture should be placed.[4] If there is inadequate or poor quality bone at the stem, then use of cement should be considered.

Intraoperative extensor tendon lacerations usually occur while raising the extensor retinaculum, especially in a previously operated wrist where scarring to the overlying skin is common.[3] Raising the skin and retinaculum together in a single flap can prevent tendon lacerations from occurring.[3,4,6] If tendon laceration occurs, repair should be performed intraoperatively, and again the rehabilitation protocol should be adjusted accordingly.[4,6]

Infection is a rare complication in TWA and, like fusions, often coincides with wound complications. Preemptive measures to guard against hematoma formation are similar, including adequate hemostasis with the tourniquet deflated and postoperative compression dressing. It is also recommended that a closed suction drain be placed for removal 1 to 2 days postoperatively.[101,102,105] When deep infection occurs, the treatment is analogous to arthroplasty of other large joints. If cultures and sensitivities of the offending organism reveal an infection that can be effectively treated with antibiotics, then a trial of surgical débridement and appropriate antibiotic therapy may be warranted in an early postoperative infection.[105,107] Late infection should be treated with resection arthroplasty followed by total wrist fusion once the infection is deemed cleared.[101,102] Antibiotic cement may be used to maintain wrist height until definitive fusion is performed.[101,102] Although there has been some literature on comparable efficacy of serial aspirations of the septic wrist versus open irrigation and débridement, serial aspirations are not likely effective in this scenario due to seeding of the prosthesis.[107,108]

The final potential complication of TWA is pathology of the DRUJ. In the setting of a painful wrist with pancarpal arthritis, it can be difficult to elucidate any symptomatic DRUJ pathology from other causes of pain due to arthritis. In such cases, it may be most judicious to leave the DRUJ intact at the time of arthroplasty, while informing patients that additional surgery may be indicated in the future to address the DRUJ.[99] This can be particularly wise in those patients with OA with ulnar-neutral/negative variance so as not to further exacerbate the variance with removal of a portion of distal ulna.[3,4]

When DRUJ pathology develops after TWA, the most straightforward solution is simple ulnar head excision. This is the case especially in patients with RA who have a high incidence of progressing to DRUJ arthritis after TWA and in those with significant radiocarpal disease that has resulted in positive ulnar variance, because preparation of the distal radius for TWA only worsens the variance.[3,4,106] The incidence of symptomatic ulnar stump instability is much lower in patients with TWA than in those with isolated resection arthroplasties, but if needed soft tissue interposition and ECU/FCU tenodesis can be performed.[78–80] Finally, the simultaneous use of DRUJ and total wrist implants has been performed sparingly with few data at this time, but there is concern for metal on metal wear that may develop between the 2 implants.

Despite the extensive list of complications that can arise from performing wrist arthroplasty, it is accepted as a worthwhile procedure by surgeons and patients alike. Perhaps the most telling sign is that patients who have had one of each procedure typically show preference to the side with the arthroplasty.[42] Many of the complications that can arise either from arthroplasty or fusion of the wrist are preventable, and prophylactic measures combined with stringent patient selection and surgical planning can go a long way in minimizing the risks of this constantly evolving field.

REFERENCES

1. Carroll RE, Dick HM. Arthrodesis of the wrist for rheumatoid arthritis. J Bone Joint Surg Am 1971; 53A:1365–9.
2. Haddad RJ, Riordan DC. Arthrodesis of the wrist: a surgical technique. J Bone Joint Surg Am 1967; 49A:950–4.
3. Adams BD. Total wrist arthroplasty. J Am Soc Surg Hand 2001;1:236–48.
4. Anderson MC, Adams BD. Total wrist arthroplasty. Hand Clin 2005;21:621–30.
5. Ritt MJ, Stuart PR, Naggar L, et al. The early history of arthroplasty of the wrist: from amputation to total wrist implant. J Hand Surg Br 1994;19(6):778–82.
6. Rosenfeld JF, Nicholson JJ. History and design considerations for arthroplasty around the wrist. Hand Clin 2013;29(1):1–13.
7. Volz RG. The development of a total wrist arthroplasty. Clin Orthop Relat Res 1976;116:209–14.
8. McElfresh E. History of arthroplasty. In: Petty W, editor. Total joint replacement. Philadelphia (PA): WB Saunders; 1991. p. 3–18.

9. Jebson PJL, Adams BD. Wrist arthrodesis: review of current techniques. J Am Acad Orthop Surg 2001;9(1):53–60.
10. Murphy DM, Khoury JG, Imbriglia JE, et al. Comparison of arthroplasty and arthrodesis for the rheumatoid wrist. J Hand Surg Am 2003;28:570–6.
11. Hayter CL, Gold SL, Potter HG. Magnetic resonance imaging of the wrist: bone and cartilage injury. J Magn Reson Imaging 2013;37(5):1005–19.
12. Taleisnik J. Subtotal arthrodeses of the wrist joint. Clin Orthop Relat Res 1984;187:81–8.
13. Nagy L, Büchler U. Long-term results of radioscapholunate fusion following fractures of the distal radius. J Hand Surg Br 1997;22(6):705–10.
14. Stanley JK, Boot DA. Radio-lunate arthrodesis. J Hand Surg Br 1989;14(3):283–7.
15. Ishida O, Tsai TM. Complications and results of scapho-trapezio-trapezoid arthrodesis. Clin Orthop Relat Res 1993;287:125–30.
16. Watson HK, Monacelli DM, Milford RS, et al. Treatment of Kienböck's disease with scaphotrapeziotrapezoid arthrodesis. J Hand Surg Am 1996;21(1):9–15.
17. Meier R, van Griensven M, Krimmer H. Scaphotrapeziotrapezoid (STT)-arthrodesis in Kienbock's disease. J Hand Surg Br 2004;29:580–4.
18. Kleinman WB. Long-term study of chronic scapholunate instability treated by scapho-trapeziotrapezoid arthrodesis. J Hand Surg Am 1989;14(3):429–45.
19. Luegmair M, Saffar P. Scaphocapitate arthrodesis for treatment of scapholunate instability in manual workers. J Hand Surg Am 2013;38(5):878–86.
20. Luegmair M, Saffar P. Scaphocapitate arthrodesis for treatment of late stage Kienbock disease. J Hand Surg Eur Vol 2014;39(4):416–22.
21. Dacho A, Grundel J, Holle G, et al. Long term results of midcarpal arthrodesis in the treatment of scaphoid nonunion advanced collapse (SNAC—Wrist) and scapholunate advanced collapse (SLAC—Wrist). Ann Plast Surg 2006;56(2):139–44.
22. Mulford JS, Ceulemans LJ, Nam D, et al. Proximal row carpectomy vs four corner fusion for scapholunate (SLAC) or scaphoid nonunion advanced collapse (SNAC) wrists: a systematic review of outcomes. J Hand Surg Eur Vol 2009;34(2):256–63.
23. Solem H, Berg NJ, Finsen V. Long term results of arthrodesis of the wrist: a 6–15 year follow up of 35 patients. Scand J Plast Reconstr Surg Hand Surg 2006;40(3):175–8.
24. Field J, Herbert TJ, Prosser R. Total wrist fusion. A functional assessment. J Hand Surg Br 1996;21:429–33.
25. Tulipan DJ, Eaton RG, Eberhart RE. The Darrach procedure defended: technique redefined and long-term follow-up. J Hand Surg Am 1991;16(3):438–44.
26. Taleisnik J. The Sauvé-Kapandji procedure. Clin Orthop Relat Res 1992;275:110–23.
27. Slater RR Jr. The Sauvé-Kapandji procedure. J Hand Surg Am 2008;33(9):1632–8.
28. Glowacki KA. Hemiresection arthroplasty of the distal radioulnar joint. Hand Clin 2005;21(4):591–601.
29. Murray PM. Current concepts in the treatment of rheumatoid arthritis of the distal radioulnar joint. Hand Clin 2011;27(1):49–55.
30. Scheker LR. Implant arthroplasty for the distal radioulnar joint. J Hand Surg Am 2008;33(9):1639–44.
31. Szabo RM. Distal radioulnar joint instability. J Bone Joint Surg Am 2006;88(4):884–94.
32. De Witte PB, Wijffels M, Jupiter JB, et al. The Darrach procedure for posttraumatic reconstruction. Acta Orthop Belg 2009;75(3):316–22.
33. Ahmed SK, Cheung JP, Fung BK, et al. Long term results of matched hemiresection interposition arthroplasty for DRUJ arthritis in rheumatoid patients. Hand Surg 2011;16(2):119–25.
34. Richou J, Chuinard C, Moineau G, et al. Proximal row carpectomy: long-term results. Chir Main 2010;29(1):10–5.
35. Elfar JC, Stern PJ. Proximal row carpectomy for scapholunate dissociation. J Hand Surg Br 2011;36(2):111–5.
36. Cohen MS, Kozin SH. Degenerative arthritis of the wrist: proximal row carpectomy versus scaphoid excision and four-corner arthrodesis. J Hand Surg Am 2001;26:94–104.
37. Wyrick JD, Stern PJ, Kiefhaber TR. Motion-preserving procedures in the treatment of scapholunate advanced collapse wrist: proximal row carpectomy versus four-corner arthrodesis. J Hand Surg Am 1995;20:965–70.
38. Garcia-Elias M. Eclypse: partial ulnar head replacement for the isolated distal radio-ulnar joint arthrosis. Tech Hand Up Extrem Surg 2007;11(1):121–8.
39. Berger RA. Indications for ulnar head replacement. Am J Orthop (Belle Mead NJ) 2008;37(8 Suppl 1):17–20.
40. De Smet L, Peeters T. Salvage of failed Sauvé-Kapandji procedures with an ulnar head prosthesis: report of three cases. J Hand Surg 2003;28B:271–3.
41. Nydick JA, Greenberg SM, Stone JD, et al. Clinical outcomes of total wrist arthroplasty. J Hand Surg Am 2012;37:1580–4.
42. Vicar AJ, Burton RI. Surgical management of the rheumatoid wrist—fusion or arthroplasty. J Hand Surg 1986;11A:790–7.
43. Boeckstyns ME, Herzberg G, Merser S. Favorable results after total wrist arthroplasty: 65 wrists in

60 patients followed for 5–9 years. Acta Orthop 2013;84:415–9.

44. Culp RW, Bachoura A, Gelman SE, et al. Proximal row carpectomy combined with wrist hemiarthroplasty. J Wrist Surg 2012;1:39–46.
45. Boyer JS, Adams B. Distal radius hemiarthroplasty combined with proximal row carpectomy: case report. Iowa Orthop J 2010;30:168–73.
46. Zachary SV, Stern PJ. Complications following AO/ASIF wrist arthrodesis. J Hand Surg Am 1995; 20(2):339–44.
47. Wysocki RW, Cohen MS. Complications of limited and total wrist arthrodesis. Hand Clin 2010;26(2): 221–8.
48. Hastings H II, Weiss AP, Quenzer D, et al. Arthrodesis of the wrist for post-traumatic disorders. J Bone Joint Surg Am 1996;78:897–902.
49. O'Bierne J, Boyer MI, Axelrod TS. Wrist arthrodesis using a dynamic compression plate. J Bone Joint Surg Br 1995;77:700–4.
50. Hartigan BJ, Nagle DJ, Foley MJ. Wrist arthrodesis with excision of the proximal carpal bones using the AO/ASIF wrist fusion plate and local bone graft. J Hand Surg Br 2001;26(3):247–51.
51. Sagerman SD, Palmer AK. Wrist arthrodesis using a dynamic compression plate. J Hand Surg Br 1996;21:437–41.
52. Meads BM, Scougall PJ, Hargreaves IC. Wrist arthrodesis using a Synthes wrist fusion plate. J Hand Surg Br 2003;28(6):571–4.
53. Clayton ML, Ferlic DC. Arthrodesis of the arthritic wrist. Clin Orthop 1984;187:89–93.
54. Mikkelsen OA. Arthrodesis of the wrist joint in rheumatoid arthritis. Hand 1980;12(2):149–53.
55. Papaioannou T, Dickson RA. Arthrodesis of the wrist in rheumatoid disease. Hand 1982;14(1):12–6.
56. Masada K, Yasuda M, Takeuchi E, et al. Technique of intra-medullary fixation for arthrodesis of the wrist in rheumatoid arthritis. Scand J Plast Reconstr Surg 2003;37(3):155–8.
57. Shin AY. Four-corner arthrodesis. J Am Soc Surg Hand 2001;1:93–111.
58. Vance MC, Hernandez JD, Didonna ML, et al. Complications and outcome of four-corner arthrodesis: circular plate fixation versus traditional techniques. J Hand Surg Am 2005;30:1122–7.
59. Kendall CB, Brown TR, Millon SJ, et al. Results of four-corner arthrodesis using dorsal circular plate fixation. J Hand Surg Am 2005;30:903–7.
60. Wood MB. Wrist arthrodesis using dorsal radial bone graft. J Hand Surg Am 1987;12:208–12.
61. Weiss APC, Wiedeman G, Quenzer D, et al. Upper extremity function after wrist arthrodesis. J Hand Surg Am 1995;20A:813–7.
62. Brighton CT, Friedenberg ZB, Mitchell EI, et al. Treatment of nonunion with constant direct current. Clin Orthop Relat Res 1977;124:106–23.
63. Dimitriou R, Babis GC. Biomaterial osseointegration enhancement with biophysical stimulation. J Musculoskelet Neuronal Interact 2007;7(3): 253–65.
64. Yonemori K, Matsunaga S, Ishidou Y, et al. Early effects of electrical stimulation on osteogenesis. Bone 1996;19(2):173–80.
65. Mollon B, da Silva V, Busse JW, et al. Electrical stimulation for long-bone fracture-healing: a meta-analysis of randomized controlled trials. J Bone Joint Surg Am 2008;90(11):2322–30.
66. Saxena A, DiDomenico LA, Widtfeldt A, et al. Implantable electrical bone stimulation for arthrodeses of the foot and ankle in high-risk patients: a multicenter study. J Foot Ankle Surg 2005;44(6): 450–4.
67. Nydick JA, Watt JF, Garcia MJ, et al. Clinical outcomes of arthrodesis and arthroplasty for the treatment of post-traumatic wrist arthritis. J Hand Surg Am 2013;38:899–903.
68. Gaston RG, Kuremsky MA. Postoperative infections: prevention and management. Hand Clin 2010;26(2):265–80.
69. Gunther SF, Gunther SB. Diabetic hand infections. Hand Clin 1998;14(4):647–56.
70. Glickel SZ. Hand infections in patients with acquired immunodeficiency syndrome. J Hand Surg 1988;13(5):770.
71. Gonzalez MH, Nikoleit J, Weinzweig N, et al. Upper extremity infections in patients with the human immunodeficiency virus. J Hand Surg Am 1998;23: 348–52.
72. Zalavras CG, Marcus RE, Levin LS, et al. Management of open fractures and subsequent complications. J Bone Joint Surg Am 2007;89(4):884–95.
73. Fortin PT, Louis DS. Long-term follow-up of scaphoid-trapezium-trapezoid arthrodesis. J Hand Surg Am 1993;18:675–81.
74. Wollstein R, Watson HK. Scaphotrapeziotrapezoid arthrodesis for arthritis. Hand Clin 2005;21: 539–43, vi.
75. Watson HK, Wollstein R, Joseph E, et al. Scaphotrapeziotrapezoid arthrodesis: a follow-up study. J Hand Surg Am 2003;28:397–404.
76. Rogers WD, Watson HK. Radial styloid impingement after triscaphe arthrodesis. J Hand Surg Am 1989;14:297–301.
77. Trumble TE, Easterling KJ, Smith RJ. Ulnocarpal abutment after wrist arthrodesis. J Hand Surg Am 1988;13:11–5.
78. Breen TF, Jupiter JB. Extensor carpi ulnaris and flexor carpi ulnaris tenodesis of the unstable distal ulna. J Hand Surg Am 1989;14(4):612–7.
79. Leslie BM, Carlson G, Ruby LK. Results of extensor carpi ulnaris tenodesis in the rheumatoid wrist undergoing a distal ulnar excision. J Hand Surg Am 1990;15A:547–51.

80. Tsai TM, Stilwell JH. Repair of chronic subluxation of the distal radioulnar joint (ulnar dorsal) using flexor carpi ulnaris tendon. J Hand Surg Br 1984; 9(3):289–94.
81. Sotereanos DG, Gobel F, Vardakas DG, et al. An allograft salvage technique for failure of the Darrach procedure: a report of four cases. J Hand Surg Br 2002;27(4):317–21.
82. Sotereanos DG, Papatheodorou LK, Williams BG. Tendon allograft interposition for failed distal ulnar resection: 2- to 14-year follow-up. J Hand Surg Am 2014;39(3):443–8.
83. Greenberg JA, Sotereanos D. Achilles allograft interposition for failed Darrach distal ulna resections. Tech Hand Up Extrem Surg 2008;12(2): 121–5.
84. Papatheodorou LK, Rubright JH, Kokkalis ZT, et al. Resection interposition arthroplasty for failed distal ulna resections. J Wrist Surg 2013;2(1):13–8.
85. Ruby LK, Ferenz CC, Dell PC. The pronator quadratus interposition transfer: an adjunct to resection arthroplasty of the distal radioulnar joint. J Hand Surg Am 1996;21(1):60–5.
86. Bain GI, Heptinstall RJ, Webb JM, et al. Hemiresection of the distal ulna by means of pronator quadratus interposition and volar stabilization. Tech Hand Up Extrem Surg 2007;11(1):83–6.
87. van Schoonhoven J, Fernandez DL, Bowers WH, et al. Salvage of failed resection arthroplasties of the distal radioulnar joint using a new ulnar head prosthesis. J Hand Surg 2000;25A:438–46.
88. van Schoonhoven J, Mühldorfer-Fodor M, Fernandez DL, et al. Salvage of failed resection arthroplasties of the distal radioulnar joint using an ulnar head prosthesis: long-term results. J Hand Surg Am 2012;37(7):1372–80.
89. Scheker LR. Implant arthroplasty for the distal radioulnar joint. J Hand Surg Am 2008;33(9): 1639–44.
90. Sauerbier M, Hahn ME, Berglund LJ, et al. Biomechanical evaluation of the dynamic radioulnar convergence after ulnar head resection, two soft tissue stabilization methods of the distal ulna and ulnar head prosthesis implantation. Arch Orthop Trauma Surg 2011;131(1):15–26.
91. Savvidou C, Murphy E, Mailhot E, et al. Semiconstrained distal radioulnar joint prosthesis. J Wrist Surg 2013;2(1):41–8.
92. Fujita S, Masada K, Takeuchi E, et al. Modified Sauvé-Kapandji procedure for disorders of the distal radioulnar joint in patients with rheumatoid arthritis. J Bone Joint Surg Am 2005;87(1):134–9.
93. Lluch A. The sauvé-kapandji procedure. J Wrist Surg 2013;2(1):33–40.
94. Ross M, Thomas J, Couzens G, et al. Salvage of the unstable Sauvé-Kapandji procedure: a new technique. Tech Hand Up Extrem Surg 2007; 11(1):87–92.
95. Allende C, Allende BT. Posttraumatic one-bone forearm reconstruction: a report of seven cases. J Bone Joint Surg Am 2004;86(2):364–9.
96. Peterson CA II, Maki S, Wood MB. Clinical results of the one-bone forearm. J Hand Surg Am 1995; 20(4):609–18.
97. Jacoby SM, Bachoura A, Diprinzio EV, et al. Complications following one-bone forearm surgery for posttraumatic forearm and distal radioulnar joint instability. J Hand Surg Am 2013;38(5):976–82.
98. Lorei MP, Figgie MP, Ranawat CS, et al. Failed total wrist arthroplasty. Analysis of failures and results of operative management. Clin Orthop Relat Res 1997;34(2):84–93.
99. Divelbiss BJ, Sollerman C, Adams BD. Early results of the universal total wrist arthroplasty in rheumatoid arthritis. J Hand Surg Am 2002;27(2):195–204.
100. Younger EM, Chapman MW. Morbidity at bone graft donor sites. J Orthop Trauma 1989;3(3): 192–5.
101. Laurie SW, Kaban LB, Mulliken JB, et al. Donorsite morbidity after harvesting rib and iliac bone. Plast Reconstr Surg 1984;73(6):933–8.
102. Ferlic DC, Jolly SN, Clayton ML. Salvage for failed implant arthroplasty of the wrist. J Hand Surg Am 1992;17(5):917–23.
103. Rizzo M, Ackerman DB, Rodrigues RL, et al. Wrist arthrodesis as a salvage procedure for failed implant arthroplasty. J Hand Surg 2011;36E:29–33.
104. Beer TA, Turner RH. Wrist arthrodesis for failed implant arthroplasty. J Hand Surg 1997;22(4): 685–93.
105. Mater WY, Jafari SM, Restrepo C, et al. Preventing infection in total joint arthroplasty. J Bone Joint Surg Am 2010;92(Suppl 2):36–46.
106. Adams BD. Complications of wrist arthroplasty. Hand Clin 2010;26(2):213–20.
107. Murray PM. Septic arthritis of the hand and wrist. Hand Clin 1998;14:579–87, viii.
108. Sammer DM, Shin AY. Comparison of arthroscopic and open treatment of septic arthritis of the wrist. J Bone Joint Surg Am 2009;91:1387–93.

Management of Complications of Flexor Tendon Injuries

Nicholas Pulos, MD[a], David J. Bozentka, MD[b,*]

KEYWORDS

• Flexor tendon injury • Flexor tendon healing • Flexor tendon repair • Flexor tendon adhesion
• Joint contracture

KEY POINTS

- Tendon adhesion and joint contracture are the most common complications after flexor tendon repair.
- Management of these complications includes prevention and continues through meticulous surgical technique and thoughtful rehabilitation protocols.
- Research in the use of biologic modulators to promote scarless healing continues to show promise.

INTRODUCTION

It has been nearly a century since Bunnell published his paper entitled "Repair of Tendons in the Fingers and Descriptions of Two New Instruments."[1] At that time, complication rates after treatment of these injuries was high. In particular, Verdan zone 2 injuries have been called no man's land based on an increased likelihood of adhesion formation and poor patient outcomes. Improvements in operative techniques, biomaterials, and rehabilitation protocols, and knowledge gained from animal experiments have made treating these injuries a real possibility.[2,3] However, despite these advances, treatment of flexor tendon injuries remains challenging with a reoperation rate of 6%.[4] Fortunately, flexor tendon injuries are uncommon, representing less than 1% of all hand and wrist injuries.[5] The goals of surgical treatment are to repair accurately the tendon ends to achieve a repair that is strong enough to withstand the forces generated during a postoperative rehabilitation protocol, which includes early digit range of motion. The purpose of this review is to highlight the complications of flexor tendon injuries and review the management of these complications.

FLEXOR TENDON HEALING

Management of complications of flexor tendon injury requires a knowledge of the basic science and anatomy of flexor tendon healing. Two mechanisms of tendon healing have been proposed. Healing via the tenocytes describes the intrinsic pathway. The extrinsic pathway achieves tendon healing via synovial fibroblasts and inflammatory cells from the tendon sheath and is thought to contribute to adhesion formation. It is likely that in vivo tendon healing is a combination of both the extrinsic and intrinsic pathways.[6]

The process of flexor tendon repair is often divided into 3 sequential phases: inflammatory, fibroblastic, and remodeling.[7–9] First, inflammatory

No benefits or funds were received in support of this study.
[a] Department of Orthopedic Surgery, University of Pennsylvania, 3737 Market Street, 6th Floor, Philadelphia, PA 19104, USA; [b] Hand Surgery, Department of Orthopedic Surgery, University of Pennsylvania, 3737 Market Street, 6th Floor, Philadelphia, PA 19104, USA
* Corresponding author.
E-mail address: david.bozentka@uphs.upenn.edu

Hand Clin 31 (2015) 293–299
http://dx.doi.org/10.1016/j.hcl.2014.12.004
0749-0712/15/$ – see front matter

cells migrate to the injury site and phagocytize necrotic tissue. Then, fibroblasts proliferate around the injury site, synthesizing collagen and other components of the extracellular matrix. Finally, collagen fibers organize along the axis of the tendon.[6] The extrinsic pathway is thought to predominate early in tendon healing, with the intrinsic pathway becoming increasingly more active after 21 days.[10] Preoperative, intraoperative, biologic, and postoperative factors, which enhance the intrinsic pathway while suppressing the extrinsic pathway, have been studied to improve outcomes in the treatment of these injuries.

The mechanism of injury may be an important preoperative factor. Patients who present with tearing-type injuries, such as those created by saws, have been shown to have poorer outcomes compared with patients with sharp flexor tendon injuries.[11] Other preoperative factors have been proposed including patient age, general health and motivation.[12] Intraoperatively, several principles of flexor tendon repair have been developed in an effort to improve outcomes. These include the use of core sutures with nonabsorbable or semiresorbable braided suture material of the largest caliber technically possible, an epitendinous suture, and delicate soft tissue handling.[2,13,14] Postoperatively, Gelberman and colleagues[15] demonstrated that early motion resulted in greater ultimate load and excursion in flexor tendons than those managed with an immobilization protocol in a canine model.

A newer area of research in flexor tendon healing investigates biologic modulation of tendon repair. Several cytokines including transforming growth factor-beta (TGF-β), connective tissue growth factor, growth differentiation factor 5, vascular endothelial growth factor, insulinlike growth factor, platelet-derived growth factor, and basic fibroblast growth factor (bFGF) have been found to be involved in tendon healing.[16]

TGF-β has been implicated in the pathogenesis of excessive scar formation. Chang and colleagues[17] found upregulation of TGF-β in both tendon and sheath fibroblasts and, subsequently, that the use of antibodies to neutralize TGF-β increased digital range of motion in a rabbit model.[18] Zhang and colleagues[19] demonstrated that TGF-β inhibition via its neutralizing antibody significantly reduced collage I production. Using microRNA, Chen and colleagues[20] were able to significantly downregulate collagen III expression without affecting collagen I expression. Although type I collagen is known to be an essential component of tendon strength, the authors speculate that downregulation of type III collagen is beneficial in decreasing adhesion formation. The precise role of TGF-β in flexor tendon healing has yet to be fully elucidated.[16]

Administration of growth differentiation factor 5 a member of the TGF-β superfamily via injection of adenovirus particles was shown to result in significantly thicker Achilles tendons and a trend toward greater strength.[21] Further, Henn and colleagues[22] demonstrated an early, beneficial effect on tendon healing in zone II flexor tendon injuries using sutures coated with growth differentiation factor 5.

The most promising in vivo results have been seen with bFGF. In tenocytes, bFGF induces type I collagen production and cellular proliferation. Tang and colleagues[23] were able to perform a gene transfer of bFGF to digital flexor tendons using the adeno-associated viral vector 2 to promote healing strength without increasing adhesion formation. Although the roles of various cytokines is yet to be fully elucidated, continued research in this field may allow us to one day use cytokine modulation to reduce tendon adhesions while improving repair strength.

TENDON ADHESION

Tendon adhesion is the most common complication of flexor tendon repair and reconstruction. The rate of adhesion formation was found to be between 4% and 10% in systematic[4] and nonsystematic reviews.[24] It has been proposed that the most important factor contributing to adhesion formation after flexor tendon repair is iatrogenic injury from poor tissue handling in the setting of an already traumatized wound bed.[25,26] A systematic review discussing the use of a modified Kessler repair technique with an epitendinous suture found that, compared with all other techniques, this technique was shown to decrease the likelihood of developing adhesions.[4] Neither age, gender, nor zone of injury were predictive of adhesion formation after flexor tendon injury.[4]

Mechanical barriers to adhesion formation have also been studied. Physical barriers made from silicone, polyethylene membranes, alumina sheaths, and polytetrafluoroethylene theoretically prevent adhesions around the repaired tendon.[6] A carbohydrate polymer ALCON-T/N was studied in a double-blind, randomized trial and was shown to lead to shorter time to final range of motion. However, total active motion at final follow-up was not improved significantly and ADCON-T/N–treated patients had a higher rupture rate.[27] The use of mechanical barriers to prevent adhesion formation is not yet routine in clinical practice.

Achieving a successful outcome requires a balance between immobilization, which can ensure integrity of the repair, and postoperative mobilization, which can prevent the formation of adhesions, stiffness, and joint contractures.[6] In a canine model, Silva and colleagues[28] found that 1.7 mm of tendon excursion was sufficient to prevent adhesion formation. Therefore, early motion protocols have been used clinically for several decades to achieve tendon excursion. In 1977, Lister and colleagues[29] showed good to excellent results with an early motion protocol for 75% of patients with zone II injuries and 84.4% of patients with flexor tendon injuries in other zones. This led to the development of several postoperative protocols emphasizing early passive motion.[30,31]

More recently, active motion protocols have been shown to improve clinical outcomes after flexor tendon repair.[32–34] In a level I prospective, randomized study, Trumble and colleagues[35] compared passive motion rehabilitation programs with early active motion with place-and-hold rehabilitation programs. Patients treated with early active range of motion when compared with passive program had greater interphalangeal joint motion, fewer flexion contractures, and greater satisfaction scores.

A systematic review of flexor tendon repair rehabilitation protocols published between 1980 and 2011 was performed by Starr and colleagues.[36] They found that, compared with early passive motion protocols, early active motion protocols resulted in higher risk of tendon rupture (4% vs 5%), but better postoperative digit range of motion. Over the time period studied, there was a statistically significant trend toward decreased rupture. The authors attribute this to better surgical techniques, materials, and a greater understanding of the effects of rehabilitation protocols.

Some patients fail to regain range of motion after several months of therapy and a tenolysis procedure may be necessary. The indication for this procedure is a failure to show improved active digital motion after at least 3 months of supervised therapy.[12] Because a vigorous and closely monitored postoperative rehabilitation protocol is necessary after tenolysis, selected patients must be well-motivated with a supple digit and subcutaneous tissues. Those who had much more passive motion than active have tendon adhesions that will benefit from tenolysis.[37]

The effectiveness of therapy after tenolysis is often limited by pain; therefore, a local anesthetic may be used to facilitate the patient to perform active flexion. An indwelling polyethylene catheter, which infuses local anesthetic, has been described.[12,38] The release of restrictive adhesions must preserve the pulley system as much as possible. Passing a small elevator through windows created in the least critical portions of the tendon sheath has been described.[12,39]

The major complication of tenolysis is tendon or graft rupture. The management of this complication requires a staged tendon reconstruction with initial implantation of a Hunter rod. Other complications include edema, pain, and injury to neurovascular structures. Skin grafting may be required for patients with long-standing contractures with inadequate skin coverage.[12]

INTERPHALANGEAL JOINT CONTRACTURE

Interphalangeal joint contracture is the most common late complication after flexor tendon repair with a reported incidence of 17%.[40] Joint contracture can result from scarring of the volar plate, tendon bowstringing owing to pulley disruption, fracture, neurovascular injury, splinting difficulties, collateral ligament contracture, skin contracture or flexor tendon adhesions, and poor nutrition.[39,41,42] Seiler[14] states that joint contracture may be more common among patients treated with dynamic flexion splinting with elastic traction.

Prevention starts with postoperative orthoses, which are used routinely by placing the wrist at flexion angle varying from 0° to 30°, metacarpophalangeal joint flexion varying from 50° to 90° and allows the interphalangeal joints to achieve full extension.[36] Early identification of interphalangeal joint contracture postoperatively starts treatment consisting of splinting the interphalangeal joints in extension between therapy sessions and at night. Increasing metacarpophalangeal joint flexion, relaxes the intrinsic mechanism, helping to resolve proximal interphalangeal joint contracture.[39,42]

Recalcitrant contractures can be considered for small joint release 4 to 6 months after tendon repair.[14] The decision to proceed with surgery is based on the patient's functional limitations and goals.[39] Surgery is aimed at first identifying extrinsic structures contributing to interphalangeal joint contracture, including the volar skin, fascia, tendon sheath, and flexor tendon adhesions. Then, intrinsic causes may be identified and treated, including the volar plate, and accessory and proper collateral ligaments. Finally, bony abnormalities blocking motion are released until full extension is achieved.[41]

RUPTURE

The rate of rupture in a systematic review was found to be 4%.[4] Surgical factors contributing to tendon rupture include weak suture material, poor repair technique with gapping that heals by scarring rather than from tenocytes, and strength not sufficient to undergo aggressive postoperative rehabilitation protocols. The results of biomechanical testing showed that repairs using 3-0 suture was 2 to 3 times stronger than repairs using 4-0 suture.[43] Additionally, a locking suture technique has been shown to increase tensile strength compared with grasping techniques.[43,44] The number of strands to use in the core suture continues to be debated. However, a meta-analysis of 29 studies failed to show superiority of one core suture technique over another.[4] Further, although the use of an epitendinous suture had an 84% lower chance of reoperation compared with repairs that did not have an epitendinous repair, it did not influence the rate of rupture.[4] Although biomechanical testing on cadaveric models demonstrated increasing the number of strands increases the fatigues strength of a tendon repair,[45] a recent systematic review failed to show a difference in clinical outcomes or rupture rates between 2-strand and multistrand core sutures.[46] It should be noted, however, that there was a trend toward lower re-rupture rate in the multistrand group[46] and no gold standard for the optimal repair has been established.[47]

In their systematic review, Chesney and colleagues[48] found no difference in rupture rates when comparing rehabilitation protocols, although tendon rupture occurs most frequently when patients are noncompliant with their rehabilitation protocol.[49] In 1 study of 23 tendon ruptures in 440 patients, approximately one-half the cases of rupture were a result of patient noncompliance, including removing the splint, lifting heavy objects, or attempting strong grasp. The authors were unable to find a relationship between age, sex, smoking, or delay between injury and tendon repair, most likely because rupture events are infrequent and the sample size is small.[50]

The preferred treatment for tendon repair rupture is reexploration and repair. Tendon repairs are weakest on postoperative days 6 through 12, with most ruptures reported around day 10.[12] Early rupture may be repaired primarily. However, ruptures that occur more than 3 weeks postoperatively are less likely to be successfully repaired and may require grafting or staged tendon reconstruction.[14]

PULLEY DISRUPTION

Pulley disruption manifests with flexor tendon bowstringing and loss of range of motion. The increased flexion force owing to bowstringing may lead to a flexion contracture. The increased linear excursion required for angular rotation may lead to a limitation in active flexion. The A2 and A4 pulleys are most critical for active digital flexion and should be repaired or reconstructed. While awaiting surgical treatment, support of the flexor tendon using the contralateral hand, a wooden block, or external ring helps to maintain tendon gliding.[42] Several techniques for pulley reconstruction have been proposed.[12] Nishida and colleagues[51] found that use of the extensor retinaculum for pulley reconstruction produced the least resistance to tendon gliding. Biomechanical analysis has shown that the volar plate "belt loop" and multiple tendon loop reconstruction is biomechanically stronger than reconstructions, which weave split tendon through the fibrous rim of the remnant pulley.[52] However, the mechanical strength required for postoperative rehabilitation and normal human hand use is unknown. Ultimately, pulley reconstruction requires a balance between strength to provide enough tension without inhibiting tendon gliding.[53]

TRIGGERING

The A2 pulley overlies the proximal two-thirds of the proximal phalanx and is a common site of flexor tendon injury. A bulbous tendon or tightly repaired tendon sheath may cause triggering at the site of repair. Tang and colleagues[54] in a healing tendon model demonstrated that incision or enlargement of the A2 pulley after tendon repair resulted in improved tendon gliding and reduced resistance during digital flexion. However, biomechanical studies have shown the A2 pulley to be the most important for flexor tendon function, followed by A4.[55] Proximal partial pulley excision may have a greater effect on digit range of motion than distal partial pulley excision.[56] To avoid the sequelae of A2 resection, reduction flexor tenoplasty has been reported.[57] Other authors have suggested "venting" of the A2 and A4 pulleys, either to facilitate repair or allow free gliding of the flexor tendons.[58] One group demonstrated that excision of up to 25% of the A2 and 75% of the A4 pulley could be performed without deleterious effects on finger range of motion or tendon excursion[59,60] and after 75% excision, mean tendon forces were sufficient to withstand activities of daily living.[61]

Intraoperatively, tendon gliding should be assessed to identify any potential sites of triggering. A partial pulley release or excision may need to be performed at the time of the repair, both for visualization and to prevent triggering. Triggering that develops after repair may be treated with scar massage, ultrasound, or corticosteroid injection.[39]

INFECTION

Infection is a rare but devastating complication after flexor tendon injury repair or reconstruction. A retrospective review of 140 patients treated for flexor tendon injuries demonstrated an infection rate of 2.1%. In this series, all wounds were treated initially with irrigation and/or scrubbing of the hand with cleansing agent followed by rinsing with sterile saline solution. Wound edges were loosely reapproximated with simple sutures, covered with sterile dressing, and immobilized with splint or bulky dressing. All patients received tetanus toxoid as indicated. Patients were treated with either early (within 12 hours) or late repair and with or without perioperative antibiotics covering gram-positive organisms. Infection was seen in 2 patients who received perioperative antibiotics, 1 treated with early repair and 1 treated in a delayed fashion. A third infection was seen in a patient treated without antibiotics, repaired more than 12 hours after injury. The authors conclude that timing of surgical repair did not seem to be a significant factor with regard to wound infection and that antibiotics should be reserved for established infections or more serious hand injuries.[62] For flexor tendon reconstructions, infection after stage I necessitates silicone rod removal followed by a healing period with appropriate antibiotic coverage before placement of a new implant if possible.[42]

HYPEREXTENSION OF THE PROXIMAL INTERPHALANGEAL JOINT

Isolated flexor digitorum superficialis rupture and volar plate injury may cause a swan neck deformity, in which there is hyperextension of the proximal interphalangeal joint with flexion of the distal interphalangeal joint.[39] Absence of the flexor digitorum superficialis tendon in a grafted finger may also result in hyperextension deformity at the proximal interphalangeal joint. The functional deficit is minimal with difficulty initiating flexion at that joint. Prevention of the swan neck deformity requires correction of volar plate injuries at the time of tendon repair and limiting hyperextension forces on the joint postoperatively. Treatment for the hyperextension deformity involves a figure-of-eight splint or tenodesis with 1 slip of the flexor digitorum superficialis across the proximal interphalangeal joint.[39,42]

QUADRIGIA

Quadrigia takes its name from the classic 4-horse chariot driven by 1 charioteer through a common rein and refers to the inability of uninjured digits to fully flex after repair. Profound cases can been seen clinically and more subtle cases may be identified with grip strength measurements. Anatomically, this complication is caused by shortening of the injured flexor digitorum profundus (FDP) tendon, which, as a result of the common muscle belly to the middle, ring, and small fingers, results in decreased proximal excursion of the uninjured tendons. Prevention of this complication relies on proper setting tendon tension during repair and reconstruction.[39] The goal of treatment is to allow the normal adjacent fingers to regain full flexion by lengthening, tenolysis or severing of the shortened tendon.[42]

LUMBRICAL PLUS FINGER

Lumbrical plus deformity is the reverse of the quadrigia effect. It is described as paradoxical extension at the interphalangeal joints of the injured digit when the patient attempts finger flexion. The lumbricals arise from the FDP and insert on the extensor mechanism. Mechanically, lengthening or laceration of the FDP tendon distal to lumbrical origin pulls the origin proximally, placing more tension on the muscle. With further proximal shift of the profundus tendon, the lumbrical exerts traction on its origin, causing interphalangeal joint extension. This complication is also seen with amputation through the middle phalanx or avulsion of the insertion of the FDP. Prevention of this complication requires placement of an appropriate length graft. Later, lumbrical muscle release relieves the paradoxical extension, allowing the patient to flex the interphalangeal joints.[63]

SUMMARY

Innovations in operative techniques, biomaterials, and rehabilitation protocols have improved the outcomes after treatment of flexor tendon injuries. Management of these complications begins with prevention through meticulous operative technique and thoughtful rehabilitation protocols. Still, complications do occur and the treatment of many of these injuries remains controversial. With the goal of preventing the most common complications after flexor tendon repair, namely, adhesions and joint contractures, research in the use of biologic modulators to promote scarless healing continues to show promise.

REFERENCES

1. Bunnell S. Repair of tendons in the fingers and description of two new instruments. Surg Gynecol Obstet 1918;26:103–10.

2. Kleinert HE, Kutz JE, Ashbell TS, et al. Primary repair of lacerated flexor tendons in "no man's land". J Bone Joint Surg Am 1967;49:577.
3. Verdan CE. Half a century of flexor-tendon surgery: current status and changing philosophies. J Bone Joint Surg Am 1972;54:472–91.
4. Dy CJ, Hernadez-Soria A, Yan M, et al. Complications after flexor tendon repair: a systematic review and meta-analysis. J Hand Surg Am 2012; 37:543–51.
5. Hill C, Riaz M, Mozzam A, et al. A regional audit of hand and wrist injuries. A study of 4873 injuries. J Hand Surg Br 1998;23:196–200.
6. Beredjiklian PK. Biologic aspects of flexor tendon laceration and repair. J Bone Joint Surg Am 2003; 85:539–50.
7. Gelberman RH. Flexor tendon physiology: tendon nutrition and cellular activity in injury and repair. Instr Course Lect 1985;34:351–60.
8. Gelberman RH, Manske PR, Akeeson WH, et al. Flexor tendon repair. J Orthop Res 1986;5:119–28.
9. Gelberman RH, Vandeberg JS, Manske PR, et al. The early stages of flexor tendon healing: a morphologic study of the first fourteen days. J Hand Surg Am 1985;10:776–84.
10. Kakar S, Khan U, McGrouther DA. Differential cellular response within the rabbit tendon unit following tendon injury. J Hand Surg Br 1998;23:627–32.
11. Starnes T, Saunders RJ, Means KR. Clinical outcomes of zone II flexor tendon repair depending on mechanism of injury. J Hand Surg Am 2012;37: 2532–40.
12. Taras JS, Gray RM, Culp RW. Complications of flexor tendon injuries. Hand Clin 1994;10:93–109.
13. Moriya T, Zhao C, An KN, et al. The effect of epitendinous suture technique on gliding resistance during cyclic motion after flexor tendon repair: a cadaveric study. J Hand Surg Am 2010;35:552–8.
14. Seiler JG. 3rd flexor tendon injury. In: Wolf SW, Hotchkiss RN, Pederson WC, et al, editors. Green's operative hand surgery, vol. 1, 6th edition. New York: Churchill Livingstone; 2011. p. 189–207.
15. Gelberman RH, Woo SL, Lothringer K, et al. Effects of early intermittent passive mobilization on healing canine flexor tendons. J Hand Surg Am 1982;7: 170–5.
16. Mostofi A, Palmer J, Akelman E. Flexor tendon injuries. In: Chung KC, Murray PM, editors. Hand surgery update 5. Rosemont (IL): American Society for Surgery of the Hand; 2011. p. 181–92.
17. Chang J, Most D, Stelnicki E, et al. Gene expression of transforming growth factor beta-1 in rabbit zone II flexor tendon wound healing: evidence for dual mechanisms of repair. Plast Reconstr Surg 1997; 100:937–44.
18. Chang J, Thunder R, Most D, et al. Studies in flexor tendon wound healing: neutralizing antibody to TGF-beta 1 increase postoperative range of motion. Plast Reconstr Surg 2000;105:148–55.
19. Zhang AY, Pham H, Ho F, et al. Inhibition of TGF-beta-induced collagen production in rabbit flexor tendons. J Hand Surg Am 2004;29:230–5.
20. Chen CH, Zhou YL, Wu YF, et al. Effectiveness of microRNA in down-regulation of TGF-b gene expression in digital flexor tendon of chickens: *in vitro* and *in vivo* study. J Hand Surg Am 2009; 34:1777–84.
21. Rickert M, Wang H, Wieloch P, et al. Adenovirus-mediated gene transfer of growth and differentiation factor-5 into tenocytes and the healing rat Achilles tendon. Connect Tissue Res 2005;46:175–83.
22. Henn RF III, Kuo CE, Kessler MW, et al. Augmentation of zone II flexor tendon repair using growth differentiation factor 5 in a rabbit model. J Hand Surg Am 2010;35(11):1825–32.
23. Tang JB, Cao Y, Zhu B, et al. Adeno-associated virus-2-mediated bFGFgene transfer to digital flexor tendons significantly increases healing strength: an in vivo study. J Bone Joint Surg Am 2009;34:900–6.
24. Tang JB. Clinical outcomes associated with flexor tendon repair. Hand Clin 2005;21:199–210.
25. Potenza AD. Tendon healing within the flexor digital sheath in the dog. J Bone Joint Surg Am 1962;44: 49–64.
26. Potenza AD. Critical evaluation of flexor-tendon healing and adhesion formation within artificial digital sheaths. J Bone Joint Surg Am 1963;45:1217–33.
27. Golash A, Kay A, Warner JG, et al. Efficacy of ADCON-T/N after primary flexor tendon repair in zone II: A controlled clinical trial. J Hand Surg Br 2003;28:113–5.
28. Silva MJ, Brodt MD, Boyer MI, et al. Effects of increased *in vivo* excursion on digital range of motion and tendon strength following flexor tendon repair. J Orthop Res 1999;17:777–83.
29. Lister GD, Kleinert HE, Kutz JE, et al. Primary flexor tendon repair followed by immediate controlled mobilization. J Hand Surg Am 1977;2:441–51.
30. Chow JA, Thomes LF, Dovelle S, et al. A combined regiment of controlled motion following flexor tendon repair in "no man's land." Plast Reconstr Surg 1987; 79:447–53.
31. Horii E, Lin GT, Cooney WP, et al. Comparative flexor tendon excursions after passive mobilization: an in vitro study. J Hand Surg Am 1992;17:559–66.
32. Bainbridge LC, Robertson C, Gillies D, et al. A comparison of post-operative mobilization of flexor tendon repairs with "passive flexion-active extension" and "controlled active motion" techniques. J Hand Surg Br 1994;19:517–21.
33. Osada D, Fujita S, Tamai K, et al. Flexor tendon repair in zone II with 6-strand techniques and early active mobilization. J Hand Surg Am 2006; 31:987–92.

34. Kitis PT, Buker N, Kara IG. Comparison of two methods of controlled mobilization of repaired flexor tendons in zone 2. Scand J Plast Reconstr Surg Hand Surg 2009;43:160–5.
35. Trumble TE, Vedder NB, Seiler JG 3rd, et al. Zone-II flexor tendon repair: a randomized prospective trial of active place-and-hold therapy compared with passive motion therapy. J Bone Joint Surg Am 2010;92:1381–9.
36. Starr HM, Snoddy M, Hammond KE, et al. Flexor tendon repair rehabilitation protocols: a systematic review. J Hand Surg Am 2013;38:1712–7.
37. Strickland JW. Flexor tenolysis. Hand Clin 1985;1: 121–32.
38. Feldscher SB, Schneider LH. Flexor tenolysis. Hand Surg 2002;7:61–74.
39. Lilly SI, Messer TM. Complications after treatment of flexor tendon injuries. J Am Acad Orthop Surg 2006; 14:387–96.
40. Kulick MI, Brazlow R, Smith S, et al. Injectable ibuprofen: preliminary evaluation of its ability to decrease peritendinous adhesions. Ann Plast Surg 1984;13:1459–67.
41. Fischer LH, Abzug JM, Osterman AL, et al. Complications of common hand and wrist surgery procedures: flexor and extensor tendon surgery. Instr Course Lect 2014;63:97–103.
42. Taras JS, Kaufmann RA. Flexor tendon reconstruction. In: Wolf SW, Hotchkiss RN, Pederson WC, et al, editors. Green's operative hand surgery, vol. 1, 6th edition. New York: Churchill Livingstone; 2011. p. 207–38.
43. Barrie KA, Tomak SL, Cholewicki J, et al. Effect of suture locking and suture caliber on fatigue strength of flexor tendon repairs. J Hand Surg Am 2001;26:340–6.
44. Hatanaka H, Zhang J, Manske PR. An in vivo study of locking and grasping techniques using a passive mobilization protocol in experimental animals. J Hand Surg Am 2000;25:260–9.
45. Barrie KA, Tomak SL, Cholewicki J, et al. The role of multiple strands and locking sutures on gap formation of flexor tendon repairs during cyclical loading. J Hand Surg Am 2000;25:714–20.
46. Hardwicke JT, Tan JJ, Foster MA, et al. A systematic review of 2-strand versus multistrand core suture techniques and functional outcome after digital flexor tendon repair. J Hand Surg Am 2014;39: 686–95.
47. Chauhan A, Palmer BA, Merrell GA. Flexor tendon repairs: techniques, eponyms, and evidence. J Hand Surg Am 2014;39:1846–53.
48. Chesney A, Chauhan A, Kattan A, et al. Systematic review of flexor tendon rehabilitation protocols in zone II of the hand. Plast Reconstr Surg 2011;127: 1583–92.
49. Strickland JW. Flexor tendon injuries: II. Operative technique. J Am Acad Orthop Surg 1995;3:55–62.
50. Harris SB, Harris D, Foster AJ, et al. The aetiology of acute rupture of flexor tendon repairs in zones 1 and 2 of the fingers during early mobilization. J Hand Surg Br 1999;24:75–80.
51. Nishida J, Amadio PC, Bettinger PC, et al. Flexor tendon-pulley interaction after pulley reconstruction: a biomechanical study in a human model in vitro. J Hand Surg Am 1998;23:665–72.
52. Lin GT, Amadio PC, An KN, et al. Biomechanical analysis of finger flexor pulley reconstruction. J Hand Surg Br 1989;14:278–82.
53. Dy CJ, Daluiksi A. Flexor pulley reconstruction. Hand Clin 2013;29:235–42.
54. Tang JB, Wang YH, Gu YT, et al. Effect of pulley integrity on excursions and work of flexion in healing flexor tendons. J Hand Surg Am 2001;26:347–53.
55. Peterson WW, Manske PR, Bollinger BA, et al. Effect of pulley excursion on flexor tendon biomechanics. J Orthop Res 1986;4:96–101.
56. Chow JC, Sensinger J, McNeal D, et al. Importance of proximal A2 and A4 pulleys to maintaining kinematics in the hand: a biomechanical study. Hand 2014;9:105–11.
57. Seradge H, Kleinert HE. Reduction flexor tenoplasty: treatment of stenosing flexor tenosynovitis distal to the first pulley. J Hand Surg Am 1981;6:543–4.
58. Kwai Ben I, Elliot D. "Venting" or partial lateral release of the A2 and A4 pulleys after repair of zone 2 flexor tendon injuries. J Hand Surg Eur 1998;23:649–54.
59. Tomaino MM, Mitsionis G, Bastidas JA, et al. The effect of partial excision of the A2 and A4 pulleys on the biomechanics of finger flexion. J Hand Surg Eur 1998;23:50–2.
60. Mitsionis G, Bastidas JA, Grewal R, et al. Feasibility of partial A2 and A4 pulley excision: effect on finger flexor tendon biomechanics. J Hand Surg Am 1999; 24:310–4.
61. Mitsionis G, Fischer KJ, Bastidas JA, et al. Feasibility of partial A2 and A4 pulley excision: residual pulley strength. J Hand Surg Eur 2000;25:90–4.
62. Stone JF, Davidson JS. The role of antibiotics and timing of repair in flexor tendon injuries of the hand. Ann Plast Surg 1998;40(1):7–13.
63. Parkes A. The "lumbrical plus" finger. J Bone Joint Surg Br 1971;53:236–9.

Management of Complications of Extensor Tendon Injuries

Kristina Lutz, MD[a], Joey Pipicelli, MScOT, CHT, OT Reg (Ont)[b], Ruby Grewal, MSc, MD, FRCSC[c,*]

KEYWORDS

• Extensor tendon • Injuries • Complications • Rehabilitation • Swan neck deformity
• Boutonnière deformity • Tendon adhesions

KEY POINTS

- Extensor tendon injuries are common and early recognition and treatment are key to the management of such injuries.
- Rehabilitation differs according to zone of injury and is important in preventing complications associated with injuries to the extensor mechanism.
- Surgical treatment of complications must be used in conjunction with rehabilitation by hand therapy.

INTRODUCTION

The management of complications of extensor tendon injuries will be discussed based on the zone of injury (**Fig. 1**).

ZONE I (MALLET FINGER)

Treatment and prognosis of acute mallet finger injuries depend on associated tissue injury and chronicity of injury. These injuries can be open or closed, with or without associated fracture or dislocation. Conservative treatment with splint immobilization is sufficient to restore tendon continuity in most cases. The distal interphalangeal (DIP) joint should be splinted in 0° of extension or slight hyperextension with an aluminum-padded splint, commercially available Stack splint, or custom-molded thermoplastic splints for 6 to 8 weeks continuously. After this, we recommend a gradual weaning-off period for an additional 6 weeks; however, the splint should continue to be worn at night until 3 months after treatment initiation.

In order to prevent complications, during the immobilization phase it is imperative that the splint fits well and is adjusted accordingly to ensure that an extensor lag does not develop and that proximal interphalangeal (PIP) range of motion (ROM) is maintained. Once tendon/bone healing has been confirmed, a structured mobilization protocol prevents overstretching of the terminal tendon and recurrence. Patients are instructed to perform active tendon gliding every 2 to 3 hours for 10 to 20 repetitions while monitoring for signs of extension lag. During the first week of mobilization, 20° to 30° of active flexion of the DIP joint is permitted, 40° to 45° at week 2, followed by a gradual increase over the following few weeks. Overzealous patients may benefit from a template exercise splint with specific angles of motion during the first 2 weeks of mobilization to prevent overstretching of the terminal tendon. If an

Disclosures: The authors have no disclosures.

[a] Division of Plastic Surgery, Department of Surgery, Roth|McFarlane Hand and Upper Limb Centre, St. Joseph's Health Care, Western University, Room D1-204, 268 Grosvenor Street, London, Ontario N6A 4L6, Canada; [b] Division of Hand Therapy, Faculty of Rehabilitation Sciences, Roth|McFarlane Hand and Upper Limb Centre, St. Joseph's Health Care, Western University, Room D3-148, 268 Grosvenor Street, London, Ontario N6A 4L6, Canada; [c] Division of Orthopedic Surgery, Roth|McFarlane Hand and Upper Limb Centre, St. Joseph's Health Care, Western University, 268 Grosvenor Street, London, Ontario N6A 4L6, Canada
* Corresponding author.
E-mail address: rgrewa@uwo.ca

Hand Clin 31 (2015) 301–310
http://dx.doi.org/10.1016/j.hcl.2014.12.006
0749-0712/15/$ – see front matter

hand.theclinics.com

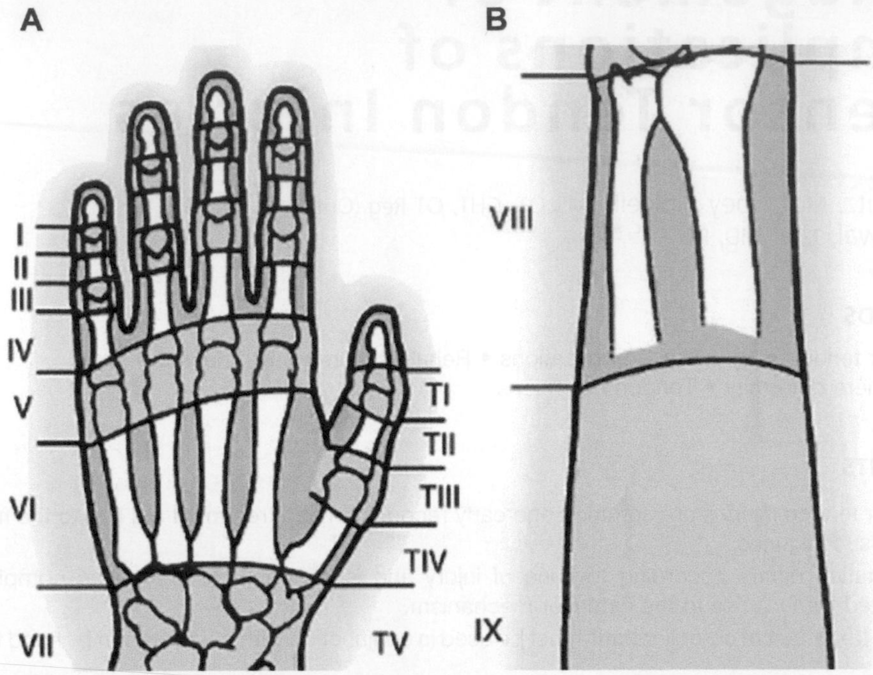

Fig. 1. (*A, B*) Extensor tendon zones of injury. (*Adapted from* Baratz M, Schmidt C, Hughes T. Extensor tendon injuries. In: Green DP, Hotchkiss RN, Pederson WC, editors. Green's operative hand surgery. 5th edition. New York: Churchill Livingstone; 2005. p. 190; with permission.)

extensor lag recurs, it is recommended that mobilization be discontinued and the patient should return to continuous full-time splinting for up to an additional 3 months.

This nonoperative method has been shown to be successful in up to 80% of patients, with success largely depending on patient compliance with the splint. Transient skin-related changes from splint use have been described in up to 45% of patients.[1] These changes are best managed with protective dressings.

There is a subset of patients with zone 1 injuries in which open reduction internal fixation may be indicated: those with open injuries, those who are not compliant with or who are unable to tolerate splinting, and/or those with injuries consisting of a large dorsal fragment with volar subluxation of the distal phalanx. Various techniques have been described and include primary repair with K-wire, pullout suture/button repair of terminal tendon, and pinning the DIP in extension for mallet fractures.[2] Complications (52%) related to K-wire fixation include pin site infection, nail deformity, joint incongruity, implant failure, residual pain, and osteomyelitis.[1]

Acute Mallet Finger with Secondary Swan Neck Deformity

The swan neck deformity is any primary disorder that causes excessive tension on the extensor apparatus, leading to PIP joint hyperextension and flexion of the DIP joint. Secondary swan neck deformity following the mallet finger is a common cause of such an imbalance. This deformity can occur with chronic mallet injuries or immediately following injury, especially in patients who present with laxity in other digits.

In order to prevent such kinematic chain imbalances, we advocate an alternative to the splinting protocol described earlier. Patients can be positioned in splints, which place the PIP joint in 40° to 60° of flexion with the DIP joint in full extension. This position encourages the volar plate to tighten and allows the lateral bands to lie closer to the anatomic axis of rotation, thereby decreasing tension at the repair site and allowing for gapless healing (**Fig. 2**).[3] This method was first introduced by Smillie[3] in 1937 and was common practice until the Stack splint was popularized in 1986.[3,4] However, a dorsal splint should be used, which allows for frequent PIP joint exercises within the confines of the splint to prevent stiffness and restrict DIP joint motion. The wearing schedule for such splints is similar to what was previously described for mallet injury.

Chronic Mallet Finger

Patients who do not seek medical attention acutely or who fail initial treatment regimens may be left with a chronic extensor lag at the DIP joint.

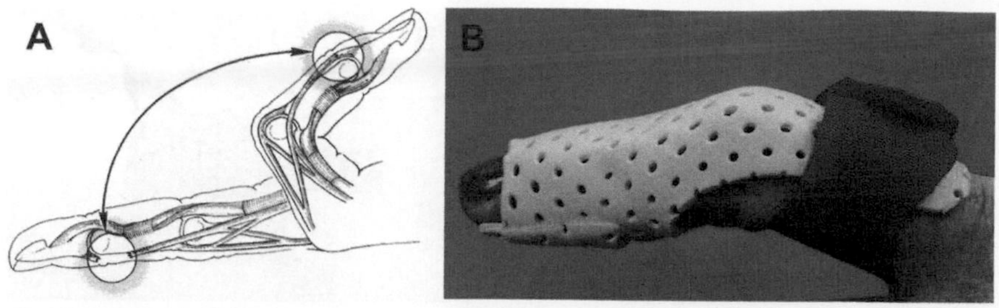

Fig. 2. (*A*) Mallet fingers with secondary swan neck deformity should be managed with the PIP joint positioned in 40° to 60° of flexion to decrease tension on the terminal tendon and allow gapless healing. (*B*) A simple dorsal splint allows complete DIP joint extension and permits frequent PIP joint active flexion exercises within the confines of the splint. ([*A*] *From* Tubiana R. The Hand, Vol. III. Philadelphia: WB Saunders; 1988; with permission.)

The resultant deformity does not interfere with function and most of these patients are asymptomatic. These patients occasionally seek medical attention because of appearance, pain at the DIP joint, or secondary swan neck deformity.

The management of a chronic extensor lag as a complication of terminal tendon injury should begin with nonoperative options. In all cases, splinting the DIP joint in neutral to 10° of hyperextension for 6 to 12 weeks should be considered first-line therapy.[5,6] If there is a secondary swan neck deformity, the splint should be extended to include the PIP joint in 40° to 60° of flexion. Surgery to rebalance the finger should not be considered until the joint deformities are passively correctable and the articular surfaces are determined to be healthy.

Operative treatment options include immobilization with transarticular K-wire fixation; excision of tendon-scar unit and fixation in hyperextension; Fowler central slip tenotomy, which attempts to rebalance the extensor mechanism by transecting the insertion of the central slip at the base of the middle phalanx, thereby transmitting increased extensor force excursion to the terminal tendon[7]; and spiral oblique retinacular ligament reconstruction.[8,9] Salvage procedures include DIP arthrodesis or amputation at the DIP.

ZONE II (MIDDLE PHALANX)

Injuries in zone II usually result from sharp lacerations, saw injuries, and crush injuries to the middle phalanx. For partial injuries involving less than 50% of the tendon (ie, 1 functioning lateral band), full extension of the DIP can be achieved and therefore treatment with a short course of splinting the DIP in extension is appropriate. Complete tendon injuries should be treated with primary repair. Several options exist, including dermadesis, figure-of-eight, or running suture techniques.[10] All techniques should be supplemented by a 6-week course of DIP joint splinting in extension or alternatively by longitudinal K-wire fixation through an extended DIP joint. Rehabilitation protocols encourage active and passive ROM of the PIP and metacarpophalangeal (MCP) to prevent stiffness.

COMPLICATIONS

Chronic zone II injuries may be treated with tendon grafts to reconstruct the spiral oblique retinacular ligament (ORL). In this procedure an ORL is created using a free palmaris or plantaris tendon graft. The graft is fixed to the distal phalanx with a pull-out button and passed between the flexor sheath and the neurovascular bundles volar to the PIP joint in a spiral fashion. The graft tension is then set and anchored into the proximal phalanx with a pull-out button.[8] An axial K-wire can be used to pin the DIP joint in a neutral position and an oblique K-wire can be used to pin the PIP joint in 10° to 15° of flexion.[9]

ZONE III (PROXIMAL INTERPHALANGEAL JOINT)

Suspicion for central slip disruption is necessary for injuries in zone III because initial findings may be subtle, including only swelling of the PIP, mild extensor lag, or weakness in extension of the PIP. The Elson test is useful in establishing the diagnosis[11] and is positive before a clear deformity is evident. With the PIP at 90° of flexion, the middle phalanx is extended against resistance. If the central slip is injured, PIP extension is weak and the DIP is immobile in extension and rigid because the lateral bands are being activated.

Tendon injury at the PIP joint must be closely monitored to achieve favorable results. Most injuries can be managed nonoperatively, consisting of continuous PIP joint extension splinting (with DIP free) for 6 weeks followed by a gradual weaning period. Immobilization can be achieved through the use of splints (**Fig. 3**) or cylinder

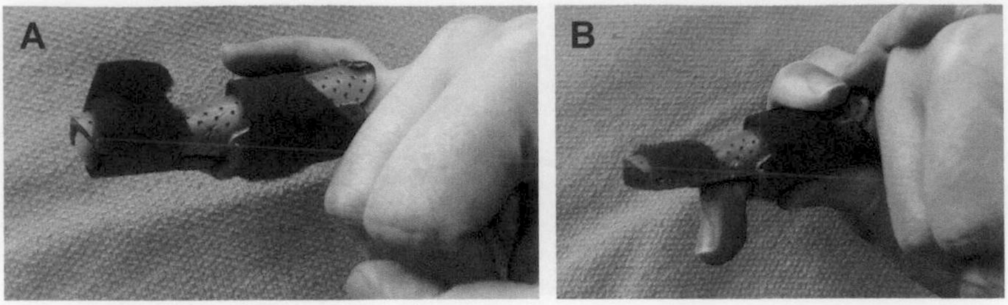

Fig. 3. Custom-made thermoplastic splint used for zone III and IV extensor tendon injuries. (*A*) This splint maintains the PIP and DIP joint in full extension. (*B*) Isolated active DIP joint flexion and extension can easily be performed in this splint, preventing loss of extensibility of the ORLs and helping to draw the lateral bands dorsal to correct alignment dorsal to the axis of rotation of the PIP joint.

plaster casts. During the initial 6 weeks, patients are instructed only to perform active DIP joint flexion and extension exercises every 1 to 2 hours for 10 to 25 repetitions. This exercise allows for distal gliding of the lateral bands and central slip and also draws the lateral bands into correct alignment slightly dorsal to the axis of rotation of the PIP joint. This process allows the triangular ligament to tighten to prevent volar migration of the lateral bands, thereby preventing the development of boutonnière deformity.

After 6 weeks of splinting, the patient is permitted to gradually wean off the splint during the day; however, the patient must wear the splint at night for an additional 6 weeks. During the first week of mobilization, we begin a short arc of active PIP joint motion to 50°, and progress to 70° during the second week of mobilization. Passive PIP joint flexion is permitted at 10 weeks as required. Grip strengthening exercises are initiated at this time. If PIP joint stiffness is a complication, patients may be placed in a dynamic or static-progressive PIP joint flexion splint at 12 to 14 weeks. If an extensor lag develops, the patient is instructed to return to full-time splint wear for an additional 4 to 6 weeks and continue with frequent DIP joint exercises.

Open injuries, displaced avulsion fractures of the dorsal middle phalanx, and nonsurgical treatment failure warrant surgical exploration and fixation in addition to splinting for 6 weeks. Avulsion fractures can be treated operatively with suture anchor repair; base of middle phalanx fractures can be treated with mini-screws; and if there is a deficiency of the extensor tendon, central slip reconstruction may be necessary.

Acutely repaired central slip injuries immobilized full time for 6 weeks postoperatively often develop complications, with impaired tendon gliding resulting in extensor tendon lag, dorsal joint capsular tightness, and joint stiffness causing significant limitations in overall hand function. In order to prevent such complications, we recommend the initiation of a controlled immediate active short-arc PIP joint motion program (**Table 1**) in the first 2 days postoperatively. This program minimizes tension to the repair during active tendon gliding exercises by permitting proximal and distal excursion of the involved tendons. For the first 6 weeks, the finger is splinted (DIP and PIP joints in full extension) full time and removed only for ROM exercises (see **Table 1**). For the following 6 weeks, the splint is worn nightly, and only intermittently during the day. At any time, if a lag develops during ROM exercises, the exercises are discontinued until 6 weeks after repair. The exercises are to be performed in the splint hourly for 10 to 20 repetitions.

Boutonnière Deformity

The major complication of untreated central slip injuries is the formation of a boutonnière deformity (**Fig. 4**). Acute (flexible) boutonnière deformities can be treated with splinting the PIP in extension

Table 1
Short-arc PIP joint ROM program

	Exercise Regime
Weeks	**Joint Position**
1[a]	Splint to permit 30° PIP flexion and 20°–25° DIP joint flexion
2[a]	Splint modified to permit 40° PIP flexion and 25° DIP flexion
3[a]	Splint modified to permit 50° PIP flexion and 35° DIP flexion
4[a]	Splint modified to permit 70°–80° PIP flexion and 50° DIP flexion
5–6	Full composite digital flexion and extension permitted

[a] Exercises are performed with the wrist in 30° of flexion and MCP joint in neutral.

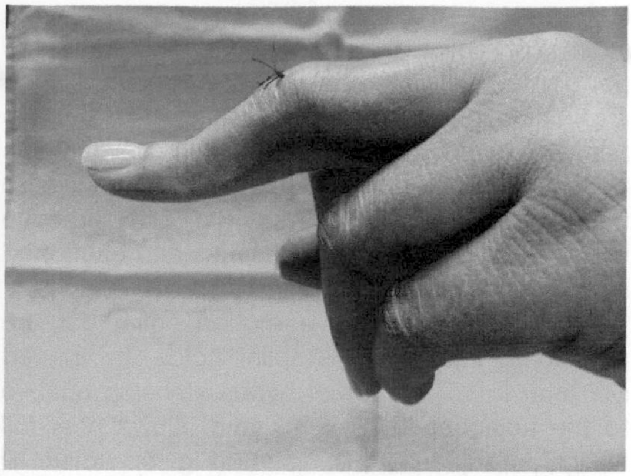

Fig. 4. Boutonnière deformity following acute zone 3 injury.

for 6 weeks followed by 6 weeks of nighttime splinting. Flexion exercises of DIP while the PIP is extended are performed throughout the treatment course, which promotes the lateral bands to pull dorsally from their volarly subluxed position.

Chronic injuries to the central slip that did not receive or failed acute treatment often evolve into a fixed (or chronic) boutonnière deformity. Burton[12] classified chronic boutonnière deformity into 3 stages to guide treatment, which is outlined in **Table 2**.

Once full passive PIP joint extension is achieved, patients are immobilized in a static PIP joint extension splint for 6 to 8 weeks full time, performing frequent DIP joint active flexion and extension exercises. The purpose of such exercises is to encourage distal gliding of the lateral bands and to draw them dorsal to the axis of rotation of the PIP joint to allow the triangular ligament to tighten. The triangular ligament assists with minimizing the amount of volar migration of the lateral bands during digital flexion following the immobilization period.

ZONE IV (PROXIMAL PHALANX)

Acute injuries of the extensor mechanism at the level of the proximal phalanx are most often secondary to dorsal lacerations and may be seen in conjunction with fractures of the proximal phalanx. The extensor mechanism at this level wraps around the proximal phalanx and so injuries are frequently partial. If the injury to the extensor tendon results in no functional loss or if the tendon is explored and there is less than 50% involvement, then management with splinting in extension and early ROM should be implemented. Hand therapy is similar to therapy following zone III injuries. If the injury results in a functional loss of extension, management with surgical exploration and repair should

Table 2
Burton classification of boutonnière deformities

Stage	Description	Treatment	Treatment Goal
1	Passively correctable deformity	Serial casting, splinting, dynamic, and/or static-progressive splinting to encourage PIP extension plus nighttime serial progressive static extension splinting	Gain full passive PIP joint extension and full active and passive DIP joint flexion, night splint to maintain extension achievement made during the day
2	Fixed contracture, contracted lateral bands	As in stage 1. If PIP joint extension is not achievable, surgical release of PIP joint is needed (note: deformities ≤30° difficult to improve with surgery)	As above
3	Fixed contracture, joint fibrosis, contractures of collateral ligament and volar plate	Terminal tendon tenotomy (distal Fowler or dolphin tenotomy) Tendon grafts Lateral band mobilization and relocation Curtis staged reconstruction	To convert from a fixed to a flexible deformity
4	Stage 3 + PIP joint arthritis	PIP arthroplasty or arthrodesis	Control pain Optimize function

From Burton RI. Extensor tendons – late reconstruction. In: Green DP, editor. Operative Hand Surgery. New York: Churchill Livingstone; 1988. p. 2073–116; with permission.

be implemented. The increased strength of core suture repairs or running interlocking horizontal mattress sutures allows early ROM protocols, which protect the repair and prevent tendon adhesions.

Complications

Extensor tendon adhesions may form after primary tendon repair and result in a stiff finger, with inability to fully flex the PIP and DIP joints. A full 6-month trial with hand therapy should be exhausted before operative interventions are considered. Ideally, full passive ROM should be achieved before embarking on operative extensor tenolysis. This condition is not a contraindication to surgery; however, if there is joint involvement requiring a concomitant joint release, patients should be aware that outcomes are not as favorable. Creighton and Steichen[13] reported the results of tenolysis after fracture, and found only a 31% improvement in total active motion overall, 50% improvement in extensor lag if only a tenolysis was required, and 21% improvement in total active motion if a dorsal capsulotomy was required with no improvement of active extensor lag.

ZONE V (METACARPOPHALANGEAL JOINT)

Sharp injuries involving the MCP joint are often the result of a clenched fist striking the tooth of another person (ie, human fight bite). The main concern acutely for these patients is the high risk of infection,[14] with associated tendon injuries a secondary concern. If localized or systemic infection develops, the treatment involves surgical debridement, broad-spectrum antibiotics, and splinting in extension.

Non–fight bite injuries include closed sagittal band ruptures with resulting subluxation of the extensor tendon. Radial sagittal band ruptures of the middle and ring fingers are most common and can occur secondary to direct trauma to the dorsal metatarsophalangeal (MP) joint or resisted extension. Patients complain that, during MCP joint flexion, the extensor digitorum communis (EDC) slips into the ulnar valley between the metacarpal heads and causes swelling, pain, difficulty achieving full MCP flexion, and possibly snapping with either tendon subluxation or relocation. If such injuries are not managed correctly and the extensor tendon remains subluxated in the ulnar valley, MCP joint extension will be limited, leading to an extensor quadriga.[15]

Acute sagittal band rupture with tendon subluxation within 3 weeks or less from the time of injury can be treated nonoperatively. In the past, such injuries have been immobilized for 6 to 8 weeks in a hand-based or forearm-based MCP joint static extension splint. The patient is instructed to perform active interphalangeal (IP) joint flexion and extension exercises exclusively 4 to 8 times per day for 10 to 20 repetitions. Following this period of MCP joint immobilization, patients are transitioned to buddy taping and gradual increase in hand use over the next 6 weeks and cautioned not to perform forceful resistive gripping.

Alternatively, a relative motion splint can be applied to injuries. This splint holds the injured MP joint in 15° to 20° of hyperextension relative to the adjacent MCP joints and allows near-full flexion of adjacent MCP joints (**Fig. 5**). Active IP motion is not restricted in this design.[16,17] This splint should be worn full time for 8 weeks. Patients who fail immobilization or who present late (>3 weeks after injury) are considered for surgical repair. Primary repair of the radial sagittal band with possible release of the ulnar sagittal band to allow the tendon to centralize is the first-line treatment. If this is not achievable, sagittal band reconstruction may be considered using a distal slip of extensor tendon, juncturae tendineae, or lumbrical muscle transfer.[18] In the past, following such procedures, a period of immobilization was instituted for 4 to 6 weeks. This immobilization often produces dense adhesion formation, limiting active and passive MCP joint flexion and active digital extension. Our preference is to apply a relative motion splint as previously described following acute injuries. Progression of rehabilitation is the same following both acute and chronic injury management.

ZONE VI (DORSAL HAND)

Acute injuries over the dorsum of the hand have a good prognosis. Dorsal hand injuries resulting from lacerations through or distal to juncturae tendineae can be difficult to diagnose because of minimal extensor lag (patients can still extend MCP via extensor indicies proprius [EIP], extensor digiti minimi [EDM] and/or juncturae tendineae). Injuries in proximal zone VI can result in retraction of the proximal tendon stump, making repair more challenging. Extensor tendon lacerations of greater than 50% at this level are amenable to repair using a core suture. The increased overlying subcutaneous tissue lessens the degree of adhesion formation and increased excursion of the tendon at this level makes it amenable to dynamic splinting.

Complications

Typical complications include rerupture, adhesion formation, and joint stiffness. In the case of extensor tendon rerupture or chronic injuries in

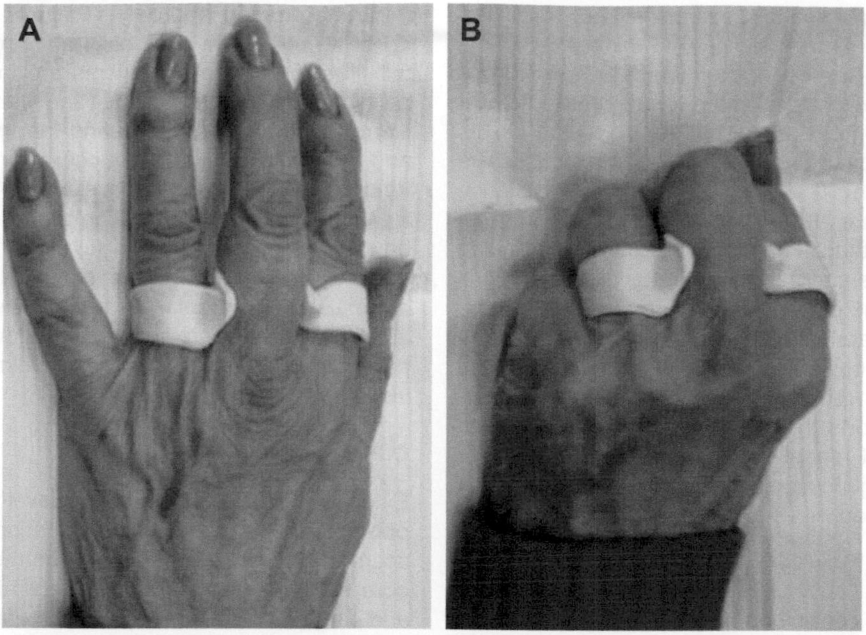

Fig. 5. The relative motion splint can be used to treat acute sagittal band injuries with tendon subluxation. This splint can also be used following acute or chronic sagittal band reconstruction. This splint allows early controlled mobilization of the affected digit and minimizes tension placed on the sagittal band during extension (*A*) and flexion (*B*). (*From* Catalano LW, Gupta S, Ragland R, et al. Closed treatment of non-rheumatoid extensor tendon dislocations at the metacarpophalangeal joint. J Hand Surg 2006;31(2):242–5; with permission.)

zone IV, side-to-side tendon transfers, intercalary tendon grafts, or 2-stage tendon reconstruction are viable treatment options. In long-standing cases of tendon loss, scar tissue may intervene and some patients may have adequate function even with total loss of EDC over the dorsum of the hand.

The primary goal is to prevent complications by ensuring adherence to a structured therapy program. Extensor tendon repairs in zones V and VI can be managed postoperatively by immobilization, controlled passive motion, or through immediate controlled active motion.[19–21]

Immobilization of the wrist and metacarpophalangeal joints

Immobilization following simple zone V and VI extensor tendon repairs has been shown to produce excellent outcomes at 6 months after repair.[22] However, in complex injuries with multiple tendon involvement and/or metacarpal fractures, immobilization produces dense adhesion formation, which limits active and passive tendon glide during both digital flexion and extension. Immobilization should be reserved for noncompliant patients or children.

To prevent complications such as tendon adhesions and joint stiffness, we recommend that patients are referred to hand therapy within the first 2 to 5 days after repair. Custom splint fabrication with the wrist positioned in 25° of extension and the MCP joints in full extension allows the patient to flex and extend the PIP and DIP joints during the day. We recommend the use of a removable component that places the IP joints in full extension for night use. The purpose of this component is to prevent PIP joint flexion contractures. At 4 weeks after repair, the splint can be discontinued and the patient instructed in active composite digital flexion and extension exercises. At 8 weeks, gentle resistance exercises are instituted as needed to enhance both proximal and distal extensor tendon excursion.

Early passive motion

Controlled early passive motion programs should be reserved for complex injuries to minimize postoperative joint stiffness and allow controlled proximal and distal tendon excursion. Such patients are typically referred to hand therapy within the first 3 days after repair for custom dynamic splint fabrication. The wrist should be positioned in approximately 25° of extension with the MCP and interphalangeal joints positioned in neutral in dynamic extension slings. This splint is worn continuously for 4 weeks. MCP joint flexion can be controlled by stoppers and can be adjusted by the therapist. Intrinsic-plus exercises are performed to allow 40° of MCP joint flexion during the first week, increasing by 10° to 15° on a weekly basis. Intrinsic-minus exercises are also performed by simply sliding the extension slings proximal to the PIP joints. These exercises produce minimal tension at the repair site. This splint is worn continuously for 4 to 6 weeks. On its removal, active and passive ROM exercises are instituted. At 8 weeks, progressive resistance exercises are added to the therapy program as needed, with full unrestricted hand use beginning at 12 weeks after repair or as the injury permits.

This form of rehabilitation remains common. However, fabrication of such splints is expensive and time consuming for therapists because the splints often require frequent adjustment. The literature supports their use; however, we think that this form of rehabilitation should be reserved for complex injuries because clinical outcomes can be maximized with simpler rehabilitation and splint designs.

Immediate controlled active motion

Early, protected, active motion of extensor tendon repairs using low-profile splints is recommended for zone V and VI injuries.[16] The splint (**Fig. 6**) consists of 2 components, one that holds the wrist in approximately 15° to 25° extension, and another (the yoke component) that holds the affected MCP joint in 15° to 20° of hyperextension relative to the adjacent MCP joints while allowing near-full MCP joint flexion. The yoke links the injured digit to the noninjured digits and functions to unload the repair and harness extension forces during active motion through the juncturae tendineae, which are on both sides of the digit. The ideal injury for this rehabilitation approach is the long or ring finger extensor tendon, with the index and small finger extensor tendons theoretically not suitable for this rehabilitation approach. Patients are placed in the 2-part splint with both components worn full time for 4 weeks. Patients are instructed to perform active intrinsic-plus and intrinsic-minus exercises every 2 hours during the first 4 weeks and are not permitted to use their hands for functional activity during this time. At 4 weeks the forearm component can be discontinued; however, the yoke is worn full time for an additional 2 weeks. At 8 weeks, resistance exercises are initiated. This splint design and rehabilitation approach has been shown to be safe and to produce excellent ROM with minimal therapy visits.[19,20]

ZONE VII (WRIST)

Extensor tendon injuries at this level can have a poor prognosis because of formation of tendon scarring and adhesions. We recommend using a core suture repair method to maximize strength and early postoperative dynamic splinting to minimize adhesion formation. The extensor retinaculum must also be taken into consideration with injuries in this zone. It is important to preserve enough retinaculum to prevent bowstringing, and to excise the portion over the repair site to prevent adhesions.

Zone VII injuries can result in reduced gliding amplitude of the tendon proximally as well as distally because the tendons can become tethered in the fibro-osseous sheath. This tethering can contribute to limitations of digital and wrist motion in both flexion and extension. Distal zone VII injuries can result in loss of combined wrist and digital flexion caused by intertendinous as well as peritendinous adhesions. Independent digital flexion can also be diminished because these

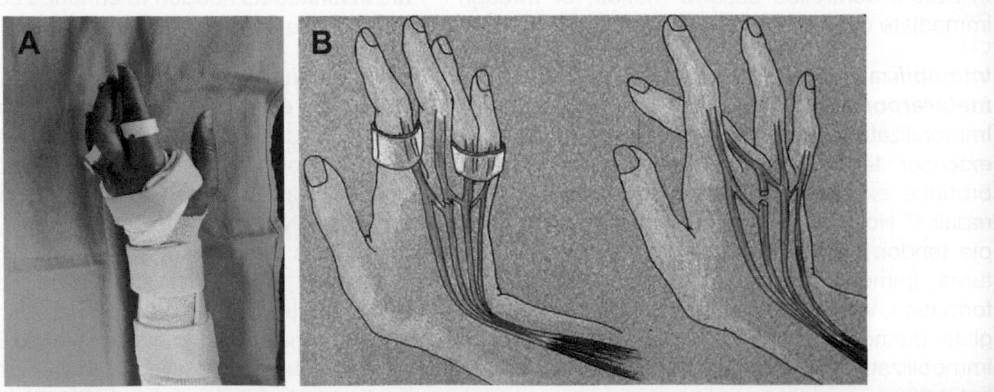

Fig. 6. (*A*) Immediate controlled active motion orthosis suing wrist support and yoke. This low-profile splint design allows early protective motion. (*B*) Immediate controlled active motion yoke links the injured digit to the noninjured digits. The yoke may function to unload the repair and harness extension forces during active motion. (*From* Howell JW, Merritt WH, Robinson SJ. Immediate controlled active motion following zone 4–7 extensor tendon repair. J Hand Ther 2005;18(2):182; with permission.)

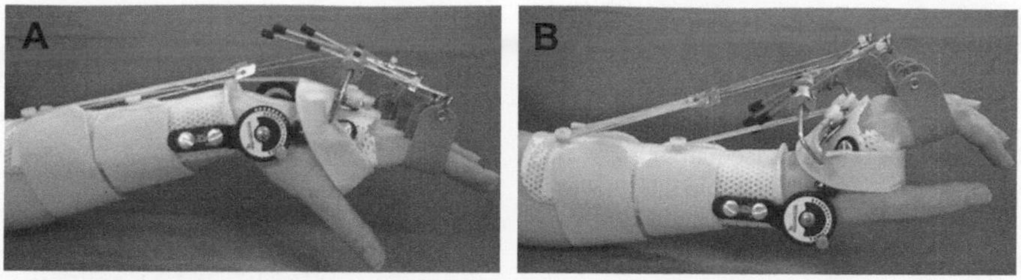

Fig. 7. Wrist tenodesis splint for early controlled motion of the extensor tendons. (*A*) Wrist flexion–finger extension. (*B*) Wrist extension–finger flexion. (*From* Chinchalkar SJ, Pipicelli JG. Complications of extensor tendon repairs at the extensor retinaculum. J H Microsurg 2010;2(1):3–12; with permission.)

adhesions result in impaired tendon gliding through the fibro-osseous sheath during flexion. Combined extension of the wrist and digits are most often unrestricted because the tendons glide proximally. On flexion of the wrist the digits can be strongly pulled into extension, showing a strong extensor-plus. Extensor-plus is a condition that shortens the excursion of the extensor hood mechanism over the MCP joint and proximal phalanx, causing a strong extension tendency of the fingers when the wrist is flexed.

Rehabilitation

It is our opinion that EDC repairs within or in close vicinity to the extensor retinaculum should be managed postoperatively using a controlled active and passive mobilization program.[23] This program can be achieved by using traditional dynamic splinting, incorporating wrist tenodesis, and differential tendon gliding exercises. This treatment approach maximizes EDC excursion, minimizes gliding resistance, provides differential tendon excursion, places minimal tension at the repair site, and prevents postoperative complications.

Wrist tenodesis following zones VI to VIII tendon repair is a well-established concept.[24–26] Two articles have addressed early controlled motion of the wrist and digits using a tenodesis motion program following injuries in close vicinity to the extensor retinaculum. Chinchalkar and Yong[24] (2004) recommend a dynamic wrist hinge splint, whereas Eissens and colleagues[25] (2007) recommend an early controlled active motion program. The goal of treatment is to maximize independent as well as combined mobility of the wrist and digits. Wrist tenodesis can begin during the inflammatory phase of wound healing within 3 to 5 days following tenorrhaphy. Wrist joint flexion may be limited between 0° and 10° initially and then gradually increased by 10° per week. Tenodesis can be performed out of the traditional dynamic splint or within a double reverse Kleinert splint, which includes a hinged wrist component and dynamic digital outriggers (**Fig. 7**).[24,26] Multiple EDC repairs may benefit from differential tendon gliding exercises beginning during the inflammatory phase of healing, which can be accomplished by actively flexing 1 digit at a time while the other digits are maintained in dynamic traction extension. The MCP joints can be moved from 30° to 40° during the first week, which can be increased by 10° to 15° weekly.

The principles of management of extensor tendon adhesions in zone VII parallel those of more distal zones. At least 6 months of nonoperative techniques of extrinsic excursion and splinting must be exhausted before consideration of surgery. Tenolysis is appropriate when tenodesis is secondary to scarring with no loss of tendon length. If tendon is shortened, the Littler technique of extensor tendon release may be performed.

In the case of attritional ruptures (eg, following distal radius fractures or rheumatoid arthritis) primary repair is usually not possible and management includes tendon transfers or tendon reconstruction using a free tendon graft.

ZONE VIII (FOREARM)

Distal forearm injuries may involve the extensor tendon, musculotendinous junction, or muscle bellies. Extensor tendons can be repaired with core sutures and muscle injuries can be repaired with absorbable figure-of-eight sutures in the muscle. Rarely, injuries occur at the musculotendinous junction. These injuries are difficult to repair because the muscle fascia is often too flimsy to hold a core stitch. In this case, side-to-side tendon transfer is a good option.

REFERENCES

1. Stern PJ, Kastrup JJ. Complications and prognosis of treatment of mallet finger. J Hand Surg Am 1988; 13(3):329–34.
2. Doyle JR. Extensor tendons – acute injuries. In: Green DF, editor. Operative hand surgery. 4th edition. New York: Churchill Livingstone; 1999. p. 195–8.

3. Smillie IS. Mallet finger. Br J Surg 1937;24:439–45.
4. Stack HG. A modified splint for mallet finger. J Hand Surg Br 1986;11:263.
5. Abouna JM, Brown H. The treatment of mallet finger. The results in a series of 148 consecutive cases and a review of the literature. Br J Surg 1968;55(9):653–67.
6. Garberman SF, Diao E, Peimer CL. Mallet finger: results of early versus delayed closed treatment. J Hand Surg Am 1994;19(5):850–2.
7. Fowler SB. The management of tendon injuries. J Bone Joint Surg Am 1959;41A(4):579–80.
8. Thompson JS, Littler JW, Upton J. The spiral oblique retinacular ligament (SORL). J Hand Surg Am 1978;3(5):482–7.
9. Kleinman WB, Petersen DP. Oblique retinacular ligament reconstruction for chronic mallet finger deformity. J Hand Surg Am 1984;9:399–404.
10. Newport ML, Blair WF, Steyers CM Jr. Long-term results of extensor tendon repair. J Hand Surg Am 1990;15(6):961–6.
11. Elson RA. Rupture of the central slip of the extensor hood of the finger: a test for early diagnosis. J Bone Joint Surg Br 1986;68:229–31.
12. Burton RI. Extensor tendons – late reconstruction. In: Green DP, editor. Operative hand surgery. New York: Churchill Livingstone; 1988. p. 2073–116.
13. Creighton JJ Jr, Steichen JB. Complications in phalangeal and metacarpal fracture management: results of extensor tenolysis. Hand Clin 1994;10:111–6.
14. Chadaev AP, Jukhtin VI, Butkevich AT, et al. Treatment of infected clenched-fist human bite wounds in the area of metacarpophalangeal joints. J Hand Surg Am 1996;21(2):299–303.
15. Chinchalkar SJ, Gan BS, McFarlane RM, et al. Extensor quadriga: pathomechanics and treatment. Can J Plast Surg 2004;12(4):174–8.
16. Merritt WH, Howell JW, Tune R, et al. Achieving immediate active motion by using relative motion splinting after long extensor repair and sagittal band ruptures with tendon subluxation. Operat Tech Plast Reconstr Surg 2000;7:31–7.
17. Catalano LW, Gupta S, Ragland R, et al. Closed treatment of non-rheumatoid extensor tendon dislocations at the metacarpophalangeal joint. J Hand Surg 2006;31(2):242–5.
18. Carroll CT, Moore JR, Weiland AJ. Posttraumatic ulnar subluxation of the extensor tendons: a reconstructive technique. J Hand Surg Am 1987;12:227–31.
19. Howell JW, Merritt WH, Robinson SJ. Immediate controlled active motion following zone 4–7 extensor tendon repair. J Hand Ther 2005;18(2):182–90.
20. Svens B, Ames E, Burford K, et al. Relative active motion programs following extensor tendon repair: a pilot study using a prospective cohort and evaluating outcomes following orthotic interventions. J Hand Ther 2014. [Epub ahead of print].
21. Burns MC, Derby B, Neumeister MW. Wyndell Merritt immediate controlled active motion (ICAM) protocol following extensor tendon repairs in zone IV-VII: review of literature, orthosis design, and case study – a multimedia article. Hand (NY) 2013;8(1):17–22.
22. Mowlavi A, Burns M, Brown RE. Dynamic versus static splinting of simple zone V and VI extensor tendon repairs: a prospective, randomized, controlled study. Plast Reconstr Surg 2005;115(2):482–7.
23. Chinchalkar SJ, Pipicelli JG. Complications of extensor tendon repairs at the extensor retinaculum. J Hand Microsurg 2010;2(1):3–12.
24. Chinchalkar S, Yong SA. A double reverse Kleinert extension splint for extensor tendon repairs in zones VI to VIII. J Hand Ther 2004;17(4):424–6.
25. Eissens MH, Schut SM, van der Sluis CK. Early active wrist mobilization in extensor tendon injuries in zones 5, 6, or 7. J Hand Ther 2007;20(1):89–91.
26. Evans RB. Clinical management of extensor tendon injuries. In: Mackin EJ, Callahan AD, Osterman AL, et al, editors. Rehabilitation of the hand and upper extremity. 5th edition. St Louis (MO): CV Mosby; 2002. p. 542–79.

Management of Complications Relating to Complex Traumatic Hand Injuries

Joel Ferreira, MD, John R. Fowler, MD*

KEYWORDS

• Complex regional pain syndrome • Stiffness • Infection

KEY POINTS

- Each injury is unique, and treatment must be individualized to achieve the best possible outcome.
- Early recognition and appropriate treatment are essential to prevent long-term morbidity.
- Complex regional pain syndrome involves an abnormal exaggerated response by the body to injury and is best treated with early recognition and hand therapy.
- The management of stiffness in the setting of complex soft tissue injury should always start with prevention.

Complex traumatic hand injuries (**Fig. 1**) present a significant challenge to the hand surgeon, as one must often manage osseous, soft tissue, neurologic, and vascular injuries in the same setting.[1] Each injury is unique, and treatment must be individualized to achieve the best possible outcome. These complex injuries result in a significant amount of energy transferred to the surrounding tissues, leading to scar tissue formation and tissue devitalization. Postoperative immobilization and swelling contributes to stiffness and pain.[2] The outcome of these complex injuries (**Fig. 2**) may depend not only on the reconstructive efforts of the surgeon but also on the patient's expectations, overall health, age, occupation, and coping skills.[2] Unlike the lower extremity for which an amputation and use of a prosthetic may result in better function than reconstruction of the mangled foot, the ability to interact and manipulate the environment with the upper extremity makes reconstruction to regain function a principal consideration.[2]

Despite the best efforts of the surgeon, patients often never regain full function of the hand, and complications may occur. Early recognition and appropriate treatment are essential to prevent long-term morbidity. Although not intended to be an exhaustive list, this review focuses on the prevention and management of 3 broad categories of complications after complex traumatic hand injuries: complex regional pain syndrome (CRPS), stiffness, and infection.

COMPLEX REGIONAL PAIN SYNDROME

CRPS is a debilitating condition that can be challenging to diagnose and treat. It involves an abnormal exaggerated response by the body to injury. Although the exact incidence and prevalence of CRPS are still unknown, risk factors for development have been found. CRPS more commonly affects the upper extremity than the lower extremity.[3] Additionally, there is an increased incidence in smokers, and the incidence is 3 to 4 times higher in women than in men,[3,4] with postmenopausal women having the highest risk of CRPS development.[5] Although trauma is the

Department of Orthopedics, University of Pittsburgh, Suite 1010, Kaufmann Building, 3471 Fifth Avenue, Pittsburgh, PA 15213, USA
* Corresponding author. Suite 1010, Kaufmann Building, 3471 Fifth Avenue, Pittsburgh, PA 15213.
E-mail address: fowlerjr@upmc.edu

Hand Clin 31 (2015) 311–317
http://dx.doi.org/10.1016/j.hcl.2014.12.005
0749-0712/15/$ – see front matter

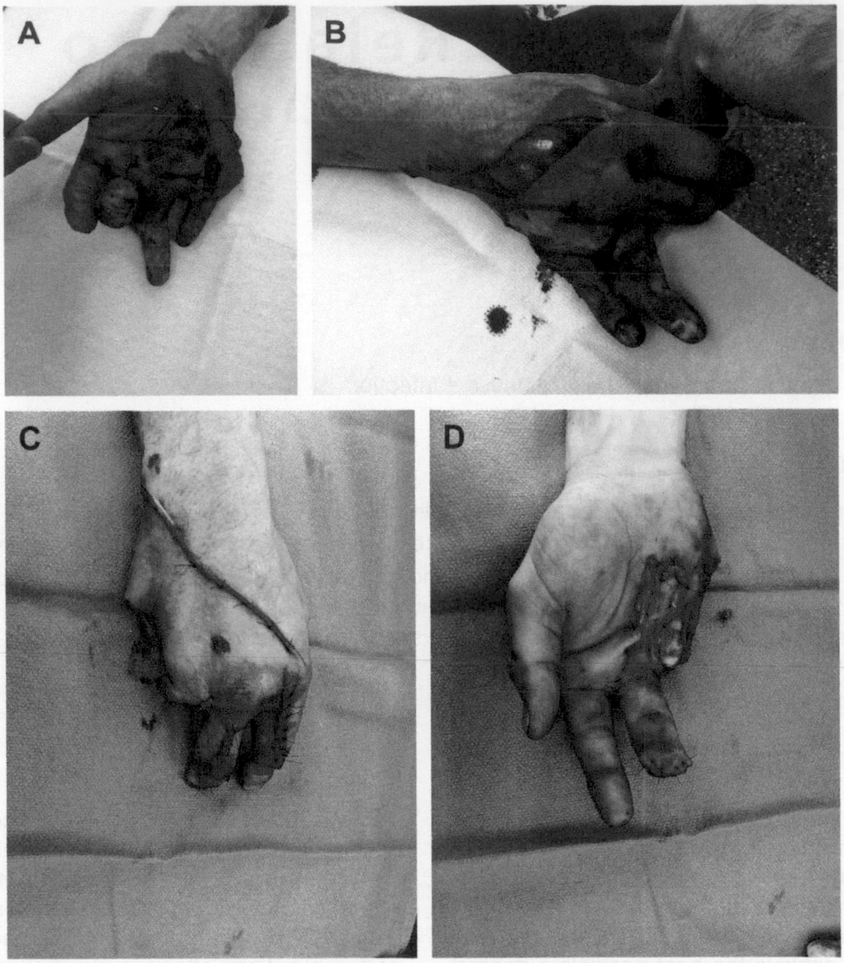

Fig. 1. (*A, B*) A 46-year-old man sustained crush injury to right hand resulting in dysvascular middle, ring, and small fingers. (*C, D*) Ray resection of the small finger and revision amputation of the ring finger were performed. Revascularization of the middle finger with open reduction and internal fixation of fractures was performed.

most frequent cause of CRPS in the upper extremity, it can also be seen postoperatively after elective procedures such as fasciectomy for Dupuytren contracture and carpal tunnel surgery.[6] Although distal radius fracture is noted to be the most common traumatic etiology,[6] CRPS may develop after other complex hand trauma such as burns and degloving injuries.[7–9]

CRPS can be classified into 2 types based on the presence or absence of identifiable nerve

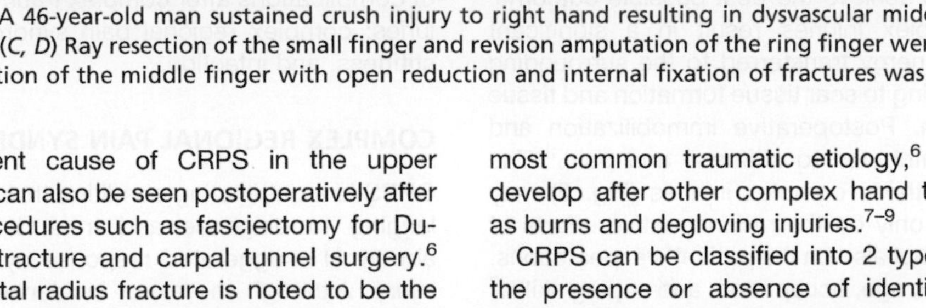

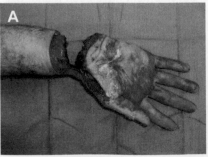

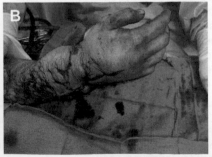

Fig. 2. (*A*) Near amputation of right hand at the wrist level by an industrial saw. (*B*) Right hand after successful revascularization.

damage. CRPS type 1 is not associated with identifiable nerve injury, whereas CRPS type 2 involves cases in which nerve injury can be immediately identified.[3,4] Regardless of the type, both syndromes are typically associated with 4 principal findings: pain, swelling, autonomic dysfunction, and stiffness. In general, pain is the most common symptom and is also the most distressing to the patient. The pain is characterized as burning or throbbing and is commonly out of proportion to the degree of the initial injury.[3,4,6] It can be associated with increased sensitivity to noxious stimuli (hyperalgesia), such as pinprick, or increased by nonnoxious stimuli (allodynia), such as light stroking of the skin or sudden loud noises.[4] The pain can be crippling in many patients and lead to insomnia. CRPS is typically unresponsive to narcotic pain medication. Autonomic dysfunction may also be present and cause discoloration of the skin, trophic changes of the skin or nails, or changes in perspiration. Vasomotor changes may lead to significant swelling of the entire hand early in the condition. This swelling, in conjunction with pain, can progress to stiffness of the affected hand and digits and contribute to further morbidity.

The lack of a single diagnostic test or specific physical findings causes difficulty in making a definitive diagnosis of CRPS. Plain radiographs are abnormal in only about 70% of cases,[3] typically showing diffuse osteopenia in association with periarticular demineralization and subchondral erosions. Three-phase bone scans have been recommended as a diagnostic tool because of their high sensitivity early in the condition (96%); however, they have poor specificity (19%).[4] Thermography and cold stress testing have been used but they lack specificity.

It can be especially difficult for the treating surgeon to differentiate CRPS from normal posttraumatic or postoperative findings in patients with complex hand trauma. CRPS is typically identified within a month of injury, but it has been documented as early as 2 weeks after injury in some patients.[10] The International Association for the Study of Pain criteria and the Budapest criteria (**Table 1**) are 2 scoring systems used to assist with the diagnosis of CRPS, but their use is limited to the pain clinic setting.[4] As a result, suspicion coupled with the patient's clinical history and examination are key factors in its diagnosis.

The main treatment goal in CRPS is restoration of function to the limb and reduction of pain. Early recognition and treatment is believed to improve patient outcomes, but studies find that despite early treatment, some patients have poor outcomes.[3] Early recognition can be difficult, especially in the milder presentations of CRPS. A multidisciplinary approach to treatment that includes hand therapists, cognitive behavioral therapists, pain clinicians, and psychological support is extremely important, as multiple modalities are used simultaneously in treatment.

Hand therapy is the mainstay of treatment and helps limit contracture and weakness. Different physiologic states exist in CRPS, and staging evaluation before initiation can guide therapy.[3] Staging involves measurements of the degree of swelling and arteriovenous shunting. High-flow extremities, characterized by a hot, swollen, and painful extremity are best treated with contrast baths and stress loading. Normal flow extremities are painful but without swelling and are best managed with contrast baths and transcutaneous electrical nerve stimulation units. Low-flow extremities, characterized by an atrophic and stiff extremity, are best managed with active and passive range of motion and transcutaneous electrical nerve stimulation units.

Cognitive behavioral therapy is also found to be beneficial in the treatment of CRPS, specifically mirror visual feedback (MVF).[4] MVF involves the

Table 1
Budapest criteria for complex regional pain syndrome

Pain out of Proportion	Symptoms	Signs	No Other Diagnosis Explaining Signs and Symptoms
	Allodynia/hypersensitivity	Hyperesthesia, allodynia to light touch	
	Temperature/color change	Temperature/color change	
	Edema/changes in sweating	Edema/sweat changes	
	Weakness, decreased motion	Tremor, dystonia, nail changes, decreased range of motion	

Patient must meet criteria from each column with 3 of the 4 symptoms and 2 of the 4 signs.
Adapted from Field J. Complex regional pain syndrome: a review. J Hand Surg Eur Vol 2013;38(6):617.

patient hiding the affected hand behind a glass mirror. As a result, when looking in the mirror the patient sees the normal hand as the affected limb. The patient then begins to exercise his or her normal hand, which the patient visualizes as exercising the affected hand. Over time, this visualization encourages the patient to move the affected hand with good effect.

Medications such as corticosteroids, antidepressants, anticonvulsants, calcium channel blockers and adrenergic agents have been used in the treatment of CRPS.[3,4,6] However, their use is off label. Despite concerns of study validity because of small sample sizes and potential side effects, pulse doses of corticosteroids are found to improve symptoms in CRPS.[3,11] Tricyclic antidepressants such as amitriptyline and nortriptyline have shown sympatholytic effects and efficacy in the treatment of neuropathic pain.[3] Anticonvulsants, such as gabapentin, have been found to be effective in the treatment of chronic pain in patients with allodynia and hyperesthesia.[4] Adrenergic agents, such as clonidine, are advocated in the early treatment of CRPS associated with hyperesthesia and allodynia. Narcotics are found to have limited efficacy in the treatment of CRPS and should be avoided.

Sympathetic blocks provide only short-term benefit in patients with sympathetically driven pain and are typically reserved for the diagnosis of sympathetically maintained CRPS rather than treatment. Blocks can allow the surgeon to perform a more thorough physical examination that is not limited secondary to the patient's pain. Invasive treatment modalities, such as spinal cord stimulators, are used in the treatment of CRPS; however, they are not found to provide any statistical decrease in pain or increase in subjective scores when compared with hand therapy alone.[4] Surgery is rarely indicated for the treatment of CRPS, unless in the setting of a known correctable cause. These causes can include treatment of a malunion or nonunion or treatment of intrinsic and extrinsic contractures and arthrofibrosis.

STIFFNESS

Stiffness of the fingers begins almost immediately after injury. The initial injury causes activation of the inflammatory cascade that causes increased capillary permeability and leads to local edema and hemorrhage.[12,13] The soft tissues expand and joint capsules distend, progressing to tightening of the surrounding ligaments. The concomitant pull of the flexor tendons causes the interphalangeal (IP) joints to be held in a position of flexion.[13,14] The opposite occurs at the metacarpophalangeal (MCP) joints, as extension of the MCP joints allows for maximal intracapsular fluid space. Given the cam effect of the metacarpal head, the collateral ligaments are shortened and prone to contracture in extension.[14] If not addressed, soft tissue contracture of the superficial fascia, flexor tendon sheath, and muscle belly may develop. As wound healing progresses, fibrosis and angiogenesis form granulation tissue. It is during this stage of wound healing that collagen cross-linking can promote the formations of adhesions and further contribute to joint stiffness. Adherence of the volar plate and retinacular ligaments to the collateral ligaments and lateral aspect of the phalanges leads to characteristic flexion contractures.[12] Fractures can further complicate matters, as adhesions can form between the overlying tendons and bone.

The management of stiffness in the setting of complex soft tissue injury should always start with prevention. Contracture of the collateral ligaments of the MCP and IP joints is a major component of stiffness; therefore, these joints need to be immobilized in a position that places the respective collateral ligaments on maximum stretch to avoid contracture. Flexion of the MCP joint to 80° to 90° lengthens the collateral ligaments and places them under tension. Conversely, the IP joint collateral ligaments are maximally stretched at approximately 10° to 15° of flexion.[15] This is the basis of the "intrinsic-plus" position for splinting of the hand. However, it should be noted that even in the setting of this position, prolonged immobilization might still lead to joint contracture and stiffness.

Determining the exact cause of contracture or stiffness can be difficult but should always begin with a thorough physical examination that focuses specifically on some key features. The clinician must determine if the contracture is fixed or flexible and also determine if the contracture is dependent on the movement of adjacent joints or muscle activation. Stiffness secondary to intrinsic or extrinsic muscle tightness can be tested easily and effectively. The Bunnell Intrinsic Tightness Test involves testing of the proximal interphalangeal (PIP) joint flexion with MCP flexion and extension. If less PIP joint flexion occurs when the MCP joint is held in extension compared with MCP joint flexion, this indicates intrinsic tightness is present. Conversely, testing for extrinsic extensor tightness is performed with the MCP joint in flexion. If less PIP joint flexion occurs in this position, then the test result is considered positive and the stiffness is caused by extrinsic muscle tightness.

The timing of diagnosis plays an important role in treatment. Early management of stiffness and contracture uses a combination of hand therapy in conjunction with therapeutic modalities such as heat or cryotherapy.[14,16] In the early stages of stiffness or contracture, immobilization of certain joints may be necessary for tissue healing, whereas other joints are allowed to move freely. It should be noted that continuous passive motion has not shown in clinical studies to be beneficial in treatment of joint stiffness once it has occurred.[17] The main issue with treating stiffness in the digits is that the muscles involved in motion cross multiple unaffected joints. Muscle contraction will result in movement of these more mobile joints before affecting the stiffer joints involved. Manual blocking of unaffected joints increases resistance in that area and transfers the muscle force to the stiff joint, which enables excursion.[18] Casting motion to mobilize stiffness can be used to treat chronic stiffness through selective immobilization of proximal joints in a desired position using casting. This technique directs all muscle force to the stiff distal joints.[18] However, there is significant controversy with this technique because of the concern for development of stiffness in previously uninvolved joints.

The current trend in hand therapy for prevention or treatment of stiffness is a focus on active motion over passive motion. Limited active range of motion restricts the effectiveness of the lymphatic system in decreasing edema and leads to excess fibrosis formation and adhesions.[18] Initially used solely for extensor tendon repairs, immediate controlled active motion (ICAM) is a type of active redirection that has gained increasing favor with hand therapists. ICAM uses low-profile orthoses to achieve immediate active motion in the compliant patient.[19]

If nonoperative treatment fails to provide functional motion in patients with normal articular joint surface, contracture release may be considered. However, this should only be performed in a motivated and compliant patient who is willing to adhere to the strict postoperative therapy treatment. A frank discussion needs to occur between the clinician and patient about realistic treatment goals and a thorough explanation of potential contracture recurrence despite adherence to therapy. Once the decision to proceed with surgery is made, the procedure should target the pathology causing the contracture.

If possible, the intervention should be done under local anesthesia with intravenous sedation for immediate evaluation of the contracture release.[14] For MCP joint contracture, capsulotomy and collateral ligament release through a volar or dorsal approach can be used. For flexion contracture of the PIP joint, a volar or midlateral incision can be used to perform the contracture release. Release of the check-rein ligaments is performed first, with careful attention to avoid damage to the transverse digital arteries. If extension is not adequate, it should be followed by successive release of the volar plate complex and accessory collateral ligament through a capsulotomy and then proper collateral ligament.[14] After each successive release, the clinician should evaluate the amount of extension to determine if adequate release has occurred. For extension contracture, a dorsal or dorsolateral approach can be performed to release the transverse retinacular ligaments and dorsal capsule. Stiffness and contracture of the distal interphalangeal (DIP) joint is frequently encountered secondary to a boutonniere or swan-neck deformity, and correction of the cause of the deformity will often resolve the DIP joint issue.[14]

INFECTION

Infection is a relatively common and potentially catastrophic complication of complex hand trauma. These injuries typically involve mechanical equipment in the home or industrial setting.[20,21] *Staphylococcus aureus* is the most commonly encountered bacteria and accounts for approximately 80% of hand infections.[22] In the last decade, the incidence of hand infections caused by methicillin-resistant *S aureus* has significantly increased from 34% to 78%.[22] Other common bacteria include *Streptococcus* species and gram-negative organisms such as *Escherichia coli* and *Pseudomonas aeruginosa*. Two studies from the Mayo Clinic found that the bacteriology of complex hand injuries differed between farm-related injuries and home/industry-related injuries.[23,24] In farm injuries, only 40% of isolates from culture were gram positive, whereas 60% were gram negative. Conversely, isolates from home-related or industry-related injuries were 70% gram positive and 30% gram negative.

A history of the patient's initial injury can be helpful in cases of atypical infections. An infection that occurred after an injury in fresh or saltwater should raise concern for a potential Mycobacterium marinum,[25] whereas an infection that occurred after a farm injury or in the setting of a significantly contaminated wound should raise concerns for anaerobic bacteria such as Clostridia. Also, the clinician should be concerned for a polymicrobial infection in patients with significant comorbidities such as intravenous drug use or a history of immunodeficiency such as diabetes or human immunodeficiency virus.

The key to treatment of hand infections is prevention. Immediate broad-spectrum intravenous antibiotics should be given in the setting of open fractures or significant soft tissue loss and should be based on the Gustilo and Anderson classification. Although initially described for open fractures of the tibia, McLain and Steyers[26] found that this classification correlated with the incidence of infection, length of hospital stay, return to work, and functional outcome in patients with open fractures of the hand. They also found that contaminated wounds are at greatest risk for infection.

The choice of antibiotics specifically for hand and upper extremity trauma is based on limited level I evidence. The general recommendation involves a first-generation cephalosporin with the addition of an aminoglycoside for significantly contaminated wounds. Despite concern of cephalosporin use in patients with penicillin allergy, studies have found a cross-reactivity of only 3% to 7%.[21] However, in patients with a severe penicillin allergy or cephalosporin allergy, vancomycin can be substituted.

Meticulous initial debridement of nonviable tissue and skeletal stabilization is paramount in preventing infection. Multiple debridements may be necessary if significant contamination is present. Swanson and colleagues[27] presented a classification system for operatively managed open fractures with soft tissue loss. Type I injuries consist of clean wounds in a patient with no history of systemic illness. Type II injuries were classified as contaminated wounds, wounds with a delay in treatment greater than 24 hours, or wounds accompanied by significant systemic illness in the patient. Fracture stabilization is based on the mechanical needs of the fracture, regardless of wound size, injury mechanism, or contamination and allows for early range of motion and prevention of stiffness.[26,27]

Infection can be prevented by a delay in soft tissue reconstruction. Swanson and colleagues[27] recommended closure of only type I injuries and using delayed closure techniques for all type II injuries. The current advent of negative-pressure wound therapy promotes granulation of wounds in the setting of a sealed vacuum environment and can be used when primary closure is not possible. Nerve and tendon repairs and any bone grafting should not be performed until adequate debridement of nonviable tissue has been performed, before definitive soft tissue coverage.[21,26,27]

Osteomyelitis is a potentially devastating complication that can occur after an open hand fracture or in the setting of previous soft tissue loss. Adequate debridement performed at the time of initial injury and appropriate delay before attempting soft tissue or bony reconstruction are important factors for prevention.[22] Presenting signs are usually limited and may only include some erythema, swelling, and pain. Systemic symptoms such as malaise and fever typically do not occur. Laboratory studies, such as erythrocyte sedimentation rate and white blood cell count, typically have normal results and are of little value. As a result, the clinician needs to be suspicious, especially in patients who report drainage after multiple soft tissue debridements. Plain radiographs are usually nonspecific and highly variable, although osteolysis of the involved bone can be seen in up to 70%. An involucrum or sequestrum is rarely visualized, typically presenting in 5% of cases.[28] MRI can detect osteomyelitis as early as 1 to 2 days after the onset of infection. Osteomyelitis is characterized on MRI as an ill-defined low signal intensity on the T1-weighted images and high signal intensity on T2-weighted and fat-suppressed sequences, such as short-tau inversion-recovery images.[29] Open biopsy and culture only yield positive cultures in 74% of patients.[28] Definitive surgical management varies greatly depending on the severity and chronicity of the infection, ranging from a simple debridement to bone resection with staged reconstruction. Regardless, the key to effective treatment is early and accurate diagnosis in combination with medical and surgical intervention.[28] In patients with persistent or recurrent drainage after multiple debridements or in patients with failed reconstructions, amputation may be necessary. Reilly and colleagues[28] found that patients who had diagnosed or were treated greater than 6 months after initial symptoms or who underwent multiple procedures had an amputation rate of 86%. In some instances, primary amputation may be considered if limb salvage is questionable but requires a lengthy discussion between the surgeon and the patient.

The treatment of soft tissue complications after complex hand trauma can be extremely challenging to manage. Regardless of the type of complication that arises, the key to successful treatment is prompt diagnosis. The physician needs to be aware of these potential complications and have a low threshold to action.

REFERENCES

1. Ciclamini D, Panero B, Titolo P, et al. Particularities of hand and wrist complex injuries in polytrauma management. Injury 2014;45(2):448–51.
2. Bueno RA, Neumeister MW. Outcomes after mutilating hand injuries: review of the literature and recommendations for assessment. Hand Clin 2003;19(1):193–204.
3. Patterson RW, Li Z, Smith BP, et al. Complex regional pain syndrome of the upper extremity. J Hand Surg Am 2011;36(9):1553–62.

4. Field J. Complex regional pain syndrome: a review. J Hand Surg Eur Vol 2013;38(6):616–26.
5. de Mos M, de Bruijn AG, Huygen FJ, et al. The incidence of complex regional pain syndrome: a population-based study. Pain 2007;129(1–2):12–20.
6. Li Z, Smith BP, Tuohy C, et al. Complex regional pain syndrome after hand surgery. Hand Clin 2010;26(2): 281–9.
7. Gokkaya NK, Karakus D, Oktay F, et al. Complex regional pain syndrome (CPRS type I) after a burn injury to the hand. Rheumatol Int 2008;28(10): 1045–8.
8. van der Laan L, Goris RJ. Reflex sympathetic dystrophy after burn injury. Burns 1996;22(4):303–6.
9. Irion G. Etiologies of common wounds. In: Irion G, editor. Complex wound management. 2nd edition. Thorofare (NJ): SLACK Incorporated; 2010. p. 73–148.
10. Żyluk A, Puchalski P. Complex regional pain syndrome: observations on diagnosis, treatment and definition of a new subgroup. J Hand Surg Eur Vol 2013;38(6):599–606.
11. Christensen K, Jensen EM, Noer I. The reflex dystrophy syndrome response to treatment with systemic corticosteroids. Acta Chir Scand 1982; 148(8):653–5.
12. Kaplan FT. The stiff finger. Hand Clin 2010;26(2): 191–204.
13. Houshian S, Jing SS, Chikkamuniyappa C, et al. Management of posttraumatic proximal interphalangeal joint contracture. J Hand Surg Am 2013;38(8): 1651–8.
14. Shin AY, Amadio PC. The stiff finger. In: Green DP, Hotchkiss RN, Pederson WC, editors. Green's operative hand surgery. 6th edition. New York: Churchill Livingstone; 1999. p. 355–88.
15. Sprague BL. Proximal interphalangeal joint contractures and their initial treatment. J Trauma 1975;15(5): 380–5.
16. Wong JM. Management of stiff hand: an occupational therapy perspective. Hand Surg 2002;7(2): 261–9.
17. Salter RB. The biologic concept of continuous passive motion of synovial joints. The first 18 years of basic research and its clinical application. Clin Orthop Relat Res 1989;(242):12–25.
18. Colditz JC. Chapter 67: therapist's management of the stiff finger. In: Skirven TM, Osterman AL, Fedorczyk J, et al, editors. Rehabilitation of the hand and upper extremity. 6th edition. Elsevier Mosby; 2011. p. 894–925.
19. Burns MC, Derby B, Neumeister MW. Wyndell merritt immediate controlled active motion (ICAM) protocol following extensor tendon repairs in zone IV-VII: review of literature, orthosis design, and case study-a multimedia article. Hand (N Y) 2013;8(1):17–22.
20. Cziffer E, Farkas J, Turchányi B. Management of potentially infected complex hand injuries. J Hand Surg Am 1991;16(5):832–4.
21. Hoffman RD, Adams BD. Antimicrobial management of mutilating hand injuries. Hand Clin 2003; 19(1):33–9.
22. McDonald LS, Bavaro MF, Hofmeister EP, et al. Hand infections. J Hand Surg Am 2011;36(8):1403–12.
23. Fitzgerald RH Jr, Cooney WP 3rd, Washington JA 2nd, et al. Bacterial colonization of mutilating hand injuries and its treatment. J Hand Surg Am 1977;2(2):85–9.
24. Cooney WP 3rd, Fitzgerald RH Jr, Dobyns JH, et al. Quantitative wound cultures in upper extremity trauma. J Trauma 1982;22(2):112–7.
25. Elhassan BT, Wynn SW, Gonzalez MH. Atypical infections of the hand. J Am Soc Surg Hand 2004; 4(1):42–9.
26. McLain RF, Steyers CM. Classification of open fractures of the hand. Iowa Orthop J 1991;11:107–11.
27. Swanson TV, Szabo RM, Anderson DD. Open hand fractures: prognosis and classification. J Hand Surg Am 1991;16(1):101–7.
28. Reilly KE, Linz JC, Stern PJ, et al. Osteomyelitis of the tubular bones of the hand. J Hand Surg Am 1997;22(4):644–9.
29. Pineda C, Espinosa R, Pena A. Radiographic imaging in osteomyelitis: the role of plain radiography, computed tomography, ultrasonography, magnetic resonance imaging, and scintigraphy. Semin Plast Surg 2009;23(2):80–9.

Management of Complications Relating to Finger Amputation and Replantation

Sang-Hyun Woo, MD, PhD*, Young-Woo Kim, MD, PhD, Ho-Jun Cheon, MD, Hyun-Je Nam, MD, Dong-Ho Kang, MD, Jong-Min Kim, MD, Hee-Chan Ahn, MD

KEYWORDS

• Finger amputation • Replantation • Complications • Management

KEY POINTS

- Management and prevention of complications relating to finger amputations according to the amputation level is described.
- Using a new classification system, replantation as well as its complications and management is described.
- Problems related to replantation of ring avulsion amputation and multiple digit amputations are discussed.
- Socioeconomic factors and cultural differences between Asian and Western countries are discussed.

INTRODUCTION

In traumatic amputation of 1 or more fingers, surgical options such as microsurgical replantation and revision amputation depend on the condition of the amputation stumps, the level of injury, and the patients' physical condition and demands. With the development of microsurgical techniques and microscope capabilities, the success rate of distal replantation in fingertip amputation cases is increasing. Moreover, Confucian moral values and the greater current emphasis on maintaining body integrity and physical appearance are reasons for performing these procedures in Asian countries. Unlike replantation, revision amputation is one of the most commonly performed procedures in hand surgery, particularly in cases of traumatic finger amputation. As an alternative to replantation, this procedure also requires serious consideration. Because the function of the traumatized finger or hand is compromised, the aim of this procedure should be to minimize disfigurement and the loss of remnant function. The hand surgeon should also consider secondary reconstruction of the amputated fingers or fitting prosthesis. Even in fingertip amputation, the initial treatment is very important. Among many options, including revision amputation, skin graft, local or distant flap, and free flap, optimal management should be determined by the age and requirements of the patient.

Conflicts of interest: None. This research received no specific grant from any funding agency in the public, commercial, or not-for-profit sectors.
Cheon & Woo's Institute for Hand & Reconstructive Microsurgery, W Hospital, 1616 Dalgubeol Daero, Dalseo Gu, Daegu 704-953, Korea
* Corresponding author.
E-mail address: handwoo@hotmail.com

Hand Clin 31 (2015) 319–338
http://dx.doi.org/10.1016/j.hcl.2015.01.006
0749-0712/15/$ – see front matter

hand.theclinics.com

Indications of Replantation

The indications for replantation in amputation of the digits have not changed significantly over the years. All indications for replantation must take into consideration the status of the amputated part (guillotine, crush, and avulsion) and the presence of systemic diseases in the patients. The indications are not based solely on viability of the replanted part but are predicated on the potential for long-term function. In cases of thumb amputation, replantation probably offers the best functional return. Even with poor motion and sensation, the thumb is useful to the patient as a post for opposition. Although single-finger replantation is generally not performed,[1–4] replantation beyond the level of the flexor digitorum superficialis (FDS) tendon insertion, and zone 1 in a flexor tendon injury, usually results in good function.[4,5] However, the replantation of a single digit amputated proximal to the insertion of the FDS is more suitable for revision amputation because this replanted digit usually leads to a stiff proximal interphalangeal (PIP) joint that interferes with overall hand function.[6,7] In cases of multiple finger amputations, hand surgeons should try to reattach the amputated digits back into their position because reconstructive procedures may be challenging. Sometimes, 1 or 2 favorable fingers that had clean-cut amputation through diaphyseal segments of bone were reattached to the more important functional position in the same manner as heterodigital or on-top replantation. Replantation of distal digital amputation is becoming more popular in special replantation centers in Asia. In the West, the loss of function in the fingertip is perceived to be negligible despite the lack of scientific evidence supporting this. Amputation of the digits in children is a clear indication for replantation, no matter whether it is single or multiple digits or proximal or distal digits involved. Digital replantation in children is no longer a challenging procedure, and survival rates are increasing. With refinement of replantation techniques, success rate is as high as with adults, and ultimate functional result is shown to be successful in long-term follow-up studies.[8,9]

This article focuses on the management and prevention of complications relating to finger amputations and replantation based on the amputation level according to the flexor zone of injury.[10] Regarding level of digital amputation, a new classification suggested by Sebastin and Chung[11] was adopted for description (**Fig. 1**). In this article, revision amputation and replantation of the thumb are excluded.

ZONE 1 DISTAL AMPUTATION: REVISION AMPUTATION

Amputation at zone 1 is distal to the FDS insertion. Zone 1 distal amputation (fingertip) is defined as the portion of the finger distal to the flexor and extensor tendon insertion. At this level of amputation, replantation may be impossible owing to severe crushing or the patient rejecting reattachment. Revision amputation with bone shortening and tension-free

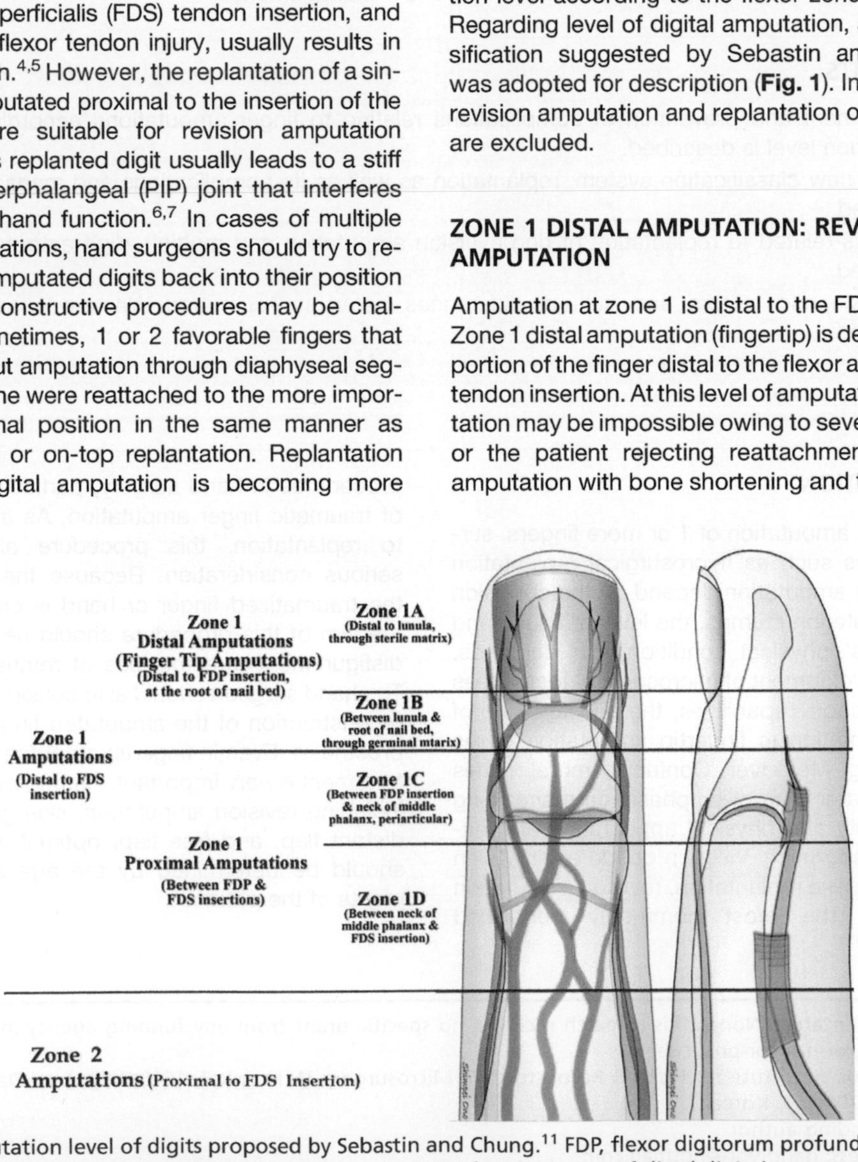

Fig. 1. Amputation level of digits proposed by Sebastin and Chung.[11] FDP, flexor digitorum profundus. (*From* Sebastin SJ, Chung KC. A systematic review of the outcomes of replantation of distal digital amputation. Plast Reconstr Surg 2011;128(3):725; with permission.)

closure is the most straightforward surgical method. At this level, this technique is indicated when preservation of the length is not important or when the remaining bone length is insufficient to support nail growth. However, there are many complications following revision amputation, including delayed wound healing, nail deformities with poor aesthetics, hypersensitivity, and residual pain.

Delayed Healing and Atrophy

Delayed healing of the wound is caused by inappropriate debridement of devitalized tissues and, more often, closure with excessive tension. This problem can occur following tissue necrosis at the wound margins. Secondary intention healing results from wound contraction and reepithelialization over time. Wound contraction leads to a scar that is significantly smaller than the initial defect, and reepithelialization results in near-normal skin coverage with unstable scar.[12] Depending on the coverage methods of amputation stumps, 60% to 70% of patients with skin grafting and 20% to 24% with flaps complained of tenderness. In addition, delayed healing of zone 1A results in atrophy of the pulp, which necessitates secondary reconstruction with flap surgery (**Fig. 2**). Hypersensitive fingertip after revision amputation tends to lessen with time, and only small percentages of patients complain of this. Constricted scar or atrophic change on the tactile pulp is usually related to delayed wound healing or inappropriate coverage. Because the presence of this discomfort makes whole digits, and sometimes the hand, functionally useless, desensitization exercises are initiated at an early stage of the rehabilitation program. To avoid this problem, flap coverage with sensate flap with proper thickness for the pulp is recommended. If possible, the scar should not be placed on the tactile portion of the pulp in the initial injury.

Nail Deformity

The reason for poor aesthetics and nail deformity is a short nail bed with inadequate bony support of the distal phalangeal bone and soft tissue deficiency.

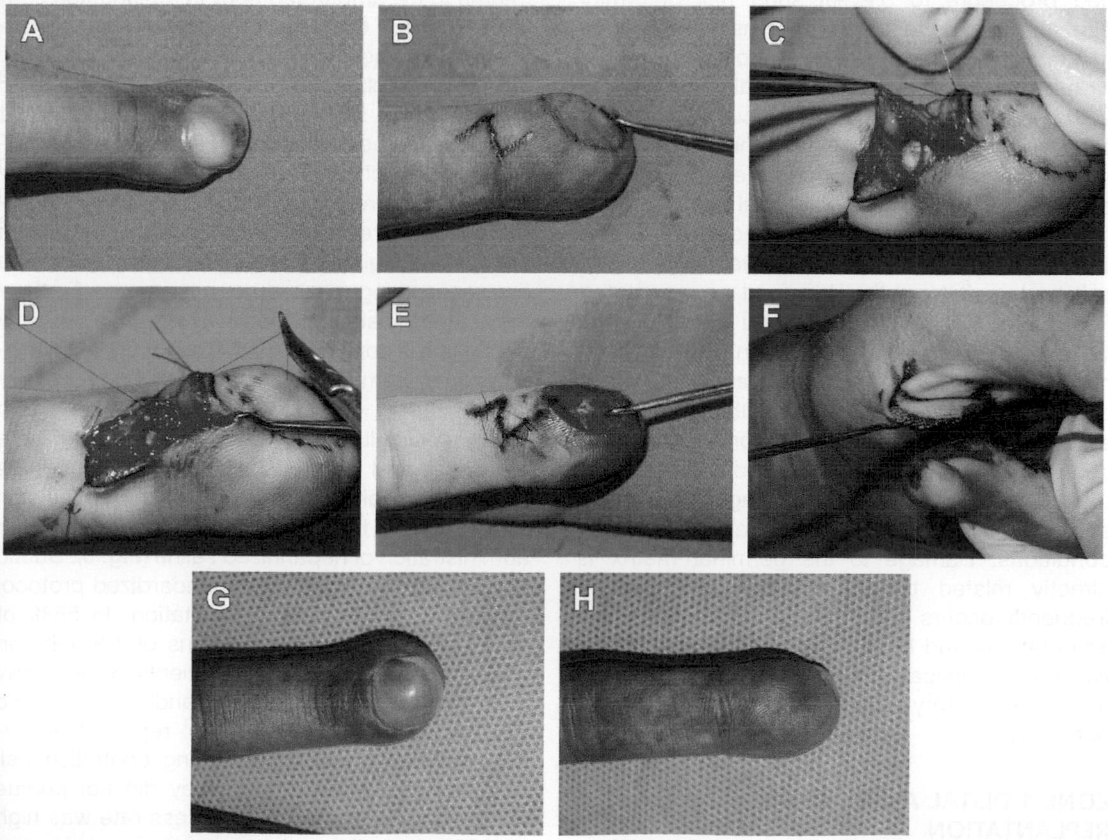

Fig. 2. (*A*) Pulp atrophy and neuroma pain of the left ring finger after crush amputation. (*B*) Preoperative design for neuroma site (*zigzag*) and deskinning area (*round*). (*C*) Neuroma in continuity of the radial digital nerve. (*D*) Direct repair of digital nerve after excision of neuroma. (*E*) Deskinning of the radial pulp area. (*F*) Elevated thenar flap to cover atrophic pulp area. (*G, H*) Postoperative views, 13 months later.

Following amputation of the fingertip, there is a loss of bone and soft tissue in the distal phalanx. The redundant nail bed folding over the tip of the terminal phalanx causes a hook nail deformity (**Fig. 3**).[13] This nail deformity is of aesthetic and functional concern, especially in young women and children. Besides the lack of pulp, fingertip discomfort or even pain may exclude the finger from daily activities. Compared with the remnant length of the distal phalangeal bone, the nail bed is overly long. According to previous reports, this deformity is highly likely if the distal two-thirds to one-half of the nail bed are without bony support.[14,15] To manage this deformity, there are many suggested surgical techniques, including the traditional antenna procedure,[16,17] composite graft from toe pulp,[18] homodigital advancement flap,[19] free toe tissue transfer,[20] and oblique triangular neurovascular osteocutaneous flap.[21] However, in the initial injury, the best way to avoid this deformity is to prevent it by excising the nail bed that extends beyond the limit of the amputated distal phalanx. In cases of amputation through the sterile matrix (zone 1A), primary eponychium folding plasty is the recommended procedure to prevent short nail deformity (**Fig. 4**). After 2 longitudinal incisions on both sides of the eponychium, the entire eponychial fold is wrapped and then sutured proximally. Pulp defect at the end of nail bed should be covered with flaps such as local or regional flaps. This technique is easy and simple.[22] In nail bed defects with intact or remaining long distal phalangeal bone, primary reconstruction of the nail bed is necessary to prevent short nail deformity. Immediate full-thickness nail bed graft from the damaged or amputated finger (**Fig. 5**)[23] or partial nail bed graft from the large toe nail represent good options.[24] Nail deformity and the occurrence of pulp atrophy are the causes of an unsatisfactory aesthetic outcome even after distal fingertip replantation. Nail regeneration after replantation is influenced by the level of the amputation, the extent of damage to the sterile and germinal matrix, and postoperative circulatory conditions. Damage to the germinal matrix is directly related to nail growth. Pulp atrophy frequently occurs after replantation of crush-type amputations and replantation with postoperative vascular complications. This condition results in an unsatisfactory appearance with hook nail deformity.[25,26]

ZONE 1 DISTAL AMPUTATION: REPLANTATION

Regarding replantation at this level of amputation, there are few published research articles in the West. Distal replantation is considered as offering little functional gain and high cost. Owing to differences in medical insurance systems and cultural backgrounds, most distal replantation research reports are from Asian countries to date. Because of the body conservation concept infused in Confucian morals, maintaining physical appearance outweighs a potential loss of function. Through the systematic review by Sebastin and Chung[11] and the retrospective study by Hattori and colleagues,[12] high success rates and good functional outcomes recently followed distal digital replantation compared with revision amputation. Despite the lack of published scientific evidence supporting this, revision amputation is perceived to be the better choice, given the minimal functional loss and reduced expense compared with replantation. Jazayeri and colleagues[27] in 2013 suggested numerous contraindications for distal replantation, including concomitant life-threatening injury or diseases, high anesthesia risk, mental instability, severely crushed or mangled body part, multilevel amputation, arteriosclerotic vessels, prolonged warm ischemia time, extreme contamination, and prior surgery or trauma to the amputated part. In replantation centers in Korea, if the patient wants to have replantation surgery, there is no absolute contraindication. This kind of replantation is usually performed using a digital nerve block or brachial plexus block. It usually takes between 1 and 2 hours for bone fixation with Kirschner wires (K-wires), 1 digital artery and/or 1 vein repair, and nail plate and skin sutures. Therefore, distal replantation is neither an overly challenging microsurgical technique nor a time-consuming procedure any more. Furthermore, the operation fee of replantation is low because it is controlled by the national medical insurance system. The most challenging procedure is vein repair. In the extreme distal zone, vein repair is difficult and sometimes impossible. There are suggested methods of salvage procedures with external bleeding with a fish mouth incision or removal of the nail bed, medical leeches, or administration of heparinized saline (**Fig. 6**). Buntic and Brooks[28] suggested a standardized protocol for artery-only fingertip replantation. In 58% of their patients, blood transfusions of 1.8 units on average were required. All patients were happy with the decision to replant and the cosmetic result. Erken and colleagues[29] reported artery-only fingertip replantations using controlled nail bed bleeding. Even though they did not pursue vein and nerve repair, the success rate was high at 88%, including adequate sensory recovery. The average blood transfusion was just 1.2 units in 68% of all patients. At Chang-Gung Memorial Hospital, continuous blood drainage from the

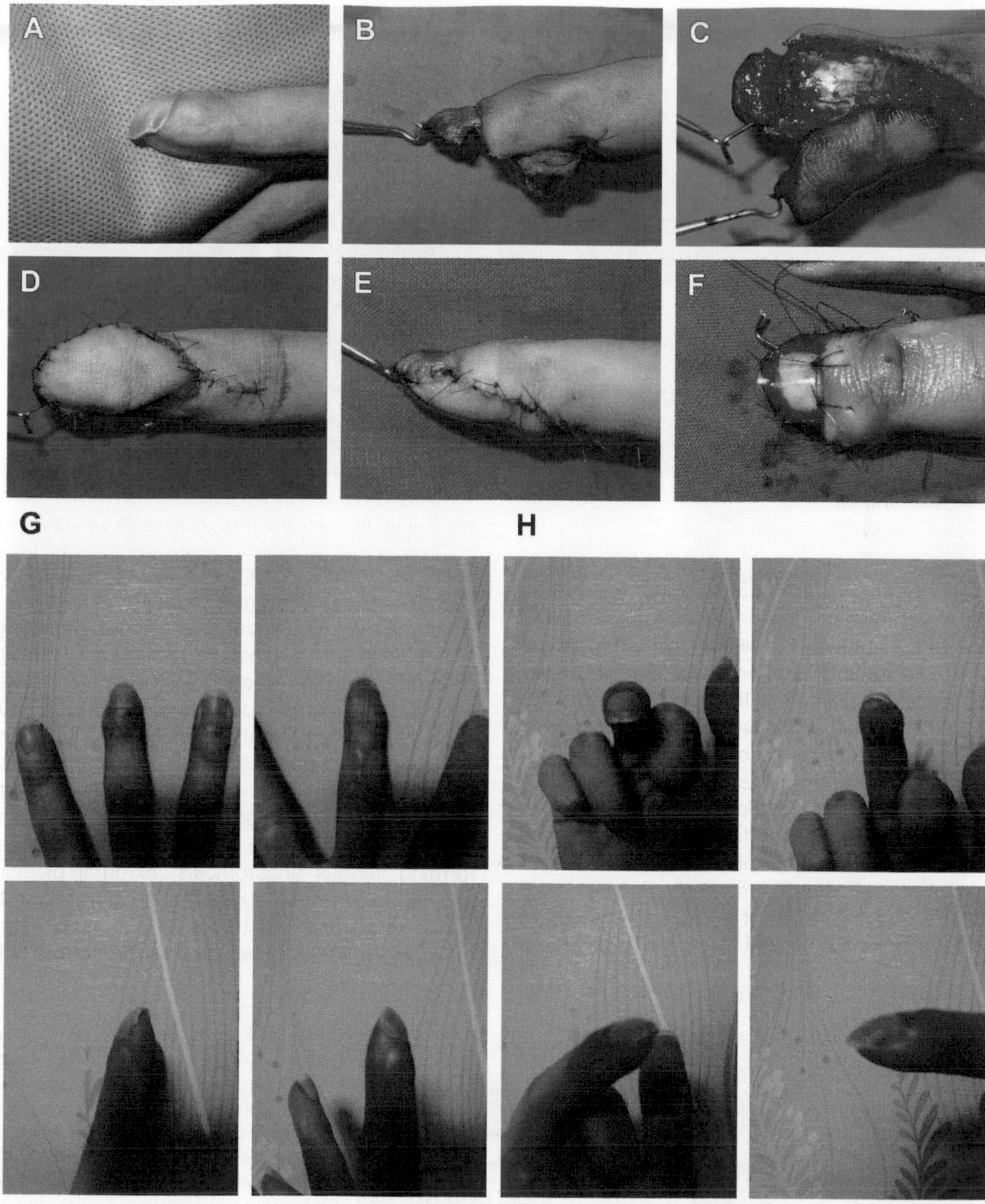

Fig. 3. Correction of hook nail deformity with open wedge osteotomy on the distal phalangeal bone and triangular pulp island flap. (*A*) Preoperative view of severe hook nail deformity of the right long finger. (*B*) Open wedge transverse osteotomy at the distal one-third of the distal phalangeal bone and pinning with 2 K-wires. (*C*) Triangular island flap advanced to cover phalangeal bone. (*D–F*) Full-thickness skin graft from hypothenar area to cover donor site of the flap and artificial nail plate fixation. (*G, H*) Postoperative view, 10 months later. (*I–K*) Preoperative and postoperative radiographs.

replanted fingertip was performed without removal of the nail plate.[30] They did not use medical leeches. With intensive monitoring of the perfusion of the replanted digits and patients' hemoglobin levels, the wound bleeding was maintained until physiologic venous outflow was restored. Survival rate was 90% and the average amount of blood transfused was 4.0 units (range, 0–16 units) for each patient or 3.29 units (range, 0–14 units) for each digit.

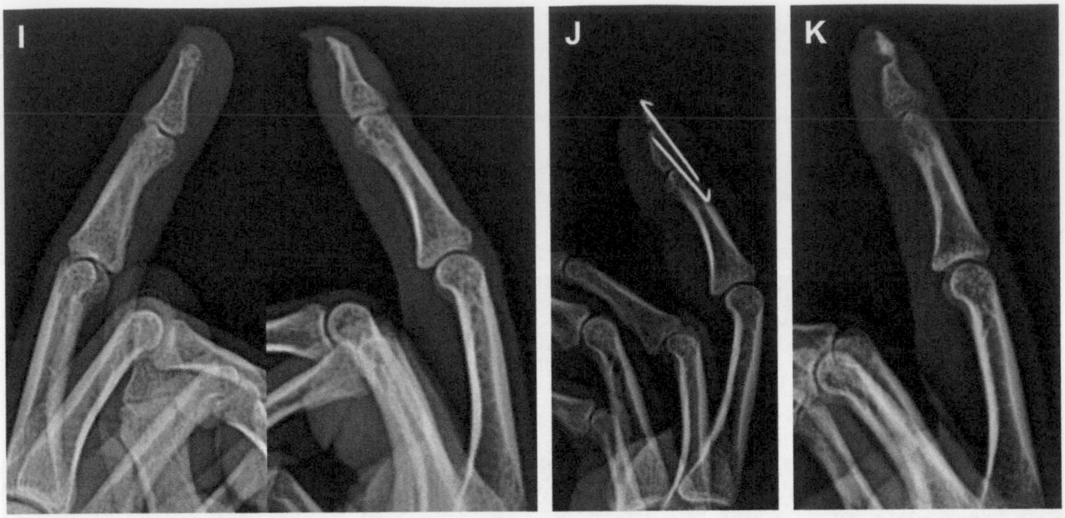

Fig. 3. (*continued*)

Importance of Vein Repair

Venous insufficiency is the most compromising cause of replantation failure in early postoperative failure. Maintenance of venous drainage is the key to successful replantation. In zone 1, venous anatomy varies greatly. At the level of the eponychium, 63% of fingers have a vein of 0.8 mm or larger, but the location of these veins is unpredictable.[31] At all levels of distal tip amputation, success is greatest when a lateral search is performed for the commissural veins, with an equal mix of vessels 0.5 mm or larger and 0.4 mm or smaller. Scheker and Becker[31] suggest repair of artery and vein using an open-book technique at the pulp. There are no absolute indications for very distal tip replantation. The procedure is contraindicated in injuries in which there is considerable tissue damage by crushing or contamination, peripheral vascular disease, or systemic conditions with associated vascular problems such as diabetes. Manual workers who require an early return to functional work should not be considered. To overcome postoperative congestion for successful fingertip replantation, the importance of venous anastomosis is impossible to overemphasize.[32] By performing venous anastomosis, external bleeding can be avoided and a higher survival rate can be achieved. Venous anastomosis for fingertip replantation is a reliable and worthwhile procedure, with

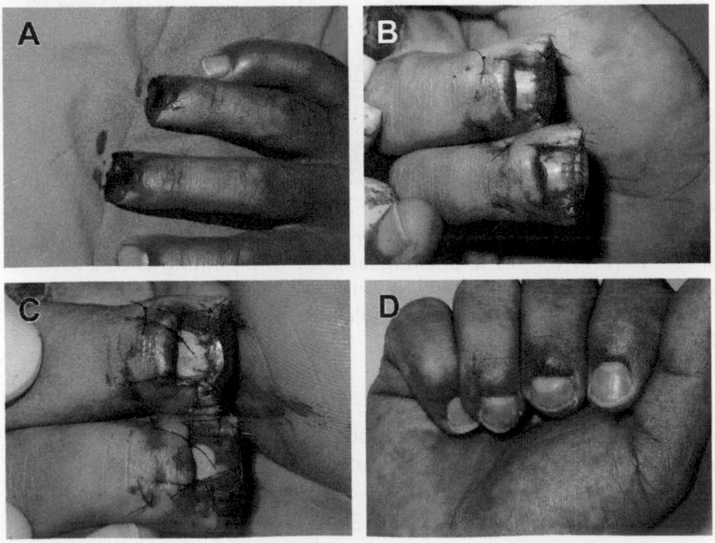

Fig. 4. Primary eponychium folding plasty. (*A*) Preoperative view of right long and ring fingertip amputation with nail bed defect. (*B*) Incision on both lateral sides of eponychium with recession of eponychial flap proximally. (*C*) Artificial nail plate insertion and fixation with skin suture. (*D*) Postoperative view showing lengthening of nail bed, 6 months later.

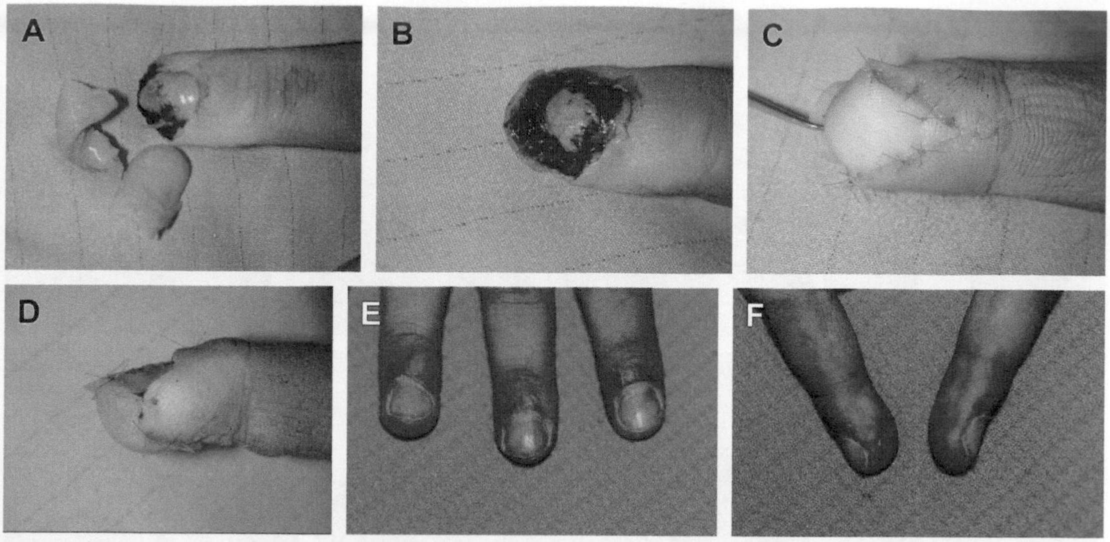

Fig. 5. Operative procedures of immediate nail bed graft with flap in acute fingertip injury with nail bed defect. (*A*) Preoperative view showing nail bed defects about 7 × 8 mm. (*B*) After debridement of wound, cortical punctuation was completed with needle or K-wire. Harvested nail bed graft from the amputated was fixed with 6-0 chromic catgut sutures on the prepared distal phalangeal bone. (*C, D*) Postoperative view of V-Y advancement flap to cover the pulp defect and reinsertion of the nail plate. (*E, F*) Postoperative view, about 18 months later.

an overall survival rate of 86%. In cases in which there is a lack of arterial perfusion after surgery, venous outflow is difficult to check. Salvage procedure should be commenced immediately following the operation. However, if there is postoperative congestion on the following day or days after the primary vascular anastomosis, dilated venules usually become larger and can easily anastomosed. Koshima and colleagues[33] tried to delay venous anastomosis with vein graft. They achieved a high success rate of 81.3% in distal phalangeal replantation. To support adequate venous drainage, external bleeding with venous anastomosis is preferable to venous anastomosis alone in the fingertip replantation of severe crush or avulsion injury.[34] When there is only 1 available solitary pulp central artery in the stump, the main trunk is used as an arterial conduit. Venous drainage was established by creating an anastomosis between the ligated branch of the solitary artery and a recipient vein from the proximal finger stump. Vein grafts, which are harvested from the volar aspect of the distal forearm, are used to aid in both arterial and venous reconstruction. This technique can save fingers without the use of leeches.[35] When vein repair is not possible, the use of external bleeding with a topical heparinized saline solution with hyperbaric oxygen therapy can overcome venous congestion. Without vein repair, Han and colleagues[36] increased the overall survival rate of fingertip replantation to 76%. In conclusion, vein repair is the most important step to attain survival of fingertip replantation.[37] It may decrease the blood loss from external bleeding and the burden of intensive nursing care in salvage procedures.

Infection and Use of Leeches

Irrespective of injury mechanism, the rate of infection after replantation surgery is low and not serious. The most serious complication of leech use is infection from *Aeromonas hydrophila*. Incidence ranges from 2.4% to 20% have been reported, with clinical presentations ranging from cellulitis and abscess, to extensive soft tissue infections causing tissue loss and systemic sepsis.[38,39] Routine antimicrobial prophylaxis with fluoroquinolone should be used.

Replantation Versus Revision Amputation: Determinants and Disability

There are many risk factors for an unsuccessful replanted fingertip, such as the patient's age, amputation level, and injury mechanism. Among these, injury mechanism, platelet count, smoking after operation, preservation method of amputated part, and the use of vein grafting were found to be the main predictors for the survival of the replanted fingertip.[34] Hattori and colleagues[12] reported the results of the study to compare the functional outcome of successful microsurgical replantation versus amputation closure for single-fingertip amputations. Active range of motion of the PIP joint was greater in the successful replantation group than in the amputation closure group. Although the existence of paresthesia and cold

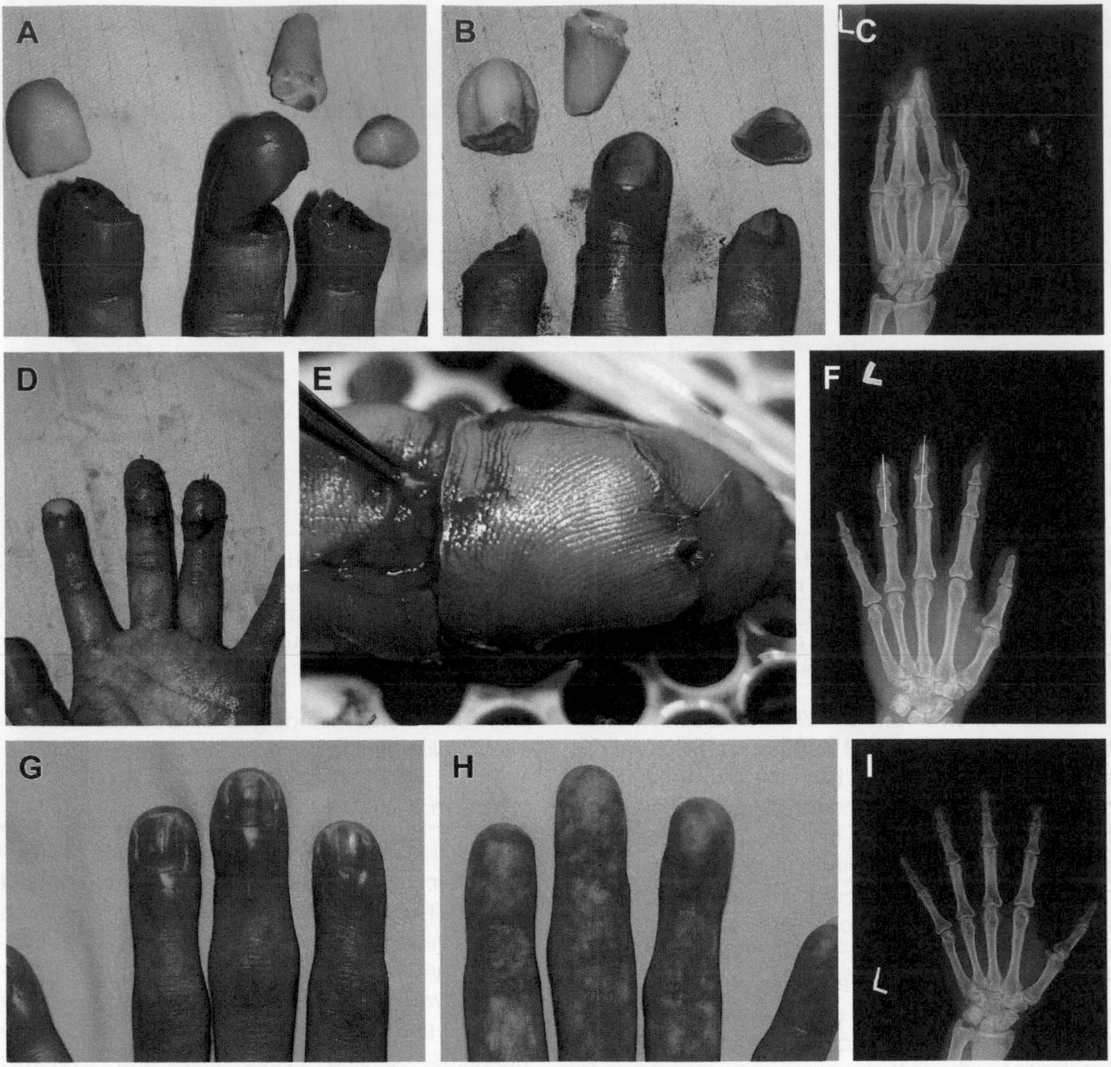

Fig. 6. Complete amputation of the left index, long, and ring fingers at zone 1A. (*A–C*) Preoperative views and radiograph. (*D, E*) Immediate postoperative view; replantation of the left index finger with 1 artery only, 1 artery and 1 vein repair for left long finger, and composite graft for ring finger. In the long finger, 1 volar vein was repaired. In the ring finger, external bleeding from the stab wound of the pulp was maintained for 6 days. (*F*) Postoperative radiograph at 2 weeks. (*G–I*) Postoperative views, about 13 months later.

intolerance were not statistically different between the two groups, pain in the affected fingers was more frequent in the amputation closure group. In spite of a longer hospital stay and the time off from work in the successful replantation group, this group was highly or fairly satisfied with the surgical results. Their conclusion was that replantation provided not only a better appearance but also a better functional outcome. However, there remains a paucity of outcomes data for comparing distal replantation with revision amputation. There are insufficient published data with which to draw conclusions that relate to the cost or the psychological or functional outcomes of one treatment versus the other.

ZONE 1 PROXIMAL AMPUTATION

Zone 1 proximal amputation is defined as the portion between flexor digitorum profundus (FDP) and FDS insertion of the finger. It is subdivided into zone 1C and 1D. Zone 1C is between the FDP insertion and the neck of the middle phalanx, where the periarticular area of the distal interphalangeal (DIP) joint can be found. Zone 1D is the area between the neck of the middle phalanx and FDS insertion. At this level of amputation, replantation is not difficult even in the repair of arteries, veins, and nerves. If replantation is not possible at this level of amputation, revision amputation is a viable alternative. The goals of amputation should be preservation of FDS insertion, durable coverage, preservation of useful sensibility, and prevention of symptomatic neuromas. Even early fitting of finger prosthesis should be applicable and early return of the patient to work, play, and other daily activities should be possible.

1C Level Amputation: Revision Amputation

When the proximal base of the distal phalangeal bone remains, it is preferable to remove this remnant bone to help prevent epidermal cyst of the nail remnant and an unexpectedly short nail. The volar and lateral condylar prominences of the middle phalangeal head should be removed. The flexor and extensor tendons should not be sutured to each other to avoid limiting digit excursion. The digital nerves should be gently pulled distally and then cut away from the scar to avoid neuroma. If bone shortening brings about detachment of FDS insertion, flap coverage is needed to retain the insertion.

Lumbrical-plus Deformity

At this level of amputation, a complication of motor dysfunction is lumbrical-plus deformity. This deformity is caused by excessive tension of the divided and retracted profundus tendon, which increases the tension in the attached lumbrical to cause a paradoxic extension of the interphalangeal joint on attempted flexion. This lumbrical-plus phenomenon occurs most commonly in the long finger. When amputation through the middle phalanx occurs distal to the insertion of FDS tendon, PIP joint flexion is markedly limited, and the middle phalanx is incapable of participating in the grasping of large objects. Dividing the lumbrical at the level of the base of the fibrous flexor sheath helps alleviate the problem.[40]

1D Level Amputation (Amputation Through the Middle Phalanx): Revision Amputation

When an amputation through the middle phalanx is distal to the superficialis insertion, the middle phalanx can participate effectively in grasping activities, although PIP flexion is virtually always limited if the middle phalanx stump is short. If amputation has occurred proximal to the insertion of the superficialis or the FDS insertion is already damaged, there will be no active flexion control of the remaining portion of the middle phalanx. In this case, revision amputation at the PIP joint is recommended. Although no flexion control of the middle phalangeal remnant is possible, the length preservation of such an amputation may be helpful in later use in preventing small objects from falling through the hand. In children or young women or in multiple digit amputation, preservation of the middle phalangeal bone is necessary for cosmetic reasons more than functional ones. Later, secondary reconstruction with toe to hand transfer may be requested; a procedure that is more common in Asian than Western countries (**Fig. 7**). At this level of amputation, at least 1 cm of middle phalangeal bone is required for toe transfer to achieve an acceptable range of proximal phalangeal joint motion. If this amount is not available, finger reconstruction options are limited. Many inexperienced surgeons in the emergency room do not give sufficient consideration to the level of amputation. In contrast with Western countries, flap coverage of the middle phalanx is chosen rather than revision amputation at the PIP joint in many situations.

Level 1C and 1D Amputation (Amputation Through the Middle Phalanx): Replantation

At this level of amputation, replantation is not technically difficult even for repair of arteries, veins, and nerves. At zone IC, artery and nerve repair is simple and vein anastomosis is possible. Around transarticular amputation at the DIP joint, arthrodesis may have a positive effect on final digit function by bone shortening. Bone shortening facilitates soft tissue closure without tension and minimizes the need for grafts of arteries, veins, nerves, and even tendons. Arthrodesis is easily performed by 2 K-wires. Until the end of 1970, it was recommended that zone ID digits amputated distal to the middle portion of the middle phalanx should not be replanted.[1] With refinement of microneurovascular techniques, replantation of an amputated digit distal to the PIP joint in select cases could be a worthwhile procedure.[41,42] May and colleagues[41] were among the first to highlight that replantation distal to the FDS insertion had a high survival rate (96%) and excellent return of function, and that patients accomplished an early return to work. Sensation was good, although all patients developed cold intolerance. In cases of multiple digit replantations at this level, sensibility is more important than motion in radial digits. Replantation of the index and long fingers in combination at this zone of amputation are strong indications to aid pinch restoration. In contrast, ulnar-sided digit replantation is more important in grip function than in sensibility. Single-digit amputation distal to the FDS insertion is an acceptable indication for replantation. Successful replantation can provide the functional length and sensation with nerve regeneration in spite of a nonfunctioning DIP joint.

Bone Fixation Methods and Malunion

Adequate fracture reduction and strong stability permitting early motion and union remain the

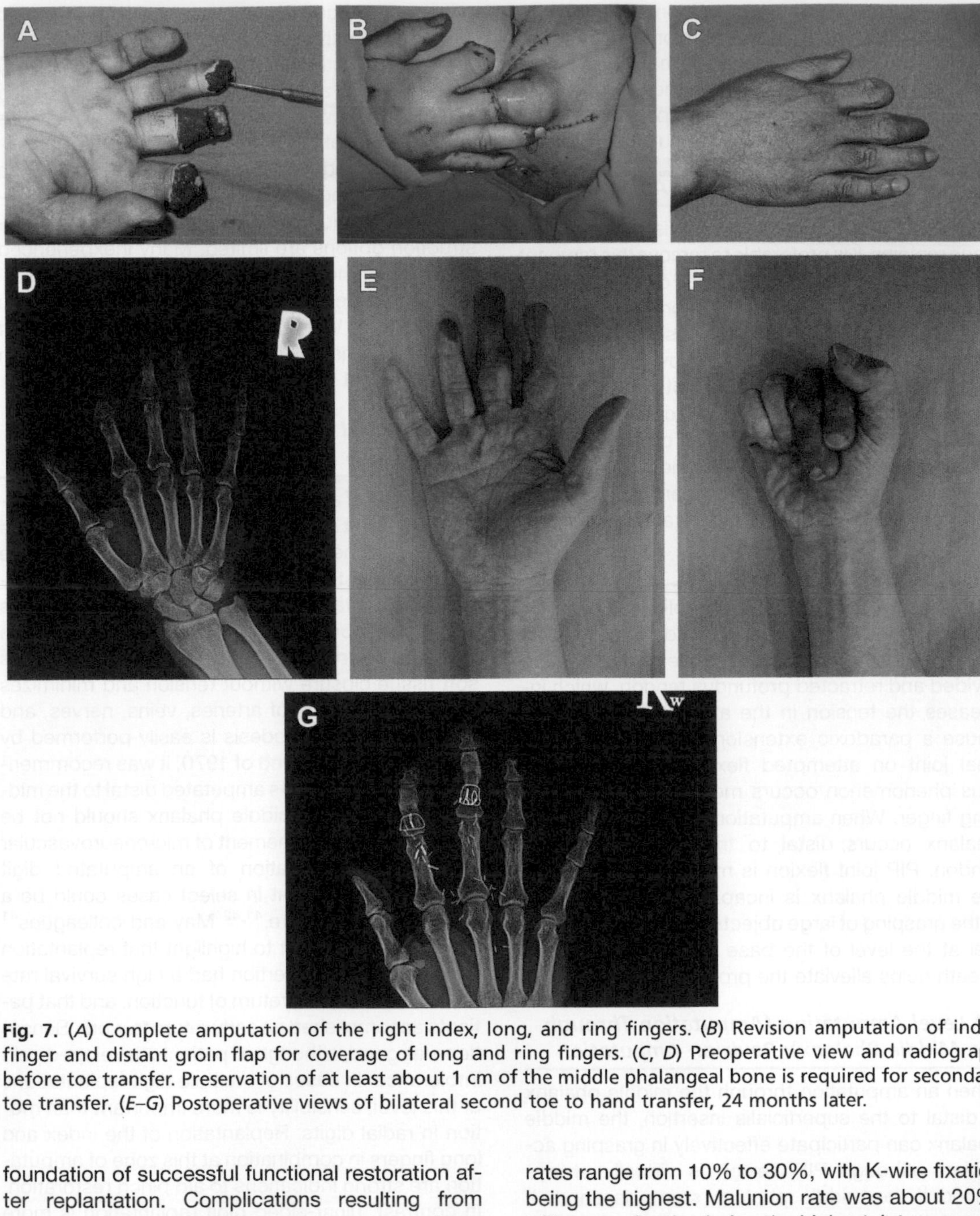

Fig. 7. (*A*) Complete amputation of the right index, long, and ring fingers. (*B*) Revision amputation of index finger and distant groin flap for coverage of long and ring fingers. (*C, D*) Preoperative view and radiograph before toe transfer. Preservation of at least about 1 cm of the middle phalangeal bone is required for secondary toe transfer. (*E–G*) Postoperative views of bilateral second toe to hand transfer, 24 months later.

foundation of successful functional restoration after replantation. Complications resulting from bony instability, malunion, and nonunion have been largely ignored. Compared with simple open fractures, bone fixation procedure during replantation should be simple and easy to apply. There are many suggested fixation methods, including use of K-wires, intraosseous wires, screws and plates, intramedullary wires or bone pegs, absorbable rods, and external fixators. Contrary to our expectations, bony problems after replantation were seen in 30% to 50% of replants.[43,44] According to the reports, nonunion rates range from 10% to 30%, with K-wire fixation being the highest. Malunion rate was about 20%, with screw fixation being the highest. Intraosseous wires alone had the lowest nonunion and complication rates. To prevent these complications, the method of fixation should be different based on the site of amputation. Transarticular amputations are usually fixed with fusion with 2 K-wires for the DIP joint and a single oblique screw for the PIP joint. Intramedullary fixation in digital replantation using bioabsorbable poly-DL-lactic acid rods showed high union with a low incidence of complications. In particular, it is a simple and effective technique for arthrodesis of the DIP or PIP joint.[45,46] Fixation of the diaphyseal fractures is recommended with 90° to 90° perpendicular intraosseous wiring and temporary additional oblique K-wire. In cases of rotational deformity or nonunion, secondary revision with corrective osteotomy and internal fixation with or without bone graft is needed (**Fig. 8**).

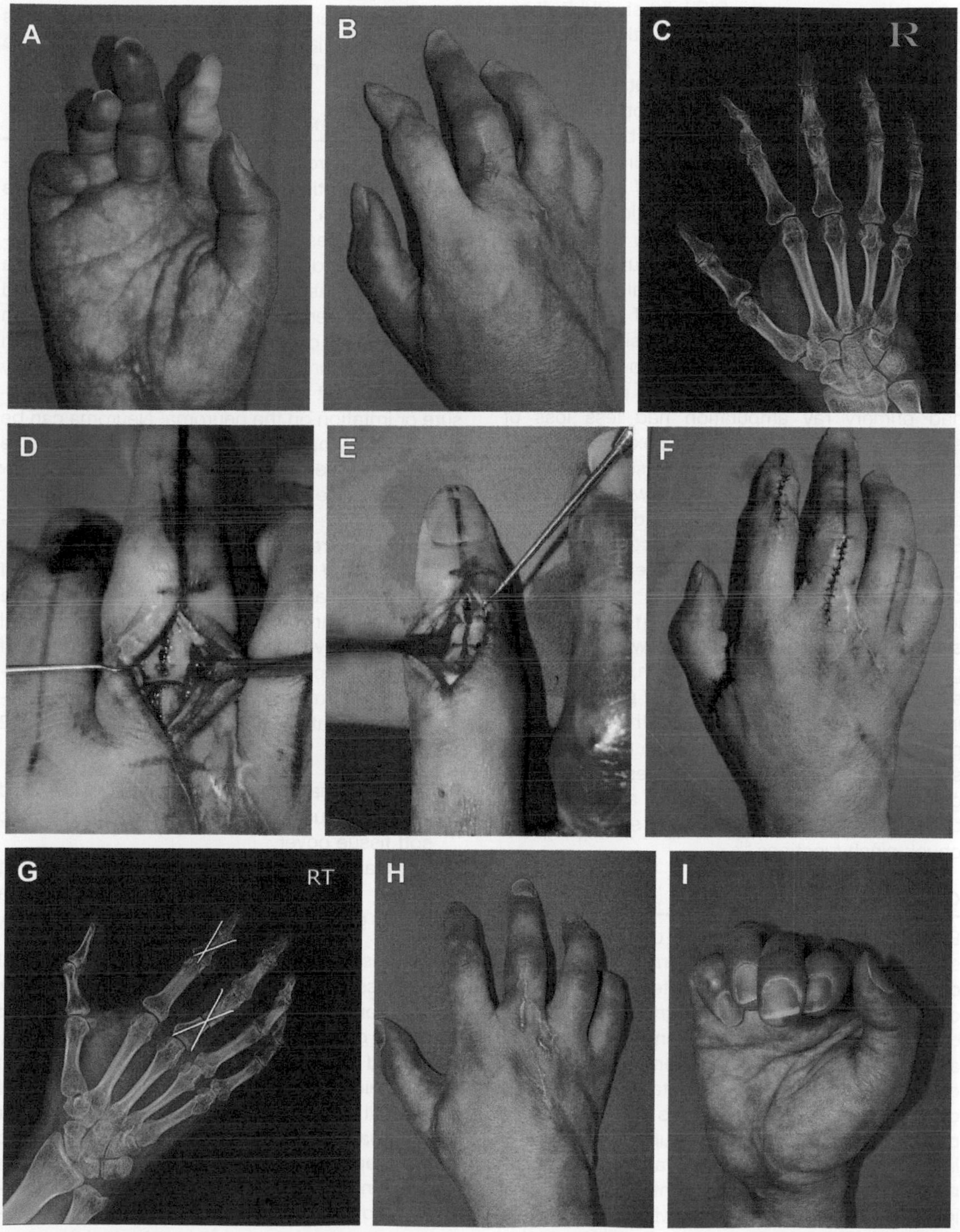

Fig. 8. (*A–C*) Rotational deformity of the right index and long fingers after replantation of right transmetacarpal and index segmental complete amputation. (*D, E*) Derotational osteotomy and internal fixation at the proximal phalanx of the long finger and middle phalanx of the index finger. (*F, G*) Immediately after operation and radiograph. (*H, I*) Postoperative views, 8 months later.

ZONE 2 AMPUTATIONS THROUGH THE MIDDLE PHALANX TO METATARSOPHALANGEAL JOINT: REVISION AMPUTATION

Amputations through the PIP joint should be performed by denuding of articular cartilage, shaping of the condyles of the proximal phalanx, and tension-free skin closure. If amputation level is proximal to the PIP joint, active motion of the remaining proximal bone is controlled by the intrinsic muscles and the extensor digitorum communis. This technique allows about 45° of active flexion in the proximal phalanx. Any remaining segment helps supports hand grip and keep small objects in the palm. However, if the amputation occurs near or at the metatarsophalangeal joint level, it is not easy to persuade patients of the suitability of ray amputation, especially in Asian countries. It is noteworthy that, although the differences were not statistically significant, patients who had primary ray amputation had less loss of strength and less diminution of dexterity. In addition, performing primary ray resection almost halves total disability, shortens work loss, and eliminates the costs of a second procedure.[47] Single-ray amputation is an effective immediate salvage procedure as well as a reasonable secondary reconstructive option to preserve and improve hand function. Long-term functional results of ring avulsion injuries showed decreased grip strength, key pinch strength, chuck pinch strength, hand circumference, and palmar volume in the ray resection group. In the amputation group, only grip strength and pulp pinch strength showed a significant decrease. These results suggest that ray resection should be avoided in patients with occupations that need strong key and chuck pinch functions.[48]

Quadriga Effect

Even with revision amputation of the digit, transient stiffness of the digits and motor dysfunction can result. Verdan[49] used the term syndrome of quadriga to describe the imbalance of the profundus tendon that occurs when this tendon is advanced and sewn to the extensor over the end of an amputation stump. Amputation of the digits causes spontaneous adhesions of the resected profundus tendon to the profundus tendons of intact fingers, which results in a decrease in the power and range of movement of the terminal joints of the uninjured fingers when they attempt full flexion. This condition is surgically correctable by release of the adherent profundus tendon of the amputated digit. Resected profundus tendons should be separated from each other in the palm interossei. If more than 1 finger is amputated, all involved profundi should be left completely free at the proximal palm.[50] To prevent this complication, profundus tendon should not be sutured over the end of the amputated bone stump. Full active flexion and extension of the intact fingers should be initiated in the early postoperative period after primary amputation.

Neuroma Formation

To prevent neuroma formation in revision amputation or replantation, nerve repair without tension is the best option. In digit amputation, injury to the digital nerve results in stump neuroma. Subsequent repair of digital nerves also causes neuroma formation in cases of excessive scarring around the repaired nerve or mismatch in size between proximal and distal segments. The pain from amputation stump neuromas can be caused by scar tissue, soft tissue or bony structures, or pressure or irritation on the neuroma. Neuroma can be diagnosed by pain and paresthesia with a positive Tinel sign as well as confirmation by ultrasonography. There are 4 suggested operative options: resection of the neuroma, use of nerve grafts to reconnect severed proximal and distal stumps, containment of the neuroma, and translocation of the nerve.[51] Laborde and colleagues[52] reported that dorsal translocation of symptomatic digital neuromas provided the most predictable relief among other options, such as excision of the neuroma, ray amputation, neurorrhaphy, or translocation. Translocation of intact neuroma serves 2 purposes:

1. The neuroma is removed from its irritating bed of scar tissue, often in an area of inadequate soft tissue cover.
2. It is placed, preferably dorsally, in an area that is not repeatedly traumatized or involved in power grip.

In cases of implantation of nerve ends into local muscle tissue, it was apparent that either muscular contraction or local pressure in gripping caused irritation of the neuroma. Boldrey[53] originally described intraosseous implantation in 1943. With this technique, the end of the neuroma is mobilized and a drill hole placed through the phalangeal or metacarpal bones. Mass and colleagues[54] showed 90% acceptable results by intraosseous relocation of digital nerve in the management of painful neuroma. Another suggested option to prevent amputation stump neuroma is centrocentral nerve repair.[55] Centrocentral nerve repair involves the coaptation of 2 nerve cords of central origin. The technique can also be applied for 1 nerve if it is split into 2 fascicles of equal size. The 2 nerves or fascicles undergo simple end-to-end repair. Belcher and Pandya[56] showed more pleasing results in centrocentral union than in simple transection of digital nerve for the prevention of neuroma formation after finger amputation. Cessation of axonal growth in this technique may be inferred from the theory that newly formed axons being under pressure in the transplantation area results in a reduction of protein production and axoplasm flow in the neuron, acting to inhibit neuroma development.

ZONE 2 AMPUTATIONS THROUGH THE MIDDLE PHALANX TO METATARSOPHALANGEAL JOINT: REPLANTATION

Circulatory Complications

In the early postoperative period, it is not difficult to detect circulatory complications by monitoring arterial insufficiency after replantation. During reexploration of the occluded artery, reanastomosis or vein graft after resection of the injured segment of artery is mandatory to maintain arterial supply. However, venous problems are more common and are tricky to detect. Compressive dressing with splinting and tight skin suture may be the reasons for venous congestion (**Fig. 9**). If the venous drainage is insufficient, surgical treatment includes resection of the thrombosed vein and reanastomosis, cross-anastomosis, and vein graft. If these methods fail, the more technical procedures, including venous free flap[57] or proximally based cross-finger flap from the dorsal aspect of the adjacent finger, may be required.[58] This venous flap provides a vessel conduit for defects of digital arteries or veins as well as soft tissue coverage. In a retrospective study by Lee and colleagues,[59] correlations between the number and the ratio of anastomosed vessels and the survival rate were verified according to the amputated digital levels. In zone II, an equal or greater number of veins than arteries repaired was an important factor in successful replantation. Repair of as many vessels as possible increases the likelihood of successful replantation. Especially in crush amputation cases, neovascularization between amputation parts is slow even though the replantation seems to be successful. In our clinical experience, some cases of replantation failed after 1 week to 10 days postoperatively. The fate of microanastomosed digital arteries after successful replantation is variable.[60] In cases of successful replantation, ultrasonography using Dopplex machines and angiography revealed no patency of anastomosed arteries in 37% of vessels after an average of 15 postoperative days. The occlusion rate was significantly different between different types of injury: 8% with guillotine and 43% with crush injuries. Amputation at the distal phalanx by crush injury increases the possibility of occlusion of microanastomosed digital arteries. In one longitudinal follow-up study, the arterial supply and reactive hyperemia of the replanted fingers were significantly reduced compared with healthy

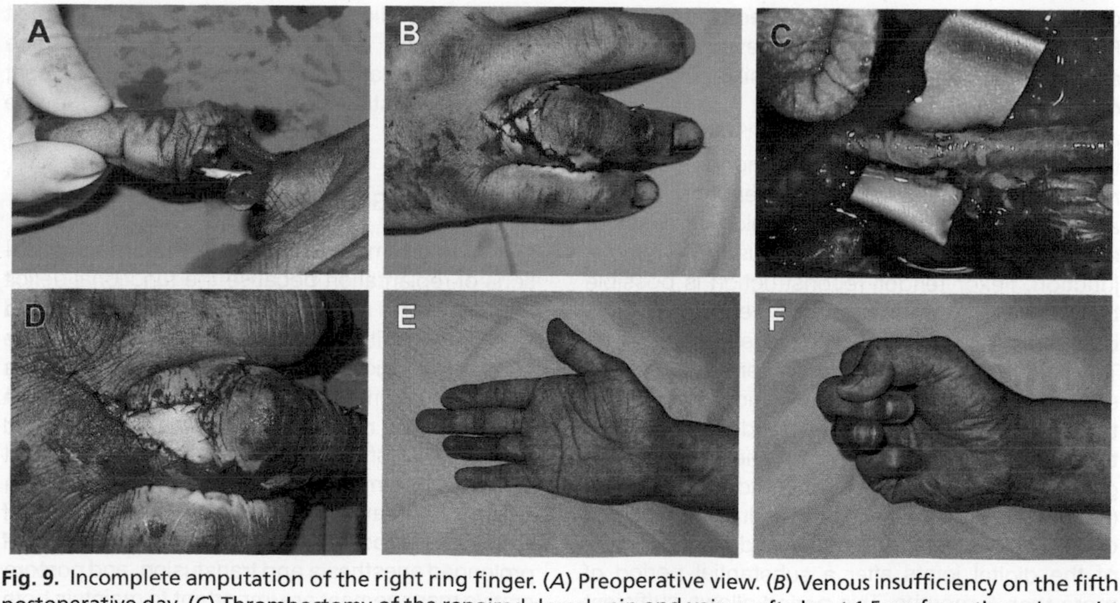

Fig. 9. Incomplete amputation of the right ring finger. (*A*) Preoperative view. (*B*) Venous insufficiency on the fifth postoperative day. (*C*) Thrombectomy of the repaired dorsal vein and vein graft about 1.5 cm from the volar wrist used to reconstruct venous drainage. (*D*) Skin graft on the skin defect of the dorsum. (*E, F*) Postoperative view 7 months later.

digits, despite the anastomosed arteries having been patent for 10 years.[61] Soft tissue atrophy or cold intolerance of surviving stumps is closely related to the type of injury and patency of microanastomosed arteries. However, a 12-year prospective study of the natural history of digital replantation concluded that cold-induced discomfort is not normalized and total blood flow improvement is not affected by late arterial occlusion.[62]

Other important factors affecting circulation in the digit are smoking and ischemic time. The patient's smoking history has minimal influence on the survival of successful replantation but, if patients continue to smoke postoperatively, they should be warned that they may be at higher risk of complications and failure. In digital replantation, although prolonged cold ischemic time does not affect survival rate and is not related to final functional outcome, more data are needed to reach a firm conclusion. Cosmetically, progressive atrophy of the replanted digits resulted from the circulatory insufficiency of cold intolerance, crush type of injury, vessel occlusion, continued smoking, neglected rehabilitation, or avoidance of daily use of replanted digits.

Tendon Repair and Adhesion

In cases of joint fusion, there are few problems caused by tendon repairs. Tendon repair should be as strong as bone fixation to allow early mobilization. In flexor tendon repair, a 4-strand (or more) core suture technique is preferred. In zone II injuries, repair of only the FDP tendon may be undertaken to avoid adhesions between the FDS and FDP tendon suture lines.[63] However, both FDP and FDS should be repaired if possible. FDS repair can provide independent PIP joint motion as well as a gliding surface for the FDP.[64] The extensor tendon is repaired next by using a horizontal mattress stitch, and the intrinsic tendons, if available, are repaired in a similar fashion. In cases of avulsed flexor tendon from musculotendinous junction, flexor tendon reconstruction is possible by interweaving the tendon into the viable muscle belly or by delayed repair with staged tendon graft. To avoid tendon complications after tendon repair, strong repair and early rehabilitation are mandatory. The indications for flexor tendon tenolysis of the replanted digits are almost the same as the general indications for flexor tendon injury only (**Fig. 10**). These indications include significant discrepancy between passive and active flexion of the digital joints after a substantial period of more than 6 months. This period allows sufficient time for wound healing and maximal rehabilitation therapy. Tenolysis after digital replantations is a useful and safe procedure to achieve an improvement in active flexion of the digit. After tenolysis of the flexor pollicis longus, avulsion amputation, significant PIP joint stiffness, and multiple digit amputations, the reconstructive outcome was less positive and represented poorer prognostic features.[65]

RING AVULSION AMPUTATION

Ring avulsion injuries have traditionally been treated by revision amputation or ray resection. Both success rates and functional results were considered unsatisfactory. Furthermore, a multistaged operation is necessary because of extensive damage of skin, nerves, and vessels. In 1989, Kay and colleagues[66] reported a 73% success rate in 55 cases of ring avulsion injury. Most patients (80%–90%) were satisfied with their functional results. According to Sears and Chung,[67] mean survival outcome in complete avulsion injuries was 66% and 78% in incomplete injuries. Mean survival outcome for 2 types of avulsion injuries was 71%, which is similar to other types of replantation. Functional outcomes of sensibility and range of motion after replantation of finger avulsion injuries are better than what is historically cited in the literature (**Fig. 11**). The results of this systematic review challenge the practice routine revision amputation of all complete finger avulsion injuries. The best indication for replantation is avulsion injuries distal to the insertion of the FDS with a functioning PIP joint.[68] Replantation needs either long reverse venous interposition grafts or transfer of a digital artery from an adjacent digit and at least 2 dorsal veins. Additional coverage with venous flap is harvested from an adjacent digit or the distal forearm, depending on the size of the defect.

MULTIPLE DIGIT REPLANTATIONS

Multiple digit amputation is one of the classic indications of replantation because the functional deficit after the loss of multiple digits is severe. Compared with single-digit or double-digit replantation, there are many considerations in replantation operations for 3 or more fingers. Complications resulting from the extensive replantation effort are not limited to functional or cosmetic problems of the hand. To avoid systemic or more serious general complications, operation techniques, preservation of stumps, method of anesthesiology, prevention of prolonged anesthesia and transfusion, and postoperative management are important to maintain both the survival of the digits and the vital signs of the patient. First, regarding anesthesia, an

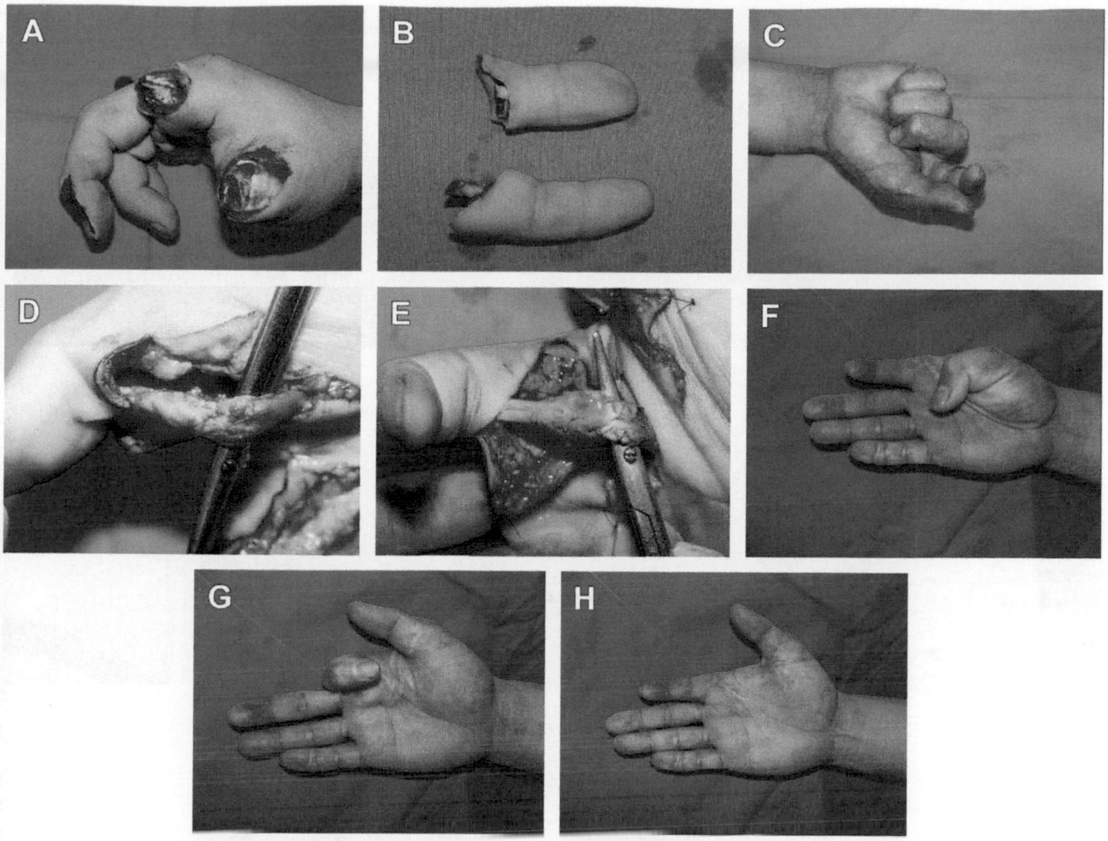

Fig. 10. (*A, B*) Complete amputation of right thumb and index finger at zone II. (*C*) Limited range of motion of both thumb and index by flexor tendon adhesion, even after successful replantation. (*D, E*) Tenolysis of flexor tendons of the thumb and index finger. (*F–H*) Recovered active range of motion of the thumb and index finger; 12 months postoperative view.

ultrasonography-guided brachial plexus block with a long-acting agent is preferred in unilateral injury. Even in busy operation rooms or operation times late in the day, surgeons should remain able to check the condition of the patient easily and verbally. Under the brachial plexus block, the sensation of postoperative pain is mitigated by maintaining the anesthetic effect even after an operation. The effect of sympathetic block by anesthetic drugs results in the vasodilatation of anastomosed vessels. However, in general anesthesia, systemic vasodilatation by inhalation agents causes severe hypovolemic shock with massive blood loss. With regard to prolonged ischemic time, it is preferable to use a digit-by-digit replantation sequence rather than structure-by-structure replantation. Digit-by-digit sequence is usually in the radial-to-ulnar direction. Because of the importance of the pinching and grasping functions of the hand, a good replantation order is the thumb first followed by the middle finger, the ring finger, index finger, and the little finger last.[69] In this way, reduction of the warm ischemic time is possible by cold storage of the remaining digits and it also limits the amount of blood loss while attaining stability of the patient's vital signs. To reduce operation time, a structure-by-structure sequence is more efficient (**Fig. 12**) because prolonged cold ischemic time at this level of amputation does not affect the survival rate and final functional results of the replanted digits.[70–73] In cases of 9-digit to 10-digit replantation by Kim and colleagues,[72] transfusions averaged 10.4 L (22 pints) from a range of 2.8 to 18.0 L (6–38 pints). Patients experienced intraoperative hypovolemic shock during operation and were managed in the intensive care unit. Furthermore, postoperative administration of multiple anticoagulants greatly increases blood loss and need for blood transfusion. Blood transfusion should be prepared before operation in cases in which 3 digits or more are being replanted. Intensive care monitoring is necessary for complications caused by massive transfusion as well as for maintaining the patient's general condition. Massive transfusion can result in transmission of viral disease as well as alteration of coagulation systems. The importance of salvaging a replanted

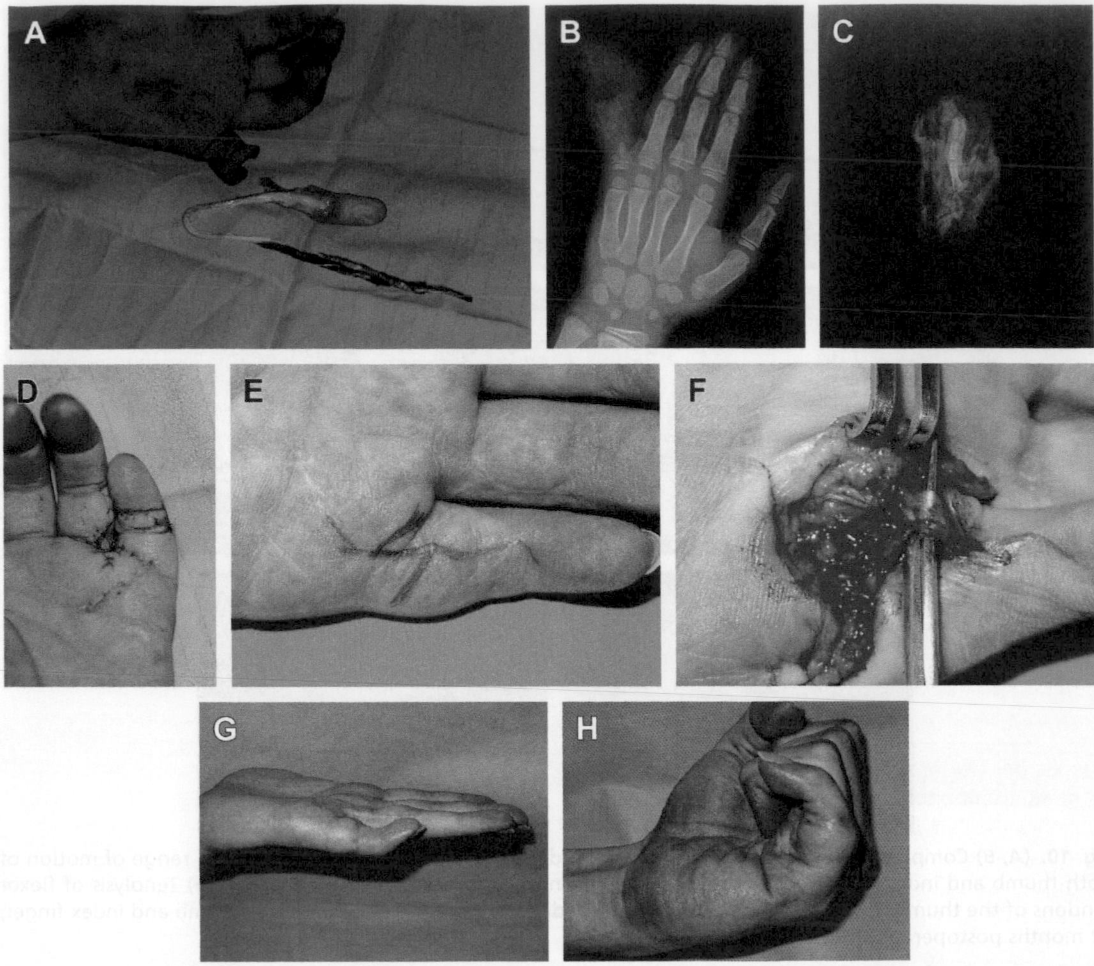

Fig. 11. Replantation of avulsion amputation of the right small finger in a 6-year-old boy. (*A*) Preoperative view shows avulsed flexor tendons from musculotendinous junction. (*B, C*) Bone fracture at base of the proximal phalanx. (*D*) Ulnar digital artery of ring finger and fourth FDS tendon was transferred to reconstruct the radial digital artery and fifth FDP remnant of the small finger. (*E, F*) After 14 years, secondary operation for tenolysis of flexor tendon and scar contracture release. (*G, H*) Ten months postoperative view.

digit or digits must be weighed against the risks of a blood transfusion.[74] Therefore, to decrease the amount of blood transfused, surgeons should consider intermittent use of pneumatic tourniquet, structure-by-structure sequence of operation, as well as brachial plexus block for anesthesia. Shortening of the phalangeal bone during osteosynthesis can also avoid the need for vessel, tendon, or skin graft. Maintenance of digital length is not a positive factor for the final functional result. If vein graft is needed, harvesting from the large venous network on the volar aspect of the forearm is better than from 1 or 2 separate veins.[75] In cases of bilateral amputation, intentionally delayed or suspended replantation is another good option to maintain a stable condition of the patient as well as to assist the medical management.[76]

ECONOMIC ANALYSIS

There are many different socioeconomic points of views on the management of digital amputations. Depending on the cultural background and insurance system of each country, treatment options vary widely. The incidence of replantation in the United States is low for finger amputation. For the years 2001, 2004, and 2007, 73% of thumb and 88% of finger traumatic amputations were treated with revision amputation.[77] Patients who underwent replantation were younger, incurred higher hospital charges, and had longer hospital stays compared with patients who did not. In hand surgery, single digit amputation proximal to the FDS insertion is traditionally not an indication for replantation. In Korea and other Asian countries, if the doctor explains this to the patient and

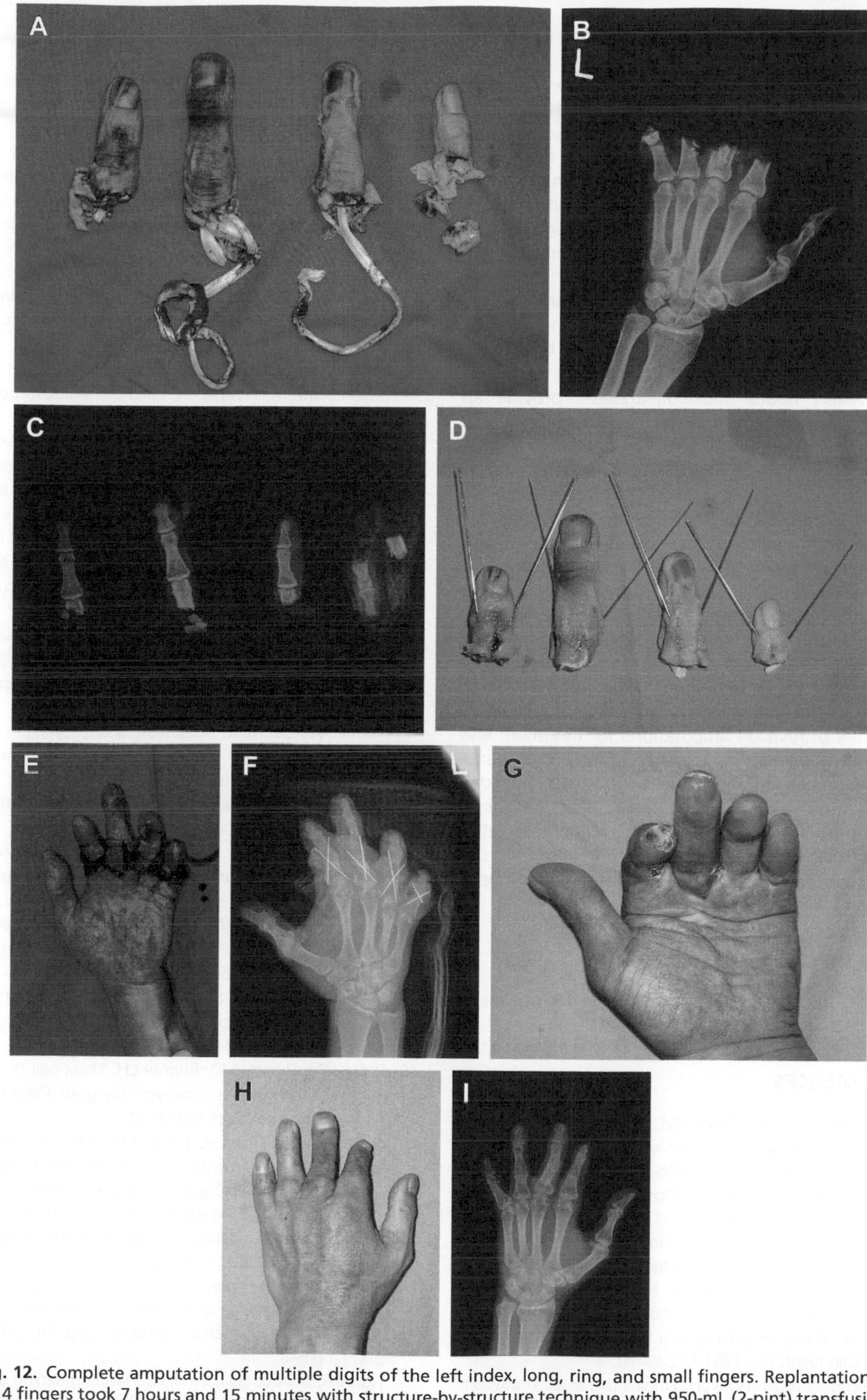

Fig. 12. Complete amputation of multiple digits of the left index, long, ring, and small fingers. Replantation of all 4 fingers took 7 hours and 15 minutes with structure-by-structure technique with 950-mL (2-pint) transfusion. (*A–C*) Preoperative view and radiographs. (*D*) Cross–K-wire fixation of the amputation stumps after identification of arteries, veins, nerves, and tendons. (*E*, *F*) Immediate postoperative view and radiograph. (*G–I*) Sixteen months postoperative views and radiograph.

recommends revision amputation, the patient is likely to be upset and leave the hospital for replantation elsewhere. Even in very distal amputation, doctors have to attempt replantation if the patient wants it. In cases in which replantation is impossible, other options, such as composite graft or secondary flap coverage, are requested to maintain the original length or shape. There are few evidence-based research articles on economic analysis in the management of digital amputation, even in the United States. The outcomes of revision amputation and replantation have been inadequately investigated and are poorly understood. However, Sears and colleagues[78] provide an essential review of the economic analysis of this topic. Replantation treatment incurred greater costs than revision amputation after adjustment for quality of life gained following surgery. The costs increased whenever indications for replantation existed, although the figures vary greatly depending on injury type. This finding highlights the variability in the value of replantation among different injury scenarios. Giladi and colleagues[79] reported outcomes and long-term disability following revision amputation in the treatment of traumatic finger and thumb amputation injuries. Despite the importance of understanding the outcomes of revision amputations for treatment and resource allocation, there has been inadequate investigation to date. However, this study provides pilot data necessary to take additional steps in comprehensively evaluating outcomes after amputation and replantation, and to improving understanding of how the treatment of finger amputation injuries affects long-term disability.

ACKNOWLEDGMENTS

The authors thank Andrew Miller for his assistance in editing this article.

REFERENCES

1. Morrison WA, O'Brien BM, MacLeod AM. Evaluation of digital replantation: a review of 100 cases. Orthop Clin North Am 1977;8:295–308.
2. Weiland AJ, Villarreal-Rios A, Kleinert HE, et al. Replantation of digits and hands: analysis of surgical techniques and functional results in 71 patients with 86 replantations. J Hand Surg Am 1977;2:1–12.
3. Zhong-Wei C, Meyer VE, Kleinert HE, et al. Present indications and contraindications for replantation as reflected by long-term functional results. Orthop Clin North Am 1981;12:849–70.
4. Urbaniak JR, Roth JH, Nunley JA, et al. The results of replantation after amputation of a single finger. J Hand Surg Am 1985;67:611–9.
5. Soucacos PN, Beris AE, Touliatos AS, et al. Current indications for single digit replantation. Acta Orthop Scand Suppl 1995;264:12–5.
6. Scott FA, Howar JW, Boswick JA Jr. Recovery of function following replantation and revascularization of amputated hand parts. J Trauma 1981;21:204–14.
7. Jones JM, Schenck RR, Chesney RB. Digital replantation and amputation—comparison of function. J Hand Surg Am 1982;7:183–9.
8. Cheng GL, Pan DD, Zhang NP, et al. Digital replantation in children: a long-term follow-up study. J Hand Surg Am 1998;23(4):635–46.
9. Shi D, Qi J, Li D, et al. Fingertip replantation at or beyond the nail base in children. Microsurgery 2010;30(5):380–5.
10. Kleinert HE, Cash SL. Current guideline for flexor tendon repair within the fibro-osseous tunnel: indication, timing and technique. In: Hunter JM, Schneider LH, Mackin EJ, editors. Tendon surgery in the hand. St. Louis (MO): CV Mosby Co; 1987. p. 117.
11. Sebastin SJ, Chung KC. A systematic review of the outcomes of replantation of distal digital amputation. Plast Reconstr Surg 2011;128(3):723–37.
12. Hattori Y, Doi K, Ikeda K, et al. A retrospective study of functional outcomes after successful replantation versus amputation closure for single fingertip amputations. J Hand Surg Am 2006;31:811–8.
13. Kumar VP, Satku K. Treatment and prevention of "hook nail" deformity with anatomic correlation. J Hand Surg Am 1993;18(4):617–20.
14. Chow SP, Ho E. Open treatment of fingertip injuries in adults. J Hand Surg Am 1982;7(5):470–6.
15. Blair JW, Moskal MJ. Revision amputation achieving maximum function and minimizing problems. Hand Clin 2001;17(3):457–71.
16. Atasoy E, Godfrey A, Kalisman M. The "antenna" procedure for the "hook-nail" deformity. J Hand Surg Am 1983;8(1):55–8.
17. Strick MJ, Bremner-Smith AT, Tonkin MA. Antenna procedure for the correction of hook nail deformity. J Hand Surg Br 2004;29(1):3–7.
18. Bubak PJ, Richey MD, Engrav LH. Hook nail deformity repaired using a composite toe graft. Plast Reconstr Surg 1992;90(6):1079–82.
19. Dumontier C, Gilbert A, Tubiana R. Hook-nail deformity: surgical treatment with a homodigital advancement flap. J Hand Surg Br 1995;20(6):830–5.
20. Yoon WY, Lee BI. Fingertip reconstruction using free toe tissue transfer without venous anastomosis. Arch Plast Surg 2012;39(5):546–50.
21. García-López A, Laredo C, Rojas A. Oblique triangular neurovascular osteocutaneous flap for hook nail deformity correction. J Hand Surg Am 2014;39(7):1415–8.
22. Adani R, Marcoccio I, Tarallo L. Nail lengthening and fingertip amputations. Plast Reconstr Surg 2003;112(5):1287–94.

23. Oh SK, Lee YJ, Woo SH, et al. Immediate full-thickness nail bed graft with various skin flaps for the acute nail bed defects of fingertip injuries. J Korean Soc Surg Hand 2007;12(4):151–7.
24. Shepard GH. Treatment of nail bed avulsions with split-thickness nail bed grafts. J Hand Surg Am 1983;8(1):49–54.
25. Nishi G, Shibata Y, Tago K, et al. Nail regeneration in digits replanted after amputation through the distal phalanx. J Hand Surg Am 1996;21(2):229–33.
26. Hattori Y, Doi K, Sakamoto S, et al. Fingertip replantation. J Hand Surg Am 2007;32(4):548–55.
27. Jazayeri L, Klausner JQ, Chang J. Distal digital replantation. Plast Reconstr Surg 2013;132(5):1207–17.
28. Buntic RF, Brooks D. Standardized protocol for artery-only fingertip replantation. J Hand Surg Am 2010;35(9):1491–6.
29. Erken HY, Takka S, Akmaz I. Artery-only fingertip replantations using a controlled nailbed bleeding protocol. J Hand Surg Am 2013;38(11):2173–9.
30. Chen YC, Chan FC, Hsu CC, et al. Fingertip replantation without venous anastomosis. Ann Plast Surg 2013;70(3):284–8.
31. Schekor LR, Becker GW. Distal finger replantation. J Hand Surg Am 2011;36(3):521–8.
32. Hattori Y, Doi K, Ikeda K, et al. Significance of venous anastomosis in fingertip replantation. Plast Reconstr Surg 2003;111(3):1151–8.
33. Koshima I, Yamashita S, Sugiyama N, et al. Successful delayed venous drainage in 16 consecutive distal phalangeal replantations. Plast Reconstr Surg 2005;115(1):149–54.
34. Li J, Guo Z, Zhu Q, et al. Fingertip replantation: determinants of survival. Plast Reconstr Surg 2008; 122(3):833–9.
35. Feng SM, Gu JX, Zhang NC, et al. Arterial and venous revascularization with bifurcation of a single central artery: a reliable strategy for Tamai zone I replantation. Plast Reconstr Surg 2010;126(6): 2043–51.
36. Han SK, Lee BI, Kim WK. Topical and systemic anticoagulation in the treatment of absent or compromised venous outflow in replanted fingertips. J Hand Surg Am 2000;25(4):659–67.
37. Oh SK, Kim KC, Woo SH, et al. A retrospective analysis of 101 cases of distal digital replantation. J Korean Soc Microsurg Surg 2007;12(4): 151–7.
38. Evans J, Lunnis PJ, Gaunt PN, et al. A case of septicaemia due to *Aeromonas hydrophila*. Br J Plast Surg 1990;43(3):371–2.
39. Lineaweaver WC, Hill MK, Buncke GM, et al. *Aeromonas hydrophila* infections following use of medicinal leeches in replantation and flap surgery. Ann Plast Surg 1992;29(3):238–44.
40. Parkes A. The "lumbrical plus" finger. J Bone Joint Surg Br 1971;53(2):236–9.
41. May JW Jr, Toth BA, Gardner M. Digital replantation distal to the proximal interphalangeal joint. J Hand Surg Am 1982;7(2):161–6.
42. Tark KC, Kim YW, Lee YH, et al. Replantation and revascularization of hands: clinical analysis and functional results of 261 cases. J Hand Surg Am 1989;14(1):17–27.
43. Hoffman R, Buck-Gramcko D. Osteosynthesis in digital replantation surgery. Ann Chir Gynaecol 1982;71(1):14–8.
44. Whitney TM, Lineaweaver WC, Buncke HJ, et al. Clinical results of bony fixation methods in digital replantation. J Hand Surg Am 1990;15(2):328–34.
45. Arata J, Ishikawa K, Sawabe K, et al. Osteosynthesis in digital replantation using bioabsorbable rods. Ann Plast Surg 2003;50(4):350–3.
46. Peiji W, Qirong D, Jianzhong Q, et al. Intramedullary fixation in digital replantation using bioabsorbable poly-DL-lactic acid rods. J Hand Surg Am 2012; 37(12):2547–52.
47. Peimer CA, Wheeler DR, Barrett A, et al. Hand function following single ray amputation. J Hand Surg Am 1999;24(6):1245–8.
48. Nuzumlali E, Orhun E, Oztürk K, et al. Results of ray resection and amputation for ring avulsion injuries at the proximal interphalangeal joint. J Hand Surg Br 2003;28(6):578–81.
49. Verdan C. Syndrome of the quadriga. Surg Clin North Am 1960;40:425–6.
50. Neu BR, Murray JF, MacKenzie JK. Profundus tendon blockage: quadriga in finger amputations. J Hand Surg Am 1985;10(6):878–83.
51. Brogan DM, Kakar S. Management of neuromas of the upper extremity. Hand Clin 2013;29(3):409–20.
52. Laborde KJ, Kalisman M, Tsai TM. Results of surgical treatment of painful neuromas of the hand. J Hand Surg Am 1982;7(2):190–3.
53. Boldrey E. Amputation neuroma in nerves implanted in bone. Ann Surg 1943;118(6):1052–7.
54. Mass DP, Ciano MC, Tortosa R, et al. Treatment of painful hand neuromas by their transfer into bone. Plast Reconstr Surg 1984;74(2):182–5.
55. Gorkisch K, Boese-Landgraf J, Vaubel E. Treatment and prevention of amputation neuromas in hand surgery. Plast Reconstr Surg 1984;73:293–9.
56. Belcher HJ, Pandya AN. Centro-central union for the prevention of neuroma formation after finger amputation. J Hand Surg Br 2000;25(2):154–9.
57. Tsai TM, Matiko JD, Breidenbach W, et al. Venous flaps in digital revascularization and replantation. J Reconstr Microsurg 1987;3(2):113–9.
58. Zhao J, Abdullah S, Li WJ, et al. A novel solution for venous congestion following digital replantation: a proximally based cross-finger flap. J Hand Surg Am 2011;36(7):1224–30.
59. Lee BI, Chung HY, Kim WK, et al. The effects of the number and ratio of repaired arteries and veins on

the survival rate in digital replantation. Ann Plast Surg 2000;44(3):288–94.
60. Lee CH, Han SK, Dhong ES, et al. The fate of microanastomosed digital arteries after successful replantation. Plast Reconstr Surg 2005;116(3):805–10.
61. Meuli-Simmen C, Canova M, Bollinger A, et al. Long-term follow up after finger and upper limb replantation: clinical, angiologic, and lymphographic studies. J Reconstr Microsurg 1998;14(2):131–6.
62. Povlsen B, Nylander G, Nylander E. Natural history of digital replantation: a 12-year prospective study. Microsurgery 1995;16(3):138–40.
63. Chung KC, Alderman AK. Replantation of the upper extremity: indications and outcomes. J Hand Surg Am 2002;2(2):78–94.
64. Lim BH, Tan BK, Peng YP. Digital replantations including fingertip and ring avulsion. Hand Clin 2001;17(3):419–31.
65. Jupiter JB, Pess GM, Bour CJ. Results of flexor tendon tenolysis after replantation in the hand. J Hand Surg Am 1989;14(1):35–44.
66. Kay S, Werntz J, Wolff TW. Ring avulsion injuries: classification and prognosis. J Hand Surg Am 1989;14(2):204–13.
67. Sears ED, Chung KC. Replantation of finger avulsion injuries: a systematic review of survival and functional outcomes. J Hand Surg Am 2011;36(4):686–94.
68. Rawles RB, Deal DN. Treatment of the complete ring avulsion injury. J Hand Surg Am 2013;39(9): 1800–2.
69. May JW Jr, Hergrueter CA, Hansen RH. Seven digit replantation: digit survival after 39 hours of cold ischemia. Plast Reconstr Surg 1986;78(4): 522–5.
70. Wei FC, Chang YL, Chen HC, et al. Three successful digital replantation in a patient after 84, 86, and 94 hours of cold ischemia time. Plast Reconstr Surg 1988;82(2):346–50.
71. VanderWilde RS, Wood MB, Zu ZG. Hand replantation after 54 hours of cold ischemia. J Hand Surg Am 1992;17(2):217–20.
72. Kim WK, Lee JM, Lim JH. Eight cases of nine-digit and ten-digit replantations. Plast Reconstr Surg 1996;98(3):477–84.
73. Kim TB, Lee YJ, Woo SH, et al. The fate of neglected vascular injury of the hand in acute hand injuries. J Korean Soc Microsurg 2007;16(1):30–8.
74. Furnas HJ, Lineaweaver W, Buncke HJ. Blood loss associated with anticoagulation in patients with replanted digits. J Hand Surg Am 1992;17(2):226–9.
75. Jones NF, Jupiter JB. The use of Y-shaped interposition vein grafts in multiple digit replantations. J Hand Surg Am 1985;10(5):675–8.
76. Woo SH, Cheon HJ, Kim YW, et al. Delayed and suspended replantation in complete amputation of digits and hands. J Hand Surg Am 2015;(40):883–9.
77. Friedrich JB, Poppler LH, Mack CD, et al. Epidemiology of upper extremity replantation surgery in the United States. J Hand Surg Am 2011;36(11):1835–40.
78. Sears ED, Shin R, Prosser LA, et al. Economic analysis of revision amputation and replantation treatment of finger amputation injuries. Plast Reconstr Surg 2014;133(4):827–40.
79. Giladi AM, McGlinn EP, Shauver MJ, et al. Measuring outcomes and determining long-term disability after revision amputation for treatment of traumatic finger and thumb amputation injuries. Plast Reconstr Surg 2014;134(5):746e–55e.

Management of Complications with Flap Procedures and Replantation

Douglas M. Sammer, MD

KEYWORDS

• Microsurgery • Microvascular • Replant • Complication • Free flap

KEY POINTS

- Vascular complications of flap procedures and replantation surgery in the upper extremity can be minimized by employing appropriate indications and thorough preoperative planning.
- Efficient surgery, with carefully performed vascular anastomoses outside the zone of injury, is paramount to the success of both replantation and free flap surgery.
- Skeletal shortening (in the case of replantation) or vein grafting may be necessary to achieve this goal. In both free flaps and pedicled flaps, careful attention to pedicle lay, with avoidance of kinking, twisting, and compression, is critical.
- Intra- and postoperative warming and hydration, pain control, and avoidance of vasopressors are important.

INTRODUCTION

Replantation and flap procedures employ microvascular techniques to salvage or reconstruct a severely damaged limb or digit. Although many types of complications can occur, the most devastating include complete or partial flap loss, or replantation failure due to vascular complications. Often, these complications can be prevented by appropriate patient selection, careful surgical planning, meticulous technique, and proper postoperative management. This article discusses complications related to replantation and flap procedures in the upper limb, focusing on the prevention and management of these complications.

REPLANTATION

Complications such as ischemia or venous congestion can result in postoperative loss of a successfully replanted part, a scenario that is frustrating for the surgeon and devastating for the patient. Reported replantation survival rates vary from as low as 66% to as high as 94%, although most recent reports are in the higher end of that range.[1–8]

The most effective way to minimize complications in replantation surgery is to establish and maintain appropriate surgical indications. Sharp amputations have a higher replantation survival rate than amputations that involve a crush or avulsion mechanism, likely because of the arterial intimal damage that accompanies these injuries.[9–12] In a landmark study of 1018 digital replantations, Waikakul and colleagues[8] found mechanism of injury to be the most important variable affecting survival rate. The replantation survival rates of sharp amputations and localized crush injuries were high, at 99.5% and 98%, respectively. However, avulsion amputations and degloving injuries had much lower survival rates of 79% and 51%, respectively. Extensive crush injuries were the least likely to survive after replantation, with a success rate of only 33%. In a subsequent meta-analysis, Dec and colleagues[7]

Department of Plastic Surgery, University of Texas Southwestern Medical Center, 1801 Inwood Road, Dallas, TX 75390, USA
E-mail address: Douglas.Sammer@UTSouthwestern.edu

Hand Clin 31 (2015) 339–344
http://dx.doi.org/10.1016/j.hcl.2015.01.008
0749-0712/15/$ – see front matter

demonstrated that sharply amputated digits have a 5 times higher replantation survival rate than crush or avulsion amputations. The importance of injury mechanism is further supported by an animal model of vascular repair, in which crush–avulsion injuries had a 25% 1-week patency rate compared with 100% patency for sharp injuries.[9] At times, replantation is clearly contraindicated owing to an obvious extensive crush mechanism. However, in some cases, intraoperative examination under the microscope must be performed to determine the suitability of the injured vessels for anastomosis. The corkscrew sign indicates severe avulsion of the artery. The red line sign on the skin overlying the course of the digital artery also indicates extensive avulsion and intimal injury (**Fig. 1**). In these circumstances, replantation is likely to fail. Although multiple patient and surgeon factors determine whether replantation is ultimately performed, a critical and realistic evaluation of the injury mechanism is the most important step in preventing replantation failure.

Other factors that affect replantation survival rates include patient age and smoking status. Young age (<13 years) has been associated with higher replantation survival rates.[8] Unlike elective free flap surgery in which tobacco use appears to have little effect, smoking does diminish

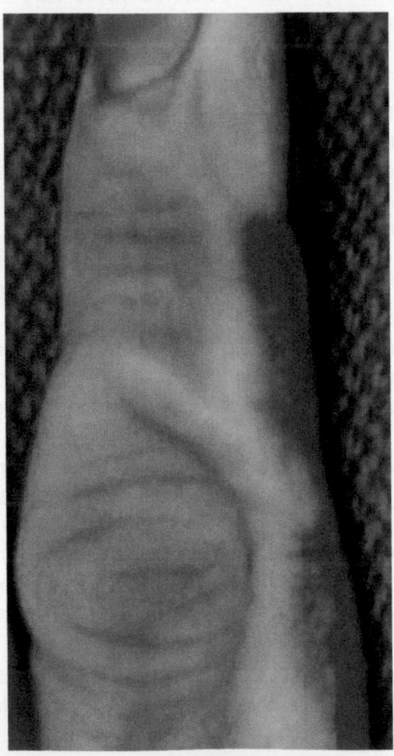

Fig. 1. The red line sign indicates an avulsion injury of the digital artery and extensive intimal damage.

replantation survival rates, reducing them from 97% in nonsmokers to 61% in smokers.[8] Another concern is ischemia time. Delayed replantation of proximal amputations that include skeletal muscle can result in limb- and life-threatening complications.[13] Irreversible damage to myocytes begins within 3 hours of warm ischemia, and complete necrosis occurs within 6 hours.[14] The time frame for re-establishing perfusion can be prolonged up to 12 hours if the amputated limb has been cooled appropriately. Beyond this time frame, replantation will not be possible due to cellular damage, muscle necrosis, and the no-reflow phenomenon. When replantation of a proximal amputation is performed, the patient must be closely monitored in the intensive care setting postoperatively. As toxic metabolites that have built up within the replanted limb during the ischemic period begin enter the systemic circulation, renal failure, cardiovascular collapse, multisystem organ failure, and in some cases death may occur.[13] Although minimizing ischemia time is critical in proximal replantations, ischemia time has little effect on the survival rate of digital amputations.[8] In fact, successful replantation of a digit after 94 hours of cold ischemia has been reported.[15]

In addition to patient and injury characteristics, intraoperative decision making can affect replant survival. In the study by Waikakul and colleagues,[8] replanted digits that underwent repair of a single artery had a 69% survival rate, compared with a 98% survival rate for those in which both arteries were repaired. Similarly, digits with a single venous anastomosis had a 56% survival rate compared with 94% for those in which 2 veins were repaired.[8] Replanted digits with a direct arterial anastomosis had a survival rate of 96% compared to an 86% survival rate when vein grafts were used.[8] It is unclear whether these findings actually indicate the importance of performing a primary repair of two arteries and two veins, or whether they simply reflect of the severity and mechanism of the injuries. Furthermore, although vein grafting was associated with lower survival rates in the study by Waikakul and colleagues,[8] other studies contradict this finding, demonstrating no effect of vein grafts on outcome.[16,17] In amputations with sharp or localized crush injuries, the most pragmatic approach is to perform skeletal shortening in order to allow tension-free primary anastomoses within minimally damaged vessels. On the other hand, the surgeon should have a low threshold for vein grafting in the case of an avulsion injury or more extensive crush injury. Because venous congestion is a common complication of replantation surgery, a minimum of 2 veins should be repaired per digit whenever possible.

Other simple steps can be taken in the operating room and postoperatively to prevent complications. The patient should be kept warm and well hydrated at all times. Efforts should be made to avoid hypotension, and to avoid the use of vasopressors. A regional block indwelling catheter can provide prolonged pain relief and peripheral vasodilation due to sympathetic blockade, which helps minimize vasospasm. Although the administration of a daily aspirin for antiplatelet properties, and chemical prophylaxis for deep venous thromboembolism (DVT) are appropriate, the use of routine postoperative anticoagulation is not indicated. Although some studies suggest that surgeons frequently use postoperative anticoagulation,[1,5] a recent study of 281 re-vascularized or replanted digits demonstrated that there was no indication for routine use of heparin following replantation.[18]

One of the most common early postoperative complications is venous congestion (**Fig. 2**). If venous congestion occurs, the first step is to remove constrictive dressings and any blood cast (dried blood over cast dressing) that may be restricting venous outflow. If this does not result in immediate resolution of congestion, skin sutures should be removed. If the congestion persists, the surgeon must decide whether to return to the operating room or manage the congestion with leech therapy. Proximal amputations that develop venous congestion should be managed like a free flap, with immediate take-back to the operating room. For digital replantations, this decision should be based on the acuity and severity of the venous congestion, and whether the surgeon believes that he or she will be able to re-establish venous outflow more successfully than at the initial operation. An acute change with severe congestion may warrant an emergent return to the operating room, with inspection and revision of the venous anastomoses. However, a more gradual onset of milder venous congestion is indicative of intact but insufficient venous outflow, which can be managed by the application of medicinal leeches. Leeches are initially applied at a rate of 1 leach per hour; after constant bleeding is established, the leeching can be performed every 4–6 hours because blood will continue to ooze from the leech bite wound because of the anticoagulant secreted by the leech. A complication of leeching is the need for blood transfusion, which requires monitoring of blood count daily. Leeching is then gradually weaned over a period of 4–6 days, based on the response of the finger. If medicinal leeches are used, prophylaxis for *Aeromonas hydrophila* should be provided. The reported infection rate during leech therapy ranges from 2.4% to 20%.[19,20] A recent study found Ciprofloxacin and Bactrim to be equally effective in preventing infection in patients treated with medicinal leeches,[21] but resistant species are not uncommon. Although *Aeromonas* species are the most common cause of infection, other organisms such as *Enterococcus*, *Serratia*, *Morganella*, and *Corynebacterium* can cause infection.

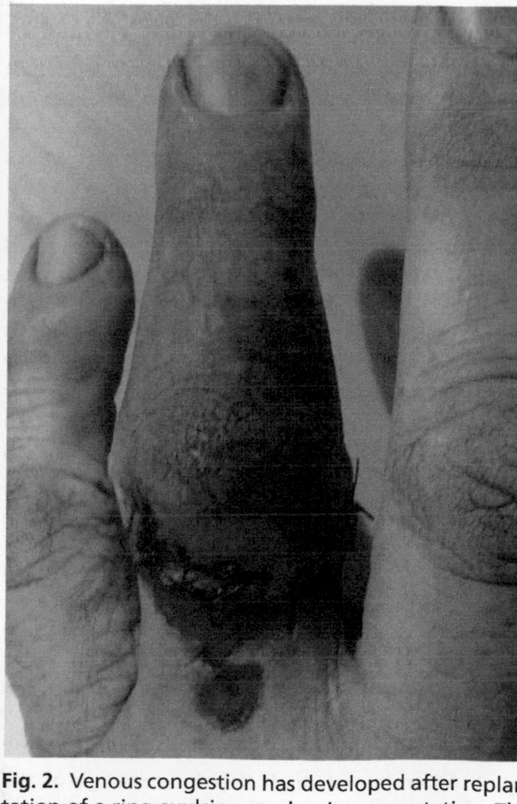

Fig. 2. Venous congestion has developed after replantation of a ring avulsion mechanism amputation. This is indicated by excessively brisk capillary refill, bluish discoloration, and brisk dark bleeding with pin prick.

Unlike venous congestion, ischemia after replantation surgery cannot be managed nonoperatively. If arterial ischemia occurs and salvage is warranted, an emergent take-back to the operating room must be performed, with inspection of the arterial anastomosis. If arterial thrombosis is observed, revision of the anastomosis with or without intraoperative thrombolysis is required. The surgeon must be prepared for the likelihood of vein grafting, either because the zone of injury is more extensive than initially appreciated, or simply because there is little redundancy of the injured artery.

FREE FLAPS

Partial or complete free flap loss in the upper extremity is an uncommon but potentially disastrous complication that can result in exposure of critical structures or even the need for amputation. The principles for preventing flap failure in the upper extremity include careful preoperative planning, minimizing time from injury to coverage, thorough debridement, placing vascular anastomoses outside of the zone of injury, minimizing ischemia time, and performing a tension-free inset. Many of these principles have been well established in the lower extremity, but are equally applicable to the upper extremity.

Godina demonstrated that flap survival was highest when open wounds were covered within 72 hours.[22] Although his work was focused on the lower extremity, his frequently cited findings have been applied to the upper extremity also. However, multiple subsequent studies contradict these findings, demonstrating that subacute or late free flap reconstruction can be performed with success rates similar to those seen in early reconstruction.[23–26] Although it is unclear what effect timing of reconstruction has on flap survival in the upper extremity, it is important to perform the reconstruction without unnecessary delay. An expeditious reconstruction allows the patient to heal, begin rehabilitation, and return to work and activity as soon as possible.

Perhaps the most important principle for preventing serious complications in free flap surgery of the upper limb is to place the vascular anastomoses completely outside the zone of injury. If a free flap is required for coverage of a soft tissue defect, the injury likely resulted in an extensive zone of vascular damage. Arteriography can be used to define the vascular anatomy of the recipient limb, which can aid in selecting a flap with appropriate pedicle length. Based on the presence and size of the recipient vessels, an end-to-end or end-to-side anastomosis may be planned. In the operating room, the anastomoses should be performed to vessels that lie within soft tissue that is not inflamed, woody, fibrotic, or friable. The vessels should have normal-appearing adventitia, no ecchymosis, and intima without swelling or damage when inspected under the microscope. Triphasic arterial signals and a brisk spurt test should be observed. After completion of the anastomosis, the vessels must lie without kinking or twisting, and compression of the vessels should be avoided. A vein graft should be performed when necessary to place the anastomosis outside the zone of injury. Although vein grafts have been associated with higher rates of flap loss, this is not consistent in all studies.[27–30] Vein grafting introduces additional complexity and may increase ischemia time, but vein grafting is preferable to performing an anastomosis to a traumatized vessel. The entire surgery must be carried out efficiently in order to minimize ischemia time. For muscle flaps, an ischemia time of more than 2 to 3 hours can result in the no-reflow phenomenon with complete flap, and this must be avoided.[31,32] After the anastomoses are completed, the flap should be inset without tension, because a tight inset can result in marginal flap loss or compression of the pedicle. This is most often an issue when a skin-to-skin closure is performed on a fasciocutaneous flap. Even if the closure is not tight at the time of surgery, it may become tight because of edema during the first 48 hours after surgery, resulting in flap compromise. It is preferable to perform a loose closure, with skin grafting of 1 subcutaneous border of fasciocutaneous flaps (**Fig. 3**) and excision of the skin graft at a later date (**Fig. 4**).

Postoperatively, the patient should be kept warm and well hydrated, and pain should be adequately controlled. Vasopressors including nicotine should be avoided. Administration of a daily aspirin and DVT prophylaxis is appropriate, but routine anticoagulation is not indicated. Careful monitoring of the free flap by an experienced nursing team in the intensive care unit (ICU) setting is critical during the first 48 hours, because most vascular complications occur within the first 24 to 48 hours after surgery.[33–35] Examination of flap turgor, capillary refill, color, temperature, and Doppler signals is performed hourly. Flap ischemia is recognized by a loss of triphasic arterial signal, coolness to touch, paleness, lack or slowing of capillary refill, or slow bleeding with pin prick. Venous congestion is indicated by excessively rapid capillary refill, flap swelling, increased turgor, mottling or bluish discoloration, and brisk dark bleeding with pin prick. When vascular compromise does occur, flap salvage rates are higher if the problem is recognized and addressed immediately.[35] Constrictive dressings should be removed, and the surgical site should be checked for

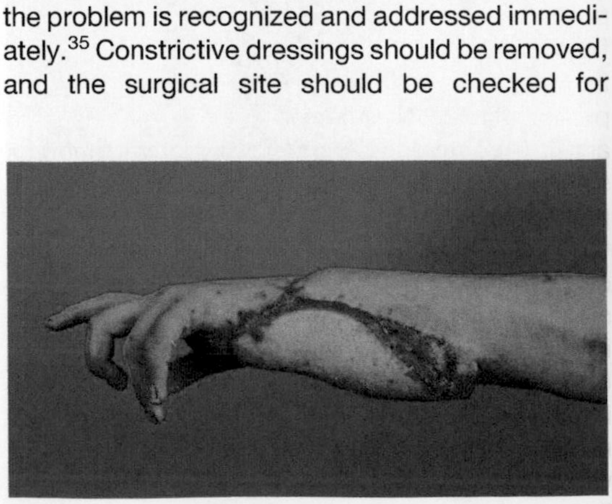

Fig. 3. Anterolateral thigh flap for coverage of the volar forearm and wrist. The subcutaneous margin of the flap has been skin grafted in order to avoid tight skin closure.

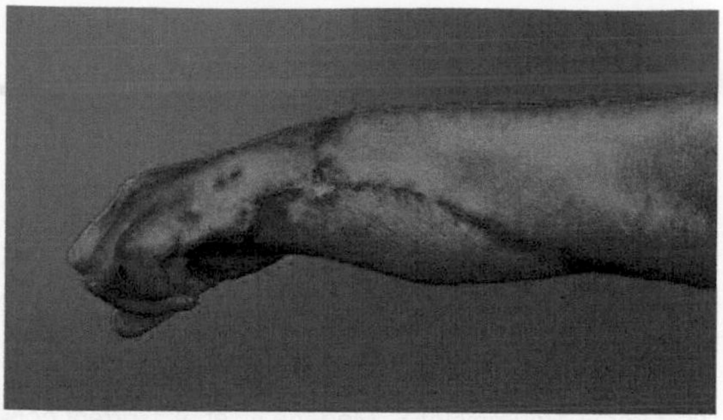

Fig. 4. Appearance of the flap after the skin grafted subcutaneous margin has been excised at a later date.

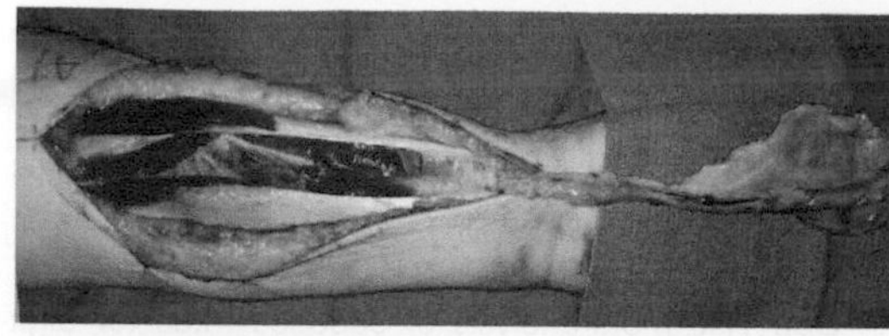

Fig. 5. Reverse radial forearm flap. Note that the radial artery and venae comitantes have not been skeletonized. A generous cuff of adipofascial tissue surrounds the vascular pedicle, minimizing the likelihood of venous congestion.

obvious sources of compression or hematoma. The patient should return to the operating room emergently for exploration of the vascular anastomoses. Any kinking, torsion, or compression of the vascular pedicle should be corrected. If this does not immediately result in normal flow and improvement in the appearance of the flap, the problematic anastomosis should be taken down and revised. If this fails, intraoperative thrombolysis with recombinant tissue plasminogen activator (TPA) or urokinase may be used to attempt flap salvage. In multiple studies, flap salvage for venous thrombosis has been more successful than for arterial thrombosis.[35,36] Although flap salvage can be achieved in most cases when vascular compromise is recognized early, a careful adherence to the previously described principles will help minimize complications.

PEDICLED FLAPS

Multiple pedicled flaps have been described for use in the upper extremity, including workhorse flaps such as the reverse radial forearm flap, the posterior interosseous artery (PIA) flap, and the first dorsal metacarpal artery flap (FDMA or kite flap). Ischemia and congestion are uncommon problems that can be avoided by careful planning and execution. First, the relationship between the skin paddle and the pedicle pivot point must be planned so that the flap can be transposed to the recipient site without undue tension or kinking of the pedicle. The pedicle should be elevated with a wide cuff of adipofascial tissue and not skeletonized, which will help minimize venous congestion (**Fig. 5**). A superficial system vein can often be identified and harvested with the flap, and anastomosed to a vein in the recipient defect to augment venous outflow if necessary. Finally, in many cases it is preferable to divide the skin overlying the pedicle and skin graft directly onto the pedicle, rather than tunnel it under a tight skin bridge. Mild congestion can be managed with suture removal and application of medicinal leeches. If severe congestion or ischemia does occur, a return to the operating room is warranted to adjust the course of the pedicle to correct any torsion, kinking, or compression.

SUMMARY

Vascular complications of flap procedures and replantation surgery in the upper extremity can be minimized by employing appropriate indications and thorough preoperative planning. Efficient surgery, with carefully performed vascular anastomoses outside the zone of injury, is paramount to the success of both replantation and free flap surgery. Skeletal shortening (in the case of replantation) or vein grafting may be necessary to achieve this goal. In both free flaps and pedicled flaps, careful attention to pedicle lay, with avoidance of kinking, twisting, and compression is critical. Intra- and postoperative warming and hydration, pain control, and avoidance of vasopressors are important. Close monitoring of the flap or replant by an experienced team in the early postoperative period, and rapid intervention in cases of vascular compromise, are keys to success.

REFERENCES

1. Salemark L. International survey of current microvascular practices in free tissue transfer and replantation surgery. Microsurgery 1991;12(4):308–11.
2. Zhang WD, Zhou GH, Zhao HR, et al. Five year digital replantation series from the frigid zone of China. Microsurgery 1993;14(6):384–7.
3. Pomerance J, Truppa K, Bilos ZJ, et al. Replantation and revascularization of the digits in a community microsurgical practice. J Reconstr Microsurg 1997; 13(3):163–70.
4. Khouri RK. Avoiding free flap failure. Clin Plast Surg 1992;19(4):773–81.

5. Glicksman A, Ferder M, Casale P, et al. 1457 years of microsurgical experience. Plast Reconstr Surg 1997;100(2):355–63.
6. Patradul A, Ngarmukos C, Parkpian V. Distal digital replantations and revascularizations. 237 digits in 192 patients. J Hand Surg Br 1998;23(5):578–82.
7. Dec WA. meta-analysis of success rates for digit replantation. Tech Hand Up Extrem Surg 2006; 10(3):124–9.
8. Waikakul S, Sakkarnkosol S, Vanadurongwan V, et al. Results of 1018 digital replantations in 552 patients. Injury 2000;31(1):33–40.
9. Gravvanis AI, Tsoutsos DA, Lykoudis EG, et al. Microvascular repair following crush-avulsion type injury with vein grafts: effect of direct inhibitors of thrombin on patency rate. Microsurgery 2003; 23(4):402–7 [discussion: 408–9].
10. Hamilton RB, O'Brien BM, Morrison A, et al. Survival factors in replantation and revascularization of the amputated thumb–10 years experience. Scand J Plast Reconstr Surg 1984;18(2):163–73.
11. Cooley BC, Gould JS. Experimental models for evaluating antithrombotic therapies in replantation microsurgery. Microsurgery 1987;8(4):230–3.
12. Han SK, Lee BI, Kim WK. Topical and systemic anticoagulation in the treatment of absent or compromised venous outflow in replanted fingertips. J Hand Surg 2000;25(4):659–67.
13. Wood MB, Cooney WP 3rd. Above elbow limb replantation: functional results. J Hand Surg 1986; 11(5):682–7.
14. Blaisdell FW. The pathophysiology of skeletal muscle ischemia and the reperfusion syndrome: a review. Cardiovasc Surg 2002;10(6):620–30.
15. Wei FC, Chang YL, Chen HC, et al. Three successful digital replantations in a patient after 84, 86, and 94 hours of cold ischemia time. Plast Reconstr Surg 1988;82(2):346–50.
16. Molski M. Replantation of fingers and hands after avulsion and crush injuries. J Plast Reconstr Aesthet Surg 2007;60(7):748–54.
17. Yan H, Jackson WD, Songcharoen S, et al. Vein grafting in fingertip replantations. Microsurgery 2009;29(4):275–81.
18. Nikolis A, Tahiri Y, St-Supery V, et al. Intravenous heparin use in digital replantation and revascularization: the Quebec provincial replantation program experience. Microsurgery 2011;31(6):421–7.
19. Evans J, Lunnis PJ, Gaunt PN, et al. A case of septicaemia due to Aeromonas hydrophila. Br J Plast Surg 1990;43(3):371–2.
20. Lineaweaver WC, Hill MK, Buncke GM, et al. Aeromonas hydrophila infections following use of medicinal leeches in replantation and flap surgery. Ann Plast Surg 1992;29(3):238–44.
21. Kruer RM, Barton CA, Roberti G, et al. Antimicrobial prophylaxis during Hirudo medicinalis therapy: a multicenter study. J Reconstr Microsurg 2014. [Epub ahead of print].
22. Godina M. Early microsurgical reconstruction of complex trauma of the extremities. Plast Reconstr Surg 1986;78(3):285–92.
23. Francel TJ, Vander Kolk CA, Hoopes JE, et al. Microvascular soft-tissue transplantation for reconstruction of acute open tibial fractures: timing of coverage and long-term functional results. Plast Reconstr Surg 1992;89(3):478–87 [discussion: 488–9].
24. Ofer N, Baumeister S, Megerle K, et al. Current concepts of microvascular reconstruction for limb salvage in electrical burn injuries. J Plast Reconstr Aesthet Surg 2007;60(7):724–30.
25. Karanas YL, Nigriny J, Chang J. The timing of microsurgical reconstruction in lower extremity trauma. Microsurgery 2008;28(8):632–4.
26. Kumar AR, Grewal NS, Chung TL, et al. Lessons from the modern battlefield: successful upper extremity injury reconstruction in the subacute period. J Trauma 2009;67(4):752–7.
27. Khouri RK, Cooley BC, Kunselman AR, et al. A prospective study of microvascular free-flap surgery and outcome. Plast Reconstr Surg 1998; 102(3):711–21.
28. Buncke HJ, Alpert B, Shah KG. Microvascular grafting. Clin Plast Surg 1978;5(2):185–94.
29. Germann G, Steinau HU. The clinical reliability of vein grafts in free-flap transfer. J Reconstr Microsurg 1996;12(1):11–7.
30. Bayramicli M, Tetik C, Sonmez A, et al. Reliability of primary vein grafts in lower extremity free tissue transfers. Ann Plast Surg 2002;48(1):21–9.
31. Ames A 3rd, Wright RL, Kowada M, et al. Cerebral ischemia. II. The no-reflow phenomenon. Am J Pathol 1968;52(2):437–53.
32. Calhoun KH, Tan L, Seikaly H. An integrated theory of the no-reflow phenomenon and the beneficial effect of vascular washout on no-reflow. Laryngoscope 1999;109(4):528–35.
33. Kroll SS, Schusterman MA, Reece GP, et al. Timing of pedicle thrombosis and flap loss after free-tissue transfer. Plast Reconstr Surg 1996;98(7): 1230–3.
34. Chen KT, Mardini S, Chuang DC, et al. Timing of presentation of the first signs of vascular compromise dictates the salvage outcome of free flap transfers. Plast Reconstr Surg 2007;120(1):187–95.
35. Bui DT, Cordeiro PG, Hu QY, et al. Free flap reexploration: indications, treatment, and outcomes in 1193 free flaps. Plast Reconstr Surg 2007;119(7): 2092–100.
36. Nakatsuka T, Harii K, Asato H, et al. Analytic review of 2372 free flap transfers for head and neck reconstruction following cancer resection. J Reconstr Microsurg 2003;19(6):363–8 [discussion: 369].

Management of Complications of Dupuytren Contracture

Kevin Cheung, MSc, MD[a], Kempland C. Walley, BSc[b], Tamara D. Rozental, MD[b,*]

KEYWORDS

• Dupuytren disease • Complications • Management • Fasciectomy • Needle aponeurotomy • Collagenase injection • Recurrence

KEY POINTS

- Current treatment options for Dupuytren contracture include fasciectomy, needle fasciotomy, and collagenase injections.
- Patient education regarding the natural history of Dupuytren disease, treatment options, outcomes, clinical course, and potential complications is paramount.
- A thorough knowledge of the pathologic anatomy of Dupuytren disease is essential to prevent complications.
- Complications may be minimized through proper patient selection and a detailed understanding of each treatment option.

INTRODUCTION

Dupuytren disease is a benign fibroproliferative disorder of the palmar digital fascia. Treatment options include collagenase injections, needle aponeurotomy, and fasciectomy. The type and rate of complications differ with each treatment method. A detailed understanding of this allows treating hand surgeons to select the most appropriate method for each patient. This evidence-based article discusses the current management options of Dupuytren disease and strategies to avoid and manage any potential complications.

NATURAL HISTORY

Fibroblast proliferation, differentiation into myofibroblasts, and subsequent involution results in the characteristic nodules and cords seen in Dupuytren disease. The pathologic stages have previously been described by Luck.[1] The typical patient is a man of northern European descent, aged 50 to 60 years, who presents with palmar nodules near the distal palmar crease. Women are affected less frequently, in a 1:2 to 1:5 ratio. The ring finger is most commonly involved, followed by the little finger, thumb, long finger, and index finger.[2]

Although the natural clinical course is unpredictable, pain is self-limited and nodules may regress or coalesce. Contracture may progress rapidly or follow a period of quiescence that is variable in duration. Of 150 untreated hands presenting with stage 0 disease, 37% of 70 hands progressed after 3 to 5 years of observation; 46% progressed after 6 to 12 years.[3]

Funding sources: None.
Conflict of interest: None.

[a] Division of Plastic Surgery, Harvard Medical School, Beth Israel Deaconess Medical Center, 330 Brookline Avenue, ST 10, Boston, MA 02215, USA; [b] Department of Orthopedics, Harvard Medical School, Beth Israel Deaconess Medical Center, 330 Brookline Avenue, ST 10, Boston, MA 02215, USA
* Corresponding author. Department of Orthopedics, Harvard Medical School, Beth Israel Deaconess Medical Center, 330 Brookline Avenue, ST 10, Boston, MA 02215.
E-mail address: trozenta@bidmc.harvard.edu

Hand Clin 31 (2015) 345–354
http://dx.doi.org/10.1016/j.hcl.2015.01.005
0749-0712/15/$ – see front matter

Dupuytren cords follow a consistent pattern involving the palmar and digital fascia.[4] Longitudinal cords over the palm and digits are referred to as pretendinous and central cords and result in flexion contracture at the metacarpophalangeal joint (MCPJ) and proximal interphalangeal joint (PIPJ), respectively. Natatory cords arise from the natatory ligaments at the margin of the web spaces, resulting in adduction contractures. Spiral, lateral, and abductor digiti minimi cords cause contracture of the PIPJ and displacement of the neurovascular bundle. Recognition of the different types of cords and understanding of the underlying pathologic anatomy are essential to avoid complications and injury to the neurovascular bundles (**Table 1**).

In addition to an anatomic description of Dupuytren cords, classifying the disease severity is important when evaluating treatment effectiveness and outcomes. Previous studies have shown a correlation between complication rates and disease severity.[5–7] Tubiana classified the severity of the disease by total passive extension deficit (TPED), which is the sum of the degrees that the MCPJ, PIPJ, and distal interphalangeal joint fall short of neutral (0°) with maximum passive extension. Staging progresses from least to most severe, with stages 1, 2, 3, and 4 corresponding with TPED less than or equal to 45°, 46° to 90°, 91° to 135°, and greater than 135° respectively. However, this classification, fails to convey the degree of MCPJ versus PIPJ contracture.

Patients with an associated history of early disease onset, bilateral hand involvement, positive family history, plantar fibromatosis (Ledderhose disease), Peyronie disease, or Garrod nodules should be recognized as having Dupuytren diasthesis.[8] These patients have a poor prognosis with high risk of disease progression and

Table 1
Pathologic anatomy of Dupuytren contracture

Cord	Origin	NVB Displacement	Contracture	Other
Pretendinous cord[a]	Pretendinous band	ND	MCPJ	Commonly extends distally to become continuous with digital cords
Vertical cord	Septa linguae and Juvara	ND	No	Not common
Spiral cord	Pretendinous band, spiral band, lateral digital sheet, Grayson ligament	Volar and medial	PIPJ	Most commonly in small finger
Natatory cord	Natatory ligament	ND	Web Space	—
Central cord	Extension of pretendinous cord in palm (no preexisting central band)	ND	PIPJ	Attaches into flexor tendon sheath near PIPJ or periosteum of middle phalanx on one side of digit
Lateral cord	Lateral digital sheet	Midline (because of its volume)	PIPJ and DIPJ	Attaches to skin or Grayson ligament
ADM	ADM tendon	Sometimes	PIPJ	Can present as isolated digital cord; insertion points vary
Distal commissural cord	Distal commissural ligament	ND	Web space	Decrease in palmar and thumb abduction
Proximal commissural cord	Proximal commissural ligament	ND	Web space	Decrease in thumb abduction
Thumb pretendinous cord	Thumb pretendinous band	ND	MPJ	—

Abbreviations: ADM, abductor digiti minimi; DIPJ, distal interphalangeal joint; ND, no displacement; NVB, neurovascular bundle.

[a] Most frequent cord.

Adapted from Vartija LK, McKnight LL, Thoma A. Dupuytren's disease. In: Bhandari M, editor. Evidence-based orthopedics. Oxford (United Kingdom): Wiley-Blackwell; 2012. p. 1032; with permission.

recurrence. Patients should have a clear understanding of their disease prognosis, and management should be planned accordingly. Intervention should be delayed until functional impairment is present, and treatment should be planned to minimize the frequency and difficulty of future procedures. In patients with severe diathesis, significant functional impairment, significant comorbidity, underlying joint changes, or multiply recurrent disease, traditional fasciectomies, aponeurotomies, or injections may not provide long-standing correction. Arthrodesis or amputation may be reasonable in these challenging cases.

TREATMENT OPTIONS

Fasciectomy

Numerous surgical procedures for Dupuytren have been described. However, aggressiveness of surgical intervention must be weighed against the clinical outcomes, potential patient morbidity, and time to recovery of each operation. Limited fasciectomy is the current standard for treatment of Dupuytren disease, involving removal of macroscopically diseased fascia from the palm and finger. Total fasciectomy involves removal of all fascia in the palm and digit. Dermatofasciectomy involves removal of both diseased fascia and the overlying skin with either skin grafting or healing by secondary intention. Segmental fasciectomy limits excision to a 1-cm segment of diseased fascia.[9] Improvements in recurrence rates have not been shown with more aggressive operations. In a randomized controlled trial (RCT) of 79 patients who underwent either fasciectomy or dermatofasciectomy, no difference in recurrence (10.9% vs 13.6%) was observed with 3-year follow-up.[10] Dermatofasciectomy may still be advocated in patients with recurrent disease or patients with extensive skin involvement.

Numerous strategies to improve the outcomes of fasciectomy have been studied. Citron and colleagues[11] performed an RCT and found no difference in recurrence rates between longitudinal incisions closed with Z-plasties and modified Bruner incisions closed with Y-V plasties. No difference was found with the adjuvant use of 5-fluorouracil or tamoxifen.[12,13] Outcomes were similar with concomitant PIPJ capsulotomy; thus, in Dupuytren resulting in significant PIPJ contracture, capsulotomy should be done to achieve complete extension following fasciectomy.[14] Night extension splinting has traditionally been advocated to maintain postoperative range of motion.[15] However, 2 recent RCTs examining the use of night extension orthoses found no benefit compared with hand therapy alone.[16,17]

Needle Fasciotomy

Needle fasciotomy or aponeurotomy is intended to correct flexion contracture through percutaneous division of palpable Dupuytren cords. Multiple fasciotomies may be made in the same cord; however, no diseased fascia is removed. This technique is less invasive than fasciectomy and can be performed as an office or clinic procedure. Compared with fasciectomy, needle fasciotomy achieves a similar initial degree of correction for Tubiana stages 1 and 2 (TPED<90°) with fewer major complications.[18] However, recurrence rates were significantly higher than with fasciectomy.[19,20]

Collagenase Clostridium Histolyticum

Collagenase *Clostridium histolyticum* enzymatically degrades the collagen-based cords, enabling correction of flexion deformity following physical manipulation.[21] In a multicentered RCT of 308 patients comparing collagenase with placebo, flexion contracture was corrected to 0° to 5° of full extension in 77% and 40% of MCPJ and PIPJ, respectively.[22] Collagenase was less successful for severely contracted digits: only 60% of digits with MCPJ contractures greater than 50° and 22% with PIPJ contractures greater than 40° met the primary outcome (vs 89%, MCPJ ≤50°, 81%, PIPJ <40°). In the study protocol, patients could receive up to 3 injections spaced 1 month apart; 61% required more than 1 injection.

COMPLICATIONS

Digital Nerve Injury

Postoperative paresthesias may be the result of traction neuropathy or iatrogenic partial or complete nerve injury. Neuropraxia without identified digital nerve injury is common following digital fasciectomy and fasciotomy, occurring in 0.4% to 46% and 1% to 6% of cases, respectively.[5,10,18,23] Symptoms are self-limited and require no intervention. Tinel sign or symptoms that persist for longer than 3 months without signs of improvement suggest a partial or complete nerve injury that warrants exploration and possible repair.

With fasciectomy, digital nerve injury occurred in 3.4% of cases (range, 0%–7.7%).[24] The incidence of nerve or arterial injury may be higher (range, 4.2%–27%) in cases of repeat fasciectomy (**Table 2**).[24] A clear understanding of the patterns of pathologic disease and potential displacement of the digital neurovascular bundles is essential to prevent intraoperative transection. Spiral, lateral, and abductor digiti minimi cords result in medial and volar displacement of the neurovascular bundle. Identification of the neurovascular bundle proximally in the palm or distally in the finger, outside the zone of disease, may prevent iatrogenic injury. Immediate primary repair is indicated for inadvertent injury.[25]

recovery of pain and touch sensibility and good localization of stimulus, but imperfect recovery of 2-point discrimination), and poor (S0–S3; >7 mm M2PD; varying degrees of sensation

Table 2
Complication rates of fasciectomy, needle fasciotomy, and collagenase

	Fasciectomy (%)	Needle Fasciotomy (%)	Collagenase Injection (%)
Digital nerve injury	3.4 (range, 0–7.7)[a,24]	0.1–4[23,26,27]	NR
Neuropraxia	0.4–46[10]	1–6[5]	NR
Arterial injury	2 (range, 0–2.6)[24]	NR	One case reported[32]
Flexor tendon injury	NR	0.05[23]	0.27[21]
Wound healing complications	Skin necrosis, 4.3 (range, 0–10)[34] Wound healing, 22.9 (range, 0–86)[24]	3–50[18,23,29,35]	11–34[2,35]
Hematoma	2.1 (range, 0–13)[24]	0.3[23]	Contusion, 51; injection-site hemorrhage, 37; ecchymosis, 25; and blood blister, 3.4[22]
Infection	2.4[24]	0.7[23]	NR[22]
Flare reactions and CRPS	5.8 (range, 1.3–13)[20,24,42]	Less than fasciectomy[20]	Less than fasciectomy[20]

[a] Incidence of nerve or arterial injury may be higher (range, 4.2%–27%) in cases of repeat fasciectomy.[24]
Data from Refs.[2,5,10,20–24,26,27,29,34,35]

With needle fasciotomy, nerve injury has been reported in 0.1% to 4% of cases.[23,26,27] Intradermal use of local anesthetic preserves sensory feedback to avoid digital nerve injury.[28] Clinical examination of the relative motion of the skin overlying the Dupuytren cord in the area between the distal palmar crease and the proximal digital crease may be helpful in avoiding iatrogenic digital nerve injury. If the overlying skin is directly adherent to the cord, there is no risk of an interposed digital nerve. Otherwise, there is the possibility of a spiral cord and needle fasciotomy should be avoided at this level.[27] For cords distal to the MCPJ, spiral cords can displace the neurovascular bundle superficially and to the midline. For cords in the proximal phalanx, Cheng and colleagues[29] advocate insertion of the needle laterally, beneath the cord, to only release the deep portion of the cord in order to protect the neurovascular bundle that runs superficially. Asking patients to flex their fingers periodically and ensuring that the needle does not move with movement may prevent flexor tendon injury.[29]

Outcomes following digital nerve repair are generally good to excellent. A recent meta-analysis showed that end-to-end digital nerve coaptation resulted in excellent (S4; 2–3 mm moving 2-point discrimination [M2PD]; complete sensory recovery), good (S3+, 4–7 mm M2PD; return) return of sensation in 28%, 50%, and 21% of cases, respectively.[30] Younger age seems to be a significant predictor of improved sensory recovery.[30,31]

Arterial Injury

Digital artery injury has been reported in 2% (range, 0%–2.6%) of patients undergoing fasciectomy.[24] With needle fasciotomy, injury to a digital artery is exceedingly rare or under recognized because of the redundant arterial supply of each digit. A single case report of digital artery injury following collagenase injection was recently published.[32] Similar to an iatrogenic digital nerve injury, most injuries are preventable with a thorough knowledge of disease characteristics and if care is taken to identify the neurovascular bundles outside the zone of disease. Doppler examination may be used to identify and avoid spiral cords before performing needle fasciotomy.[28] Injury to both digital arteries is rare but may require microsurgical revascularization.[33]

More commonly, digital ischemia may result from vasospasm. Routine management includes warm compresses, topical lidocaine, or calcium channel blockers. Recalcitrant vasospasm caused by traction may require protecting the digit in a flexed position to relieve traction on the digital arteries.

Flexor Tendon Injury

Flexor tendon injury is a recognized but rare complication, occurring at a rate of 0.05% and 0.27% following needle fasciotomy and collagenase injection, respectively.[21,23] Transection following needle fasciotomy may be amenable to primary repair; however, rupture caused by collagenase injection requires staged tendon reconstruction.

During needle fasciotomy, flexor tendon injury is avoided by asking the patient to lightly flex and extend the finger with the needle in situ. Motion of the needle with tendon excursion suggests that the needle is within the tendon sheath and the needle should be retracted.[28,29]

In the clinical trials of collagenase, all tendon ruptures occurred following injection of little finger PIPJ contractures. For central cords it is therefore not advised to inject more than 4 mm distal to the palmar digital crease. Inserting the needle horizontally (in the coronal plane) rather than vertically (in the sagittal plane) may further help to avoid flexor tendon injury.[21]

Wound Healing Complications

With fasciectomy, wound healing complications occurred in 22.9% (range, 0%–86%) of cases, although necrosis of skin, flap, or grafts was reported separately and occurred in 4.3% (range, 0%–10%).[24] Wound healing complications and skin flap necrosis can be avoided by careful incision planning, meticulous tension-free closure, and intraoperatively assessing flap viability.[25] Open wounds and flap or skin graft necrosis may be managed with local wound care or skin grafts, although treatment should be expeditious to minimize the delay in postoperative rehabilitation.

Skin fissures were the most common complication following needle fasciotomy, with rates ranging from 3% to 50%.[18,23,29,34] Eaton[35] describes multiple strategies to prevent skin fissures, including avoiding areas of nodular skin involvement, use of multiple portals to disperse tension, and sweeping the needle under the dermis tangentially to release vertical septae. Skin fissures also occurred in 11% to 34% of collagenase injections, most often with MCPJ contractures greater than 50°.[21,34] Most fissures heal with local wound care and require no further surgical intervention, although use of skin grafts has been reported.[36]

Hematoma

Postoperative hematoma may compromise the vascularity to the digit or overlying skin flaps and grafts. In this setting, prompt evacuation is required. Otherwise, hematomas can be safely monitored until resolution. Postoperative hematoma was reported in 2.1% (range, 0%–13%) of patients undergoing fasciectomy[24] compared with 0.3% for needle fasciectomy.[23] Collagenase injections are associated with a high rate of contusion (51%), injection-site hemorrhage (37%), ecchymosis (25%), and blood blister (3.4%).[22] There were no reports of patients requiring evacuation or reoperation for these complications.

Infection

Postoperative infection following fasciectomy and needle fasciotomy was reported to occur in 2.4% and 0.7% of cases, respectively.[23,24] In a large case series of collagenase injections, postoperative infection was not identified or reported.[22] Although no study has been performed examining the use of prophylactic antibiotics in fasciectomy for Dupuytren disease, current evidence does not support preoperative antibiotics to prevent surgical site infections in elective hand surgery. A pseudorandomized controlled study comparing preoperative antibiotics with placebo did not show a significant difference (3.4% vs 3.1%; $P = .759$) in postoperative infection rates in healthy patients undergoing both emergent and elective hand surgery.[37] Similarly, a retrospective cohort study of patients undergoing elective outpatient hand surgery failed to show a significant reduction in surgical site infections with prophylactic antibiotics (0.54% vs 0.26%). Predictors of infection included smoking, diabetes, and length of procedure, with odds ratios of 3.0, 2.8, and 1.02, respectively.[38] In elective hand surgeries greater than 2 hours in duration, preoperative antibiotics are beneficial.[39]

Antibiotic therapy remains the primary treatment of postoperative infection. First-generation cephalosporins cover most pathologic organisms; however, wound cultures before commencing antibiotics are essential to guide antibiotic therapy. In the rare development of a deep pyogenic infection, irrigation and debridement are required to prevent spread to the flexor tendon sheath and deep spaces of the hand.

Flare Reaction/Complex Regional Pain Syndrome

Postoperative pain disproportionate to the surgery, sudomotor activity, and/or vasomotor instability following fasciectomy, colloquially known as a flare reaction, may represent a form of complex regional pain syndrome (CRPS). Previously known as reflex sympathetic dystrophy, CRPS type 1 develops after a noxious event, not limited to the distribution of a single peripheral nerve. The Budapest diagnostic criteria include (1) continuing pain, disproportionate to the inciting event; and (2) evidence of edema, changes in skin blood flow, abnormal sudomotor activity in the region of pain, or motor disturbances and trophic changes, such as altered nail and hair growth.[40,41] Following fasciectomy for Dupuytren disease, CRPS has been reported in 5.8% (range, 1.3%–13%) of cases.[20,24,42] It is much less common following needle fasciotomy and collagenase injection.[20] The precise incidence is difficult to estimate, because diagnostic criteria are evolving.

Identifying patients at risk for CRPS is challenging. Historically, simultaneous fasciectomy and carpal tunnel release have been avoided for fear of increased risk of CRPS.[43] However, there is little evidence for this association, and the pathophysiology linking Dupuytren with CRPS is unknown. A recent case series suggested that concurrent procedures may be feasible with no increased risk of CRPS.[44]

Numerous medications and therapies for CRPS have been investigated, including nonsteroidal antiinflammatory drugs, opioids, local anesthetics, anticonvulsants, antidepressants, free radical scavengers, steroids, bisphosphonates, and calcitonin. Medications for neuropathic pain, such as tricyclic antidepressants, serotonin-norepinephrine reuptake inhibitors, and the anticonvulsants gabapentin and pregabalin, may have some benefit in patients with CRPS.[40] A recent Cochrane Review found that most of the evidence was of "low or very low quality and cannot be regarded as reliable."[45] Only intravenous ketamine, bisphosphonates, calcitonin, and programs of graded motor imagery had sufficient evidence to suggest efficacy in treating CRPS. Early diagnosis and referral to a specialized pain clinic are essential.

Recurrence

Recurrence rates of Dupuytren following fasciectomy and needle fasciotomy vary depending on the definition of recurrence, severity of disease, and length of follow-up. It is often difficult to differentiate between recurrent disease and postoperative scarring or residual joint contractures. Recurrence is often described as worsening disease or contracture compared with the initial postoperative phase. In an RCT of 111 patients, 5-year recurrence rates following limited fasciectomy and needle fasciotomy were 20.9% and 84.9% ($P<.001$), respectively. When recurrence was defined as loss of any degree of extension, recurrence rates for the MCPJ following fasciectomy and needle fasciotomy were 21% and 57%, respectively; for the PIPJ, recurrence was 21% and 70%, respectively.[19] Similar conclusions were reported in a systematic review: recurrence rates for fasciectomy ranged from 0% to 39% compared with 50% to 58% for needle fasciotomy.[20] Long-term recurrence rates following collagenase injection are still pending. In a study of patients receiving collagenase injection in one of 5 previous clinical studies, overall recurrence rate at 3 years was 35% (27% for MCPJs and 56% for PIPJs) (**Table 3**).[46]

Management of recurrent Dupuytren disease can be challenging, and treatment of primary recurrence does not preclude further recurrence. Patients undergoing fasciectomy and needle fasciotomy for recurrent disease required additional procedures in 32% and 50% within 4 years, respectively.[47,48] Patient education is paramount to establish realistic expectations.

Table 3
Recurrence rates following fasciectomy, needle fasciotomy, and collagenase

	Overall Recurrence Rate (%)	MCPJ (%)	PIPJ (%)
Fasciectomy[a,b,c]	21[19]	21[19]	21[19]
Needle fasciotomy[a,b,c]	85[19]	57[19]	70[19]
Collagenase injection[d,e]	35[46]	27[46]	56[46]

[a] Patients undergoing fasciectomy and needle fasciotomy for recurrent disease required additional procedures in 32% and 50% within 4 years, respectively.[47,48]
[b] Recurrence rates for fasciectomy and needle fasciotomy ranged from 0% to 39% and 50% to 58% respectively.[20]
[c] Recurrence was defined as an increase of total passive extension deficit of at least 30°.[19]
[d] Recurrence was defined as an increase in joint contracture of 20° or greater in the presence of a palpable cord, or the need for the joint to have further medical or surgical intervention.[46]
[e] Overall reoccurrence rate reported at 3 years following intervention.[46]
Data from Refs.[19,20,46–48]

Roush and Stern[47] described their management of patients with recurrent Dupuytren following primary fasciectomy. Patients with total active motion (TAM) less than 150° were treated with limited fasciectomy and interphalangeal arthrodesis; patients with TAM greater than or equal to 150° were treated with either fasciectomy and full-thickness skin graft or fasciectomy and local flap closure. No patient achieved restoration of full range of motion. Semmes-Weinstein monofilament evaluation revealed diminished sensation in 64% of digits at final follow-up. Two-point discrimination was greater than or equal to 7 mm in 43%

Table 4
Prevention and management of complications associated with Dupuytren contracture

		Fasciectomy	Needle Fasciotomy	Collagenase Injection
Digital nerve/artery injury	Prevention	Thorough knowledge of pathologic anatomy to protect displaced neurovascular bundles		
		Clinical and Doppler examination may help to identify spiral cords[27,28]		
		Identification of the neurovascular bundles proximally and distally outside the zone of disease	Intradermal use of local anesthetic to preserve sensory feedback[28] Distal to the MCPJ, coronal insertion of the needle and release of only the deep portion of the cord[29]	NR
	Management	Laceration: immediate primary repair		
		Vasospasm: warm compresses, topical lidocaine or calcium channel blockers, protection of digit in slight flexion to relieve traction		
Flexor tendon injury	Prevention	NR	Motion of the needle with tendon excursion suggests that the needle is within the tendon and should be retracted[23,29]	Avoid injection >4 mm distal to the palmar digital crease. Coronal insertion of the needle may further help to avoid flexor tendon injury[21]
	Management	May be amenable to primary repair		Staged tendon reconstruction
Wound healing complications	Prevention	Careful incision planning, meticulous tension-free closure, and assessing flap viability intraoperatively[25]	Avoid areas of nodular skin, use multiple portals, sweep tangentially to release dermis[35]	Occur most often in MCPJ contractures >50°
	Management	Local wound care, skin grafts, or local flaps		
Infection	Prevention	No evidence for routine preoperative antibiotics unless surgery >2 h or other risk factors[37–39]		
	Management	Wound cultures and antibiotic therapy. Rare need for irrigation and debridement		
Flare reactions and CRPS	Prevention	Early diagnosis and referral to specialized pain clinic		
	Management	IV ketamine, bisphosphonates, calcitonin, and programs of graded motor imagery[45]		
Recurrence	Prevention	Understanding of disease prognosis and effectiveness of treatment options		
	Management	May be amenable to any treatment modality		
		Potential for increased risk of nerve injury and loss of tissue planes		

Abbreviation: NR, not reported.
Data from Refs.[21,27–29,35,37–39,45]

of digits at final follow-up, including 11% that had no sensibility.

van Rijssen and Werker[48] examined the subset of their patients who underwent repeat needle fasciotomy for recurrent disease. Secondary recurrence occurred in 50% of patients after a mean of 1.4 years. Tertiary recurrences were treated with limited fasciectomy. Although cords appeared broader and more diffuse, fasciectomy was not more complicated than in primary Dupuytren.

In a survey of the surgeons participating in the initial collagenase clinical trials, the difficulty of surgical management of recurrent disease following collagenase injection was reported.[49] However, 7 of 9 surgeons rated the surgery as easier or equivalent to a primary operation. Focal areas of thinning in the cord were observed and were hypothesized to be at sites of the original collagenase injection. Abnormal thickening and adherence of the cord to surrounding tissue was also reported.

SUMMARY

Management of complications of Dupuytren contracture should first be directed at prevention of complications (**Table 4**). Understanding the natural history and the risks and benefits of the available treatment options for Dupuytren disease is essential. Patient education and setting realistic expectations are paramount. Nodules or cords that result in minimal functional impairment or flexion contracture may be safely observed, because disease progression is variable. The traditional thresholds for surgical intervention include functional impairment and flexion contracture of greater than 30° at the MCPJ and/or greater than 0° at the PIPJ. With the advent of less invasive treatment options such as aponeurotomy or collagenase injection, some physicians and patients are electing to pursue treatment at earlier stages of disease progression.[50] Although fasciectomy remains the standard, the low rates of recurrence for surgery should be weighed against the procedure's morbidity and recovery time.

Less invasive techniques of needle fasciotomy and collagenase injections may be successful in cases of less severe disease. Serious complications are rare, but even minor complications may delay a patient's rehabilitation and time to recovery. Needle fasciotomy is associated with high recurrence rates compared with fasciectomy. Almost all patients receiving collagenase injections experience a minor complication. Patients treated with collagenase may require several injections to achieve extension, and treatment is less effective for disease resulting in PIPJ contracture. Medication costs may be prohibitive, and long-term results are pending. Despite these limitations, less invasive techniques should also be considered and discussed with patients presenting with Dupuytren disease. For patients with more severe flexion contractures, fasciectomy remains the ideal treatment method.

Although this article provides a summary of the best available evidence, it is not systematic. Included studies vary in quality, and complications in the original studies were reported heterogeneously and with varying definitions. Patients' perceptions of complication rates may be significantly higher. In a survey of 1177 patients undergoing fasciectomy, patients reported a 46% overall complication rate, including 36% numbness (after 2 days), 20% wound infection, and 12% circulatory disturbance.[6]

In our practice, we prefer treatment of Dupuytren disease with limited fasciectomy through midline incisions and Z-plasty closure, minimizing skin grafts if possible. Physical therapy is started in the first postoperative week with night splinting. Hematomas are closely monitored with a low threshold for evacuation. Collagenase injection is also offered to patients with MCPJ or PIPJ involvement and a palpable cord. Injections of the small finger PIPJ are avoided because of risk of flexor rupture. Elevation and compression are used in the first 48 hours to minimize edema.

REFERENCES

1. Luck JV. Dupuytren's contracture: a new concept of the pathogenesis. J Bone Joint Surg Am 1959;41:635–64.
2. Swartz WM, Lalonde DH. Dupuytren's disease. Plast Reconstr Surg 2008;121(4):1–10.
3. Millesi H. Dupuytren's contracture. In: Bentley G, editor. European instructional lectures. Berlin; Heidelberg (Germany): Springer; 2009. p. 137–52.
4. McFarlane RM. Patterns of the diseased fascia in the fingers in Dupuytren's contracture. Plast Reconstr Surg 1974;54(1):31–44.
5. Bulstrode NW, Jemec B, Smith PJ. The complications of Dupuytren's contracture surgery. J Hand Surg 2005;30(5):1021–5.
6. Dias JJ, Braybrooke J. Dupuytren's contracture: an audit of the outcomes of surgery. J Hand Surg Br 2006;31(5):514–21.
7. Loos B, Puschkin V, Horch RE. 50 years experience with Dupuytren's contracture in the Erlangen University Hospital–a retrospective analysis of 2919 operated hands from 1956 to 2006. BMC Musculoskelet Disord 2007;8(1):60.
8. Hindocha S, Stanley JK, Watson S, et al. Dupuytren's diathesis revisited: evaluation of prognostic

indicators for risk of disease recurrence. J Hand Surg 2006;31(10):1626–34.
9. Moermans JP. Segmental aponeurectomy in Dupuytren's disease. J Hand Surg Br 1991;16(3): 243–54.
10. Ullah AS, Dias JJ, Bhowal B. Does a 'firebreak' full-thickness skin graft prevent recurrence after surgery for Dupuytren's contracture? A prospective, randomised trial. J Bone Joint Surg Br 2009;91(3): 374–8.
11. Citron ND, Nunez V. Recurrence after surgery for Dupuytren's disease: a randomized trial of two skin incisions. J Hand Surg Br 2005;30(6):563–6.
12. Bulstrode NW, Bisson M, Jemec B, et al. A prospective randomised clinical trial of the intra-operative use of 5-fluorouracil on the outcome of Dupuytren's disease. J Hand Surg Br 2004;29(1): 18–21.
13. Degreef I, Tejpar S, Sciot R, et al. High-dosage tamoxifen as neoadjuvant treatment in minimally invasive surgery for Dupuytren disease in patients with a strong predisposition toward fibrosis a randomized controlled trial. J Bone Joint Surg Am 2014;96(8):655–62.
14. Beyermann K, Prommersberger KJ, Jacobs C, et al. Severe contracture of the proximal interphalangeal joint in Dupuytren's disease: does capsuloligamentous release improve outcome? J Hand Surg Br 2004;29(3):238–41.
15. Hurst L. Dupuytren's contracture. In: Wolfe SW, Hotchkiss RN, Pederson WC, et al, editors. Green's operative hand surgery. 6th edition. Philadelphia: Elsevier Churchill-Livingston; 2010. Chapter 5. p. 141–58.
16. Collis J, Collocott S, Hing W, et al. The effect of night extension orthoses following surgical release of Dupuytren contracture: a single-center, randomized, controlled trial. J Hand Surg 2013;38(7): 1285–94.
17. Jerosch-Herold C, Shepstone L, Chojnowski AJ, et al. Night-time splinting after fasciectomy or dermo-fasciectomy for Dupuytren's contracture: a pragmatic, multi-centre, randomised controlled trial. BMC Musculoskelet Disord 2011;12(1):136.
18. van Rijssen AL, Gerbrandy FS, Linden HT, et al. A comparison of the direct outcomes of percutaneous needle fasciotomy and limited fasciectomy for Dupuytren's disease: a 6-week follow-up study. J Hand Surg 2006;31(5):717–25.
19. van Rijssen AL, ter Linden H, Werker PM. Five-year results of a randomized clinical trial on treatment in Dupuytren's disease: percutaneous needle fasciotomy versus limited fasciectomy. Plast Reconstr Surg 2012;129(2):469–77.
20. Chen NC, Srinivasan RC, Shauver MJ, et al. A systematic review of outcomes of fasciotomy, aponeurotomy, and collagenase treatments for Dupuytren's contracture. Hand (N Y) 2011;6(3): 250–5.
21. Hentz VR, Watt AJ, Desai SS, et al. Advances in the management of Dupuytren disease: collagenase. Hand Clin 2012;28(4):551–63.
22. Hurst LC, Badalamente MA, Hentz VR, et al. Injectable collagenase clostridium histolyticum for Dupuytren's contracture. N Engl J Med 2009;361(10):968–79.
23. Beaudreuil J, Lellouche H, Orcel P, et al. Needle aponeurotomy in Dupuytren's disease. Joint Bone Spine 2012;79(1):13–6.
24. Denkler K. Surgical complications associated with fasciectomy for Dupuytren's disease: a 20-year review of the English literature. Eplasty 2010;10:e15.
25. Boyer MI, Gelberman RH. Complications of the operative treatment of Dupuytren's disease. Hand Clin 1999;15(1):161–6.
26. Pess GM, Pess RM, Pess RA. Results of needle aponeurotomy for Dupuytren contracture in over 1,000 fingers. J Hand Surg 2012;37(4):651–6.
27. Foucher G, Medina J, Navarro R. Percutaneous needle aponeurotomy: complications and results. J Hand Surg Br 2003;28(5):427–31.
28. Eaton C. Percutaneous fasciotomy for Dupuytren's contracture. J Hand Surg 2011;36(5):910–5.
29. Cheng HS, Hung LK, Tse WL, et al. Needle aponeurotomy for Dupuytren's contracture. J Orthop Surg (Hong Kong) 2008;16(1):88–90.
30. Paprottka FJ, Wolf P, Harder Y, et al. Sensory recovery outcome after digital nerve repair in relation to different reconstructive techniques: meta-analysis and systematic review. Plast Surg Int 2013;2013: 704589.
31. Mermans JF, Franssen BB, Serroyen J, et al. Digital nerve injuries: a review of predictors of sensory recovery after microsurgical digital nerve repair. Hand (N Y) 2012;7(3):233–41.
32. Spiers JD, Ullah A, Dias JJ. Vascular complication after collagenase injection and manipulation for Dupuytren's contracture. J Hand Surg Eur Vol 2014; 39(5):554–6.
33. Jones NF, Huang JI. Emergency microsurgical revascularization for critical ischemia during surgery for Dupuytren's contracture: a case report. J Hand Surg 2001;26(6):1125–8.
34. Nydick JA, Olliff BW, Garcia MJ, et al. A comparison of percutaneous needle fasciotomy and collagenase injection for Dupuytren disease. J Hand Surg 2013; 38(12):2377–80.
35. Eaton C. A technique of needle aponeurotomy for Dupuytren's contracture. In: Eaton C, Seegenschmiedt MH, Bayat A, et al, editors. Dupuytren's disease and related hyperproliferative disorders. Berlin; Heidelberg (Germany): Springer; 2012. p. 267–79.
36. Hallock GG. Skin laceration as a serious adverse sequela of injectable collagenase for Dupuytren

contracture. Plast Reconstr Surg 2012;129(1): 205e–6e.
37. Aydin N, Uraloglu M, Yilmaz Burhanoglu AD, et al. A prospective trial on the use of antibiotics in hand surgery. Plast Reconstr Surg 2010;126:1617–23.
38. Bykowski MR, Sivak WN, Cray J, et al. Assessing the impact of antibiotic prophylaxis in outpatient elective hand surgery: a single-center, retrospective review of 8,850 cases. J Hand Surg 2011;36(11):1741–7.
39. Rizvi M, Bille B, Holtom P, et al. The role of prophylactic antibiotics in elective hand surgery. J Hand Surg 2008;33(3):413–20.
40. Fukushima FB, Bezerra DM, Villas Boas PJ, et al. Complex regional pain syndrome. BMJ 2014;348:g3683.
41. Harden RN, Oaklander AL, Burton AW, et al. Complex regional pain syndrome: practical diagnostic and treatment guidelines. Pain Med 2013;14(2):180–229.
42. Crean SM, Gerber RA, Le Graverand MP, et al. The efficacy and safety of fasciectomy and fasciotomy for Dupuytren's contracture in European patients: a structured review of published studies. J Hand Surg Eur Vol 2011;36(5):396–407.
43. Nissenbaum M, Kleinert HE. Treatment considerations in carpal tunnel syndrome with coexistent Dupuytren's disease. J Hand Surg 1980;5(6):544–7.
44. Lilly SI, Stern PJ. Simultaneous carpal tunnel release and Dupuytren's fasciectomy. J Hand Surg 2010; 35(5):754–9.
45. O'Connell NE, Wand BM, McAuley J, et al. Interventions for treating pain and disability in adults with complex regional pain syndrome – an overview of systematic reviews. Cochrane Database Syst Rev 2013;(4):CD009416.
46. Peimer CA, Blazar P, Coleman S, et al. Dupuytren contracture recurrence following treatment with collagenase clostridium histolyticum (CORDLESS study): 3-year data. J Hand Surg 2013;38(1):12–22.
47. Roush TF, Stern PJ. Results following surgery for recurrent Dupuytren's disease. J Hand Surg 2000; 25(2):291–6.
48. van Rijssen AL, Werker P. Percutaneous needle fasciotomy for recurrent Dupuytren disease. J Hand Surg 2012;37(9):1820–3.
49. Hay DC, Louie DL, Earp BE, et al. Surgical findings in the treatment of Dupuytren's disease after initial treatment with clostridial collagenase (Xiaflex). J Hand Surg Eur Vol 2013;39:463–5.
50. Desai SS, Hentz VR. The treatment of Dupuytren disease. J Hand Surg 2011;36(5):936–42.

Infection After Hand Surgery

Kyle R. Eberlin, MD[a,b,*], David Ring, MD, PhD[a,c]

KEYWORDS

- Perioperative antibiotics • Hand infections • Prophylactic measures • Surgical site infection
- Postoperative infection

KEY POINTS

- Prophylactic measures that may reduce the risk of postoperative infection include hand washing, skin preparation, sterile technique, and perioperative antibiotics.
- Perioperative antibiotics are indicated for operations lasting more than 2 hours, contaminated or dirty wounds, and most open fractures.
- Local, superficial infections around a suture or pin are treated with removal of the suture or pin alone when removal is appropriate and antibiotics when the suture or pin should be retained.
- More extensive superficial infections are treated with oral or parenteral antibiotics.
- Deep infections are treated with operative debridement and parenteral antibiotics.

INTRODUCTION

Deep infection after hand surgery is uncommon, but when present, can contribute to scarring, stiffness, and even amputation.[1] The incidence of infection is variable and may depend on the criteria used for diagnosis. For instance, the rate of infection after clean elective procedures such as carpal tunnel release has been reported as between 1%[2] and 11%.[3–5] In the authors' experience, deep infection is uncommon. Suture abscesses and small colonized wound separations occur more often but typically resolve without sequelae. Proposed risk factors for infection after hand surgery include diabetes, immunosuppression, severe burns, and malnutrition.[6,7] Open fractures,[3,8] animal[9] or human[10] bites, and severely crushed or contaminated wounds[11] may also predispose patients to postoperative infection.

The most common organism involved in postoperative infection is *Staphylococcus aureus*.[12,13] Some infections are caused by *Streptococci* or mixed flora.[14] Patients with diabetes or a history of intravenous drug abuse are more likely to develop infections with gram-negative organisms, although *S aureus* remains the most common.[13] Methicillin-resistant *S aureus* (MRSA) has become increasingly prevalent, community-acquired MRSA (caMRSA) in particular.[15–18] caMRSA has toxins that cause greater tissue damage than typical *S aureus* infections.

Necrotizing fasciitis can be caused by a wide spectrum of different organisms: polymicrobial infections are most common, but monomicrobial necrotizing infections are typically caused by group A *Streptococcus*.[19] Other less common organisms include enterococci, pseudomonas, vibrio species, nocardia, mycobacteria, and *Aeromonas hydrophilia*, among others.[20]

This review addresses prophylaxis, diagnosis, and treatment of postoperative infections in the hand.

[a] Hand Surgery Service, Massachusetts General Hospital, 55 Fruit Street, Boston, MA 02114, USA; [b] Division of Plastic and Reconstructive Surgery, Massachusetts General Hospital, Harvard Medical School, Wang Ambulatory Care Center 435, 15 Parkman Street, Boston, MA 02114, USA; [c] Department of Orthopedic Surgery, Massachusetts General Hospital, Harvard Medical School, Yawkey 2C, 55 Fruit Street, Boston, MA 02114, USA
* Corresponding author. Division of Plastic and Reconstructive Surgery, Massachusetts General Hospital, Harvard Medical School, Wang Ambulatory Care Center 435, 15 Parkman Street, Boston, MA 02114.
E-mail address: keberlin@mgh.harvard.edu

Hand Clin 31 (2015) 355–360
http://dx.doi.org/10.1016/j.hcl.2014.12.007
0749-0712/15/$ – see front matter

PREVENTION OF POSTOPERATIVE INFECTIONS

Adequate surgeon hand washing can result in lower bacterial counts[21,22] and may help to prevent surgical site infections.[23] Povidone iodine, chlorhexidine, and alcohol-based products can all be effective for preparation of the surgeon's hands if used properly. This entails routine cleaning of subungual areas, scrubbing the hands and fingers before the forearm, avoidance of contamination of surgical attire during hand washing, and rinsing in one direction from the fingertips to the elbow.[21,24]

The duration of washing should last for at least 90 seconds, but one study showed no difference in reduction of bacterial colony forming units between 90 and 180 seconds of surgical hand antisepsis.[25] Another study in patients undergoing hip arthroplasty demonstrated that prolonged duration of hand-scrub (10 vs 5 minutes) does not provide additional benefit.[26] There is no consensus on the optimal solution and duration for hand washing before surgery. Preoperative surgical hand preparation should last at least 90 seconds and should involve organized, meticulous scrubbing.

Preoperative prophylactic antibiotics are ideally administered at least 5 minutes but no more than 60 minutes before insufflation of an extremity tourniquet so they are present at adequate levels in the desired tissue at the time of incision.[27,28] In a study of 37 patients undergoing knee replacement, Bannister and colleagues[27] found that 61% of patients developed bactericidal levels of antibiotics 30 seconds after administration, 83% at 2 minutes after administration, and 100% at 5 minutes after administration. Antibiotics are more effective if given before bacteria have been present in the tissues longer than 3 hours.[29]

The use of preoperative prophylactic antibiotics for small elective soft tissue procedures such as trigger finger or carpal tunnel release is debated. In 1997, Kleinert and colleagues[4] described more than 2000 patients undergoing elective upper-extremity surgery and reported an overall infection rate of 1.4%, with a deep infection rate of 0.3%. Similar results were found by Hanssen and colleagues,[2] who retrospectively studied 3620 patients undergoing elective carpal tunnel release and found an overall infection rate less than 1%. These findings were further supported by Harness and colleagues,[30] who reported a similarly low rate of infection in a multicenter, retrospective review of elective carpal tunnel surgery. These authors concluded that the routine use of antibiotics in carpal tunnel surgery was not indicated, even for patients with diabetes.

In another large, retrospective review of almost 9000 patients undergoing small elective soft tissue procedures in the hand, Bykowski and colleagues[31] found that the administration of prophylactic antibiotics did not reduce the overall 1% incidence of postoperative infections. These findings were corroborated in a study by Tosti and colleagues,[32] who demonstrated an infection rate of 0.66% in 600 patients undergoing elective hand surgery procedures, with no difference between those who did and did not receive preoperative antibiotics.

In one prospective, randomized trial of 160 patients with skin, tendon, and nerve injuries without debris or devitalized tissue in the wound, there was no significant difference in the rate of infection between patients who received and did not receive antibiotics.[33] It is important to note that the overall infection rate of 10% in this study is higher than other studies, perhaps because of prospective evaluation and stringent criteria for diagnosis of infection with inclusion of suture abscesses.

Prophylactic antibiotics are routine in patients having soft tissue surgeries lasting longer than 2 hours, surgeries involving bone or implants, and patients with debris or devitalized tissue in the wound,[11,34] as well as animal or human bites.[3,9,35–37] This routine use of prophylactic antibiotics is mostly based on wisdom and rationale. There are clinical trials that address the use of antibiotics for open fractures of the distal phalanx with conflicting evidence. One study of 85 patients found an infection rate of 30% in patients who did not receive antibiotics and less than 3% in patients treated with antibiotics.[8] However, another double-blind, randomized placebo-controlled trial of 193 patients presenting to the emergency room with open fractures of the distal phalanx demonstrated similar rates of infection in patients treated with and without antibiotics (3% in the group receiving antibiotics and 4% in the group without antibiotics).[38]

Both prospective and retrospective studies have identified that operations lasting longer than 2 hours have a higher risk of postoperative infection.[37,39,40] Other factors such as the American Society of Anesthesiologists' assessment and the level of contamination may also play a role; composite risk indices incorporating such information can help in the stratification of risk for postoperative infections.[41] Although it is often difficult to predict the precise duration of an operation, those that may take longer than 2 hours may benefit from prophylactic antibiotics given the higher risk of postoperative infection (**Table 1**).

Table 1
Recommendations for prophylactic antibiotic use in hand surgery

Patient Group	Recommendations
Clean, elective procedures with an operative duration less than 2 h	Use of prophylactic antibiotics is not necessary
Clean, elective procedures longer than 2 h in duration	Preoperative and perioperative prophylactic use of antibiotics are recommended, not to exceed 24 h in duration
Elective procedures in the setting of clean, isolated hand injuries with simple lacerations	Prophylactic antibiotics are optional but not necessary
Traumatic contaminated or dirty wounds including human and animal bites	Targeted antibiotic use preoperatively and perioperatively based on type and degree of contamination, typically given for 1–2 wk
Open fractures of the phalanges or metacarpals	Prophylactic antibiotics targeting gram-positive bacteria are recommended until at least 24 h after wound closure; gram-negative coverage recommended for high-grade injuries
Patients with diabetes and other systemic diseases such as rheumatoid arthritis	Routine use of prophylactic antibiotics for elective, clean procedures less than 2 h in duration is not necessary

DIAGNOSIS OF INFECTION AFTER HAND SURGERY

A consensus is needed for diagnostic criteria for infection after hand surgery that are reliable. It will be difficult to test the accuracy of diagnostic criteria because there is no reference standard (eg, cultures are often negative).

Peel and Taylor[42] diagnosed postoperative infection based on the simultaneous presence of erythema, tenderness, edema, wound separation, and the presence of purulence—criteria most appropriate for deep infections. Some erythema and swelling can be normal postoperatively, particularly around sutures. A small wound separation may be colonized, but not necessarily infected. According to the criteria set by the Centers for Disease Control and Prevention (CDC), a surgical site infection can be superficial or deep.[30] Superficial infections occur within 30 days after the procedure and involve only the skin and subcutaneous tissue of the incision, in the presence of other cardinal signs of infection. Deep infections occur within 30 days after the operation (or 1 year if an implant has been placed) and involves the deep soft tissues, such as fascial and muscle layers.[32] Both categories require objective criteria to meet the diagnosis, or diagnosis by a surgeon or other attending physician. Given the stringency of the criteria provided by the CDC, consistent application of these definitions within the hand surgery community may contribute to more impactful and meaningful data within the literature.

TREATMENT OF INFECTION AFTER HAND SURGERY

Cellulitis (infection of the skin and subcutaneous tissues) around a wound typically occurs approximately 1 week after surgery. Patients often present with an edematous, painful hand with erythema at the incision site. This erythema may involve a small area around the suture penetration site (so-called suture abscess).[43,44] Most superficial infections resolve with suture removal with or without empiric oral antibiotics. Worsening infection or lymphangitic spread usually merits intravenous antibiotics and close monitoring, often with hospital admission.

Kirschner wires and external fixation pins protruding from the skin can become infected. In one review of 422 pins used in hand surgery, there was a 7% infection rate and a 4% rate of pin loosening without infection.[45] Stahl and Swartz[46] studied 236 patients undergoing K-wire fixation in the hand, 13 of whom (5.5%) developed pin site infection between 2 and 8 weeks after surgery. In another study of percutaneous pinning of proximal phalanx fractures, 2 of 50 patients (4%) developed pin-tract infections.[47] Factors associated with pin-tract infections may include motion at the bony interface, necrotic bone or soft tissue adjacent to the pin, and/or motion or tension on the skin. Pin infections usually resolve without antibiotics after pin removal. Oral antibiotics are used when it is too early to remove the pin, when the pin is loose or there is deep purulence, or when the pin crosses a joint. Infections with extensive cellulitis might benefit from intravenous antibiotics initially. Operative treatment is considered for pin infection associated with substantial radiolucency around the pin (so-called ring sequestrum).[1]

Patients undergoing hand or finger replantation or reconstructive flap coverage of wounds are at risk of infection because of contamination from the initial injury, leech therapy, and relative ischemia and/or vascular congestion in the tissues. If medicinal leeches are used, infection with *A hydrophila* can occur within the first day or even weeks after initiation of leech therapy.[48] A common prophylactic antibiotic choice is a fluoroquinolone such as ciprofloxacin,[49] and established infections can be treated with third-generation cephalosporins, aminoglycosides, fluoroquinolones, tetracycline, trimethoprim/sulfamethoxazole, or a combination of agents.[50] It is important to provide prophylaxis during therapy with medicinal leeches and to know the local characteristics of *Aeromonas* resistance.[51] Surgery for debridement of necrotic tissue and irrigation of involved tissues are recommended when there is deep purulence.

Deep space infections following hand surgery are uncommon. There are 4 confined spaces in the hand in which infection can develop; these include the thenar space, hypothenar space, midpalmar space, and web space.[52] For thenar and hypothenar space abscesses, a volar incision is made over the thenar or hypothenar eminence, respectively. Postoperative deep space infections in the midpalmar space are often decompressed through a direct incision; most commonly, an existing surgical incision is used for access. Web space infections typically require both a volar and a dorsal approach; longitudinal incisions are preferred to prevent contracture. Deep space infections following hand surgery are rare but most require surgical drainage.

There are no established guidelines for duration of antibiotic therapy in postoperative hand infections. In a recent article by Osterman and colleagues,[20] recommendations were made for antibiotic duration in suture abscesses (7–10 days); deep space infection (7–10 days); cat, dog, or human bites (7–14 days); tenosynovitis (2–3 weeks); septic arthritis (3–4 weeks); and osteomyelitis (6–8 weeks). In the absence of prospective data comparing multiple different regimens, these guidelines are reasonable and consistent with current practice.

DIRECTIONS FOR FUTURE RESEARCH

The study of a large, multicenter prospective cohort of patients having hand surgery would help determine risk factors for superficial and deep infection. There may be subsets of patients who benefit from specific prophylactic measures such as perioperative antibiotics, particularly those with significant systemic disease, such as diabetes and rheumatoid arthritis, among others.

Given the infrequency of deep infection after hand surgery, prospective randomized trials comparing the advantages and disadvantages of various prophylactic measures (eg, skin preparation, preoperative antibiotics) would need to be very large to detect a difference. If an acceptable rate of deep infection after hand surgery can be agreed on in terms of resource utilization, lost time from work, and the risk of permanent impairment from the infection and operative treatment, the difference in infection rate that would be meaningful can be determined. Prospective studies would then be powered to detect this difference. It is possible that we are already within the acceptable rate of infection with current practices.

In the authors' opinion, it is likely that a combination of factors, including the patient's age, nature of injury, comorbidities, type of procedure or procedures, and operative duration will provide a composite measure of risk of infection after surgery. Such a probability score might help guide perioperative patient care and inform patient and surgeon decision-making. Because the acceptable rate of infection after surgery is a balance of the risks of harm (eg, allergic reaction or colitis from prophylactic antibiotics) as well as a matter of values and preferences, a probability score would help patients and surgeons make an informed, shared decision.

REFERENCES

1. Shapiro DB. Postoperative infection in hand surgery. Cause, prevention, and treatment. Hand Clin 1998;14:669–81, x.
2. Hanssen AD, Amadio PC, DeSilva SP, et al. Deep postoperative wound infection after carpal tunnel release. J Hand Surg Am 1989;14:869–73.
3. Platt AJ, Page RE. Post-operative infection following hand surgery. Guidelines for antibiotic use. J Hand Surg Br 1995;20:685–90.
4. Kleinert JM, Hoffmann J, Miller Crain G, et al. Postoperative infection in a double-occupancy operating room. A prospective study of two thousand four hundred and fifty-eight procedures on the extremities. J Bone Joint Surg Am 1997;79:503–13.
5. Ariyan S, Watson HK. The palmar approach for the visualization and release of the carpal tunnel. An analysis of 429 cases. Plast Reconstr Surg 1977;60:539–47.
6. Gunther SF, Gunther SB. Diabetic hand infections. Hand Clin 1998;14:647–56.

7. Deitch EA. Infection in the compromised host. Surg Clin North Am 1988;68:181–97.
8. Sloan JP, Dove AF, Maheson M, et al. Antibiotics in open fractures of the distal phalanx? J Hand Surg Br 1987;12:123–4.
9. Cummings P. Antibiotics to prevent infection in patients with dog bite wounds: a meta-analysis of randomized trials. Ann Emerg Med 1994;23:535–40.
10. Zubowicz VN, Gravier M. Management of early human bites of the hand: a prospective randomized study. Plast Reconstr Surg 1991;88:111–4.
11. Hoffman RD, Adams BD. The role of antibiotics in the management of elective and post-traumatic hand surgery. Hand Clin 1998;14:657–66.
12. Hausman MR, Lisser SP. Hand infections. Orthop Clin North Am 1992;23:171–85.
13. Houshian S, Seyedipour S, Wedderkopp N. Epidemiology of bacterial hand infections. Int J Infect Dis 2006;10:315–9.
14. Tosti R, Ilyas AM. Empiric antibiotics for acute infections of the hand. J Hand Surg Am 2010;35:125–8.
15. O'Malley M, Fowler J, Ilyas AM. Community-acquired methicillin-resistant Staphylococcus aureus infections of the hand: prevalence and timeliness of treatment. J Hand Surg Am 2009;34:504–8.
16. Kiran RV, McCampbell B, Angeles AP, et al. Increased prevalence of community-acquired methicillin-resistant Staphylococcus aureus in hand infections at an urban medical center. Plast Reconstr Surg 2006;118:161–6 [discussion: 167–9].
17. Bach HG, Steffin B, Chhadia AM, et al. Community-associated methicillin-resistant Staphylococcus aureus hand infections in an urban setting. J Hand Surg Am 2007;32:380–3.
18. LeBlanc DM, Reece EM, Horton JB, et al. Increasing incidence of methicillin resistant Staphylococcus aureus in hand infections: a 3-year county hospital experience. Plast Reconstr Surg 2007;119:935–40.
19. Wong CH, Chang HC, Pasupathy S, et al. Necrotizing fasciitis: clinical presentation, microbiology, and determinants of mortality. J Bone Joint Surg Am 2003;85A:1454–60.
20. Osterman M, Draeger R, Stern P. Acute hand infections. J Hand Surg Am 2014;39:1628–35.
21. Widmer AF. Surgical hand hygiene: scrub or rub? J Hosp Infect 2013;83(Suppl 1):S35–9.
22. Widmer AF, Rotter M, Voss A, et al. Surgical hand preparation: state-of-the-art. J Hosp Infect 2010;74:112–22.
23. Awad SS, Palacio CH, Subramanian A, et al. Implementation of a methicillin-resistant Staphylococcus aureus (MRSA) prevention bundle results in decreased MRSA surgical site infections. Am J Surg 2009;198:607–10.
24. Lai KW, Foo TL, Low W, et al. Surgical hand antisepsis—a pilot study comparing povidone iodine hand scrub and alcohol-based chlorhexidine gluconate hand rub. Ann Acad Med Singapore 2012;41:12–6.
25. Weber WP, Reck S, Neff U, et al. Surgical hand antisepsis with alcohol-based hand rub: comparison of effectiveness after 1.5 and 3 minutes of application. Infect Control Hosp Epidemiol 2009;30:420–6.
26. O'Farrell DA, Kenny G, O'Sullivan M, et al. Evaluation of the optimal hand-scrub duration before total hip arthroplasty. J Hosp Infect 1994;26:93–8.
27. Bannister GC, Auchincloss JM, Johnson DP, et al. The timing of tourniquet application in relation to prophylactic antibiotic administration. J Bone Joint Surg Br 1988;70:322–4.
28. Oragui E, Parsons A, White T, et al. Tourniquet use in upper limb surgery. Hand (N Y) 2011;6:165–73.
29. Burke JF. The effective period of preventive antibiotic action in experimental incisions and dermal lesions. Surgery 1961;50:161–8.
30. Harness NG, Inacio MC, Pfeil FF, et al. Rate of infection after carpal tunnel release surgery and effect of antibiotic prophylaxis. J Hand Surg Am 2010;35:189–96.
31. Bykowski MR, Sivak WN, Cray J, et al. Assessing the impact of antibiotic prophylaxis in outpatient elective hand surgery: a single-center, retrospective review of 8,850 cases. J Hand Surg Am 2011;36:1741–7.
32. Tosti R, Fowler J, Dwyer J, et al. Is antibiotic prophylaxis necessary in elective soft tissue hand surgery? Orthopedics 2012;35:e829–33.
33. Whittaker JP, Nancarrow JD, Sterne GD. The role of antibiotic prophylaxis in clean incised hand injuries: a prospective randomized placebo controlled double blind trial. J Hand Surg Br 2005;30:162–7.
34. Amland PF, Andenaes K, Samdal F, et al. A prospective, double-blind, placebo-controlled trial of a single dose of azithromycin on postoperative wound infections in plastic surgery. Plast Reconstr Surg 1995;96:1378–83.
35. Garibaldi RA, Cushing D, Lerer T. Risk factors for postoperative infection. Am J Med 1991;91:158S–63S.
36. Griego RD, Rosen T, Orengo IF, et al. Dog, cat, and human bites: a review. J Am Acad Dermatol 1995;33:1019–29.
37. Haley RW, Culver DH, Morgan WM, et al. Identifying patients at high risk of surgical wound infection. A simple multivariate index of patient susceptibility and wound contamination. Am J Epidemiol 1985;121:206–15.
38. Stevenson J, McNaughton G, Riley J. The use of prophylactic flucloxacillin in treatment of open fractures of the distal phalanx within an accident and emergency department: a double-blind randomized placebo-controlled trial. J Hand Surg Br 2003;28:388–94.
39. Classen DC, Evans RS, Pestotnik SL, et al. The timing of prophylactic administration of antibiotics

and the risk of surgical-wound infection. N Engl J Med 1992;326:281–6.
40. Henley MB, Jones RE, Wyatt RW, et al. Prophylaxis with cefamandole nafate in elective orthopedic surgery. Clin Orthop Relat Res 1986;(209):249–54.
41. Culver DH, Horan TC, Gaynes RP, et al. Surgical wound infection rates by wound class, operative procedure, and patient risk index. National Nosocomial Infections Surveillance System. Am J Med 1991;91:152S–7S.
42. Peel AL, Taylor EW. Proposed definitions for the audit of postoperative infection: a discussion paper. Surgical Infection Study Group. Ann R Coll Surg Engl 1991;73:385–8.
43. Mangram AJ, Horan TC, Pearson ML, et al. Guideline for Prevention of Surgical Site Infection, 1999. Centers for Disease Control and Prevention (CDC) Hospital Infection Control Practices Advisory Committee. Am J Infect Control 1999;27:97–132 [quiz: 133–4; discussion: 196].
44. Robson MC. Wound infection. A failure of wound healing caused by an imbalance of bacteria. Surg Clin North Am 1997;77:637–50.
45. Botte MJ, Davis JL, Rose BA, et al. Complications of smooth pin fixation of fractures and dislocations in the hand and wrist. Clin Orthop Relat Res 1992;(276):194–201.
46. Stahl S, Schwartz O. Complications of K-wire fixation of fractures and dislocations in the hand and wrist. Arch Orthop Trauma Surg 2001;121:527–30.
47. Eberlin KR, Babushkina A, Neira JR, et al. Outcomes of closed reduction and periarticular pinning of base and shaft fractures of the proximal phalanx. J Hand Surg Am 2014;39:1524–8.
48. Lineaweaver WC, Hill MK, Buncke GM, et al. Aeromonas hydrophila infections following use of medicinal leeches in replantation and flap surgery. Ann Plast Surg 1992;29:238–44.
49. Green PA, Shafritz AB. Medicinal leech use in microsurgery. J Hand Surg Am 2010;35:1019–21.
50. Ardehali B, Hand K, Nduka C, et al. Delayed leech-borne infection with Aeromonas hydrophilia in escharotic flap wound. J Plast Reconstr Aesthet Surg 2006;59:94–5.
51. Whitaker IS, Kamya C, Azzopardi EA, et al. Preventing infective complications following leech therapy: is practice keeping pace with current research? Microsurgery 2009;29:619–25.
52. Ong YS, Levin LS. Hand infections. Plast Reconstr Surg 2009;124:225e–33e.

Management of Complications of Congenital Hand Disorders

Garet C. Comer, MD, Amy L. Ladd, MD*

KEYWORDS

• Syndactyly • Polydactyly • Thumb duplication • Radial longitudinal deficiency • Radial club hand • Thumb hypoplasia • Pollicization • Epidermolysis bullosa

KEY POINTS

- A thorough knowledge of patient presentation, natural history, and treatment options is essentially to effectively manage patients with congenital hand differences.
- Although some treatment complications are inevitable, judicious preoperative planning, meticulous technique, and knowledge of surgery-specific lessons help to decrease the risk of complications.
- Management of syndactyly, camptodactyly, ulnar polydactyly, radial polydactyly, thumb hypoplasia, radial longitudinal deficiency, and epidermolysis bullosa has evolved with refined understanding of disease processes and treatments.

INTRODUCTION

Advances in the care of patients with congenital hand differences have made dramatic progress in the modern era. These advances include refined surgical procedures, improved classifications, new technology, improved understanding of the embryology and pathogenesis of disease, and an increased understanding of the psychological implications of having a congenital hand difference This article focuses on 7 conditions frequently treated by hand surgeons: syndactyly, camptodactyly, ulnar polydactyly, radial polydactyly, thumb hypoplasia, radial longitudinal deficiency (RLD), and epidermolysis bullosa (EB). We review each topic and discuss methods to avoid complications in the treatment of patients with these conditions.

SYNDACTYLY

Syndactyly occurs in 1 in 2000 to 3000 live births, making it one of the most common congenital hand anomalies.[1] It most commonly appears in isolation, but may also be associated with congenital syndromes, such as Apert syndrome and Poland syndrome.[2] Syndactyly most commonly affects the third web space followed by the fourth, second, and first web spaces, respectively. It is frequently bilateral and is more commonly seen in males than females.[1,3–5] In addition to the hand, patients should be evaluated for foot involvement and associated syndromes.

The timing of surgical release of the digits is debatable, although surgery is most frequently undertaken at 12 to 18 months of age. Although good results have been reported with delaying

Funding Sources: None related to this topic.
Conflicts of Interest: None related to this topic.
Department of Orthopedic Surgery, Robert A. Chase Hand & Upper Limb Center, Stanford University, 450 Broadway Street, Pavilion C, Redwood City, CA 94063, USA
* Corresponding author.
E-mail address: alad@stanford.edu

Hand Clin 31 (2015) 361–375
http://dx.doi.org/10.1016/j.hcl.2015.01.011
0749-0712/15/$ – see front matter

surgery until 4 or 5 years for simple syndactyly,[1] separation is typically not delayed past 12 months for digits of unequal length to avoid deformity caused by the shorter digit tethering the longer.

The surgical treatment of syndactyly has evolved dramatically over the years. In the 19th century, digits were separated with straight dorsal and palmar incisions with attempted primary closure.[6] However, this led to unacceptable results from wound closure under tension and contracture formation.[7] Currently, surgery is based on the following principles:

1. Division of the web with zigzag incisions,
2. Achieving tension-free closure by utilizing free skin graft when primary closure is not possible, and
3. Applying dorsal flap for commissure reconstruction.

Building on these principles, subsequent reports have focused on refining these techniques and improving outcomes. Specifically, recent literature has focused on split-thickness versus full-thickness skin grafts, commissure reconstruction techniques, and the use of tissue expanders to obviate the need for skin grafting. Several authors have advocated for the superiority of full-thickness skin grafts over split-thickness grafts by citing a lower rate of contracture and web creep.[1,5,8] However, others have noted comparable outcomes with both techniques.[9]

Many commissure reconstructions techniques have been developed. These include the Flatt dorsal hourglass-shaped rotational web flap,[10,11] V-Y advancement flaps,[12,13] trilobed dorsal flaps,[14] and triangular flap designs.[15,16] Barabás and Pickford[17] reported on 144 webs reconstructions by a modified Flatt technique at a mean of 5 years follow-up. The rate of complications was low with 7 (4.9%) graft failures, 6 patients (4.2%) with web creep, and only 4 patients (2.8%) requiring reoperation. The authors recommend avoidance of longitudinal wound lines extending midaxially from the commissural flap as seen when a volar T-shaped incision is used.

Common complications include (1) web creep—losing the deep commissure performed at surgery - with an incidence of 2% to 24% (**Fig. 1**).[8] (2) Skin graft slough is common and may contribute to web creep, especially with the most proximal grafts set distal to the dorsal flap. (3) Vascular compromise is a potential challenge in complex syndactyly and polysyndactyly, such as Apert syndrome and rotational deformities owing to anomalous transverse or even absent arterial flow (**Fig. 2**). The long-held dictum in syndactyly surgery is that separating only 1 digit at a time in multiple contiguous syndactyly prevents vascular compromise and loss of a digit. We find, however, this is seldom a problem in simple syndactyly when a full complement of neurovascular structures is the rule. (4) Nail deformity is often underappreciated and seen in complex syndactyly, especially Apert syndrome and fused distal phalanx presentations.[18] (5) Finally, rotational deformity may be unmasked in complex syndactyly when the digits are freed and allowed to develop unencumbered (**Fig. 3**). However, this is less a complication and more an unanticipated outcome because deformity development may be unpredictable; nonetheless, the possibility should be reviewed with the family at the initial surgery.

Minimizing complications in the surgical treatment of syndactyly requires meticulous operative technique, tension-free closure, and reduction of shear forces across skin graft sites. Using

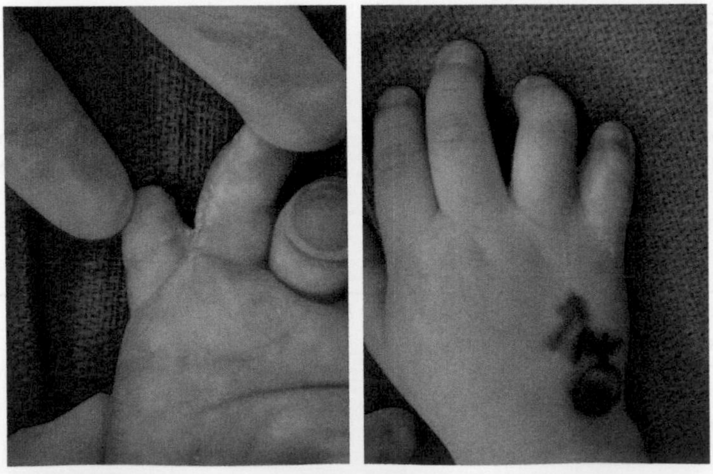

Fig. 1. Web creep after the release of a complete syndactyly.

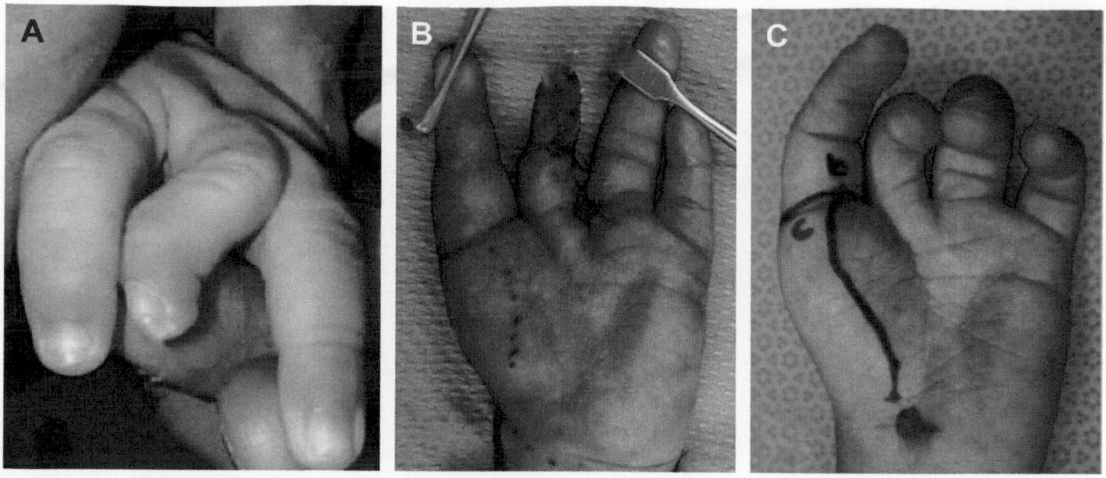

Fig. 2. (*A*) In complex syndactylies with rotational deformities, postoperative vascular compromise is a heightened concern owing to possible anomalous vascularity. (*B*) Postoperatively, the tip of the central digit became ischemic and eventually autoamputated. (*C*) Late outcome after debridement, in anticipation of a pollicization (with proposed skin incision markings shown).

compressive dressings and postoperative immobilization help to decrease flap necrosis and wound breakdown.

Authors' recommendations for avoiding and minimizing syndactyly complications

1. Meticulous surgical technique: thoroughly defat grafts, achieve complete hemostasis, and close completely tension free.
2. Place a bulky, compressive dressings and complete cast coverage for 2 weeks.
3. In complex syndactyly, obtain radiographs and acknowledge bony contribution to angular or rotational deformity and nail abnormalities.

CAMPTODACTYLY

Camptodactyly is defined as a nontraumatic flexion deformity isolated to the proximal interphalangeal (PIP) joint, typically involving the small finger. Bilateral involvement occurs around two-thirds of the time. Other digits may be affected with the ring being second most common, followed by index, then middle. Age at presentation is typically either in infancy or in adolescence, around the time of growth spurts. There is an equal sex distribution in the infantile presentation, whereas girls are more commonly affected when the disease presents in adolescence.[19,20] Most cases present sporadically without prior family history, although familial cases have been reported, as have other associated congenital disorders.[21,22]

Nearly every structure within the finger has been implicated in the pathogenesis of the condition, including skin, fascia, flexor tendon sheath, flexor tendons, lumbricals, collateral ligaments, and volar plate.[8,23–26] However, no single anatomic anomaly seems to exist in all cases. A recent theory proposes that an imbalance between flexor and extensor forces lies behind the pathogenesis of camptodactyly.[19]

Patient presentation varies significantly, and proper patient assessment is key to guiding treatment. The most common patient complaint is appearance, followed by functional limitation; pain is uncommon.[20,27,28] The degree and flexibility of deformity is variable, although progression of the deformity from supple to stiff has not been documented.[22,29] Radiographs are obtained to rule out any other source of pathology and to detect articular changes, including articular incongruity, proximal phalangeal flattening, and notching of the middle phalanx base (**Fig. 4**).[3] Other causes of flexion deformity should be ruled out, including a traumatic boutonniere injury or neurogenic clawing.

Foucher and colleagues[22] developed a classification scheme with a corresponding treatment algorithm.[30] Patients are classified as having early onset (<5 years old; type I), late onset (type II), first ray involvement (type III), or association with complex syndromes (type IV). They are subdivided into subtype a (stiff deformity) or subtype b (correctable deformity).

Nonoperative treatment is favored currently, with an emphasis on digital stretching with night splinting; surgery is generally reserved for moderate to severe deformity (>60°), functional limitation, or pain that has been refractory to nonoperative treatment.[19,22,27,28] In general, better

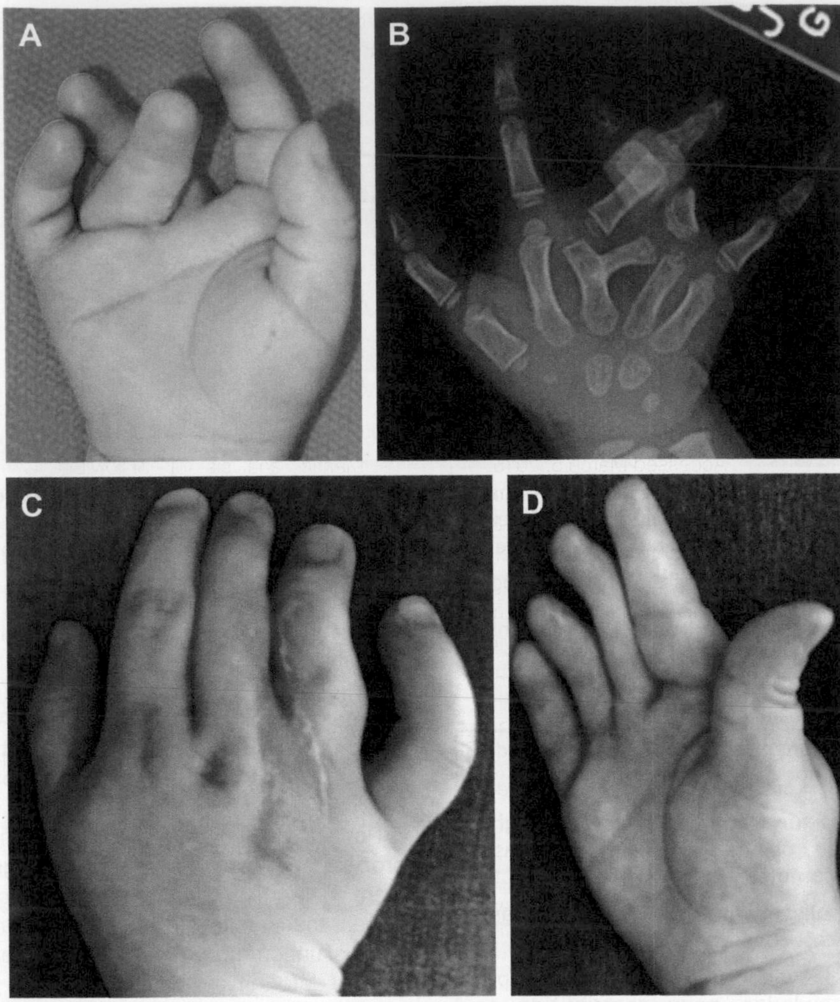

Fig. 3. (*A, B*) Postoperative rotational deformity of the third web space unmasked after syndactyly release in a complex polysyndactyly. (*C, D*), Postoperative images after subsequent multiple osteotomies and excision of the metacarpal bar. A subtle malrotation of the ring digit persists.

treatment results are seen with less severe deformity and shorter duration of deformity.[19,29,31]

Surgical treatments have focused on a variety of pathologic structures, but have failed to yield consistently good results. Some authors have recommended treatment focused on addressing specific pathologic structures, including the lumbricals,[32,33] the flexor digitorum superficialis (FDS),[34,35] and the volar skin.[36] Other authors instead view the entire digit as imperfectly developed and advocate for an all-inclusive operative approach.[8,22,34] In this regard, a step-wise, uniform approach to the disease as advocated by Foucher colleagues[22] has led to improved surgical outcomes. The authors describe a series of physical examination steps to evaluate the volar skin, FDS, and central slip, which led to a lower treatment failure rate and improved surgical outcomes.

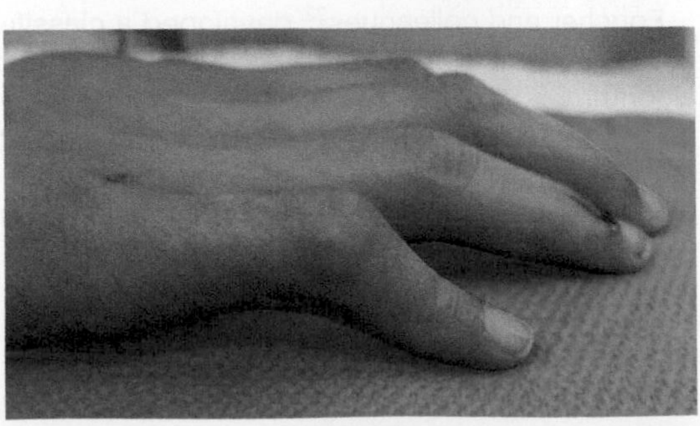

Fig. 4. Radiographic findings in camptodactyly are demonstrated with subtle joint subluxation and notching of the middle phalanx base.

Outcomes of patients treated surgically for camptodactyly remain inconsistent with surgery frequently complicated by recurrence of the deformity (**Fig. 5**). In 1 series of 53 surgically treated patients, 11% developed a worse contracture

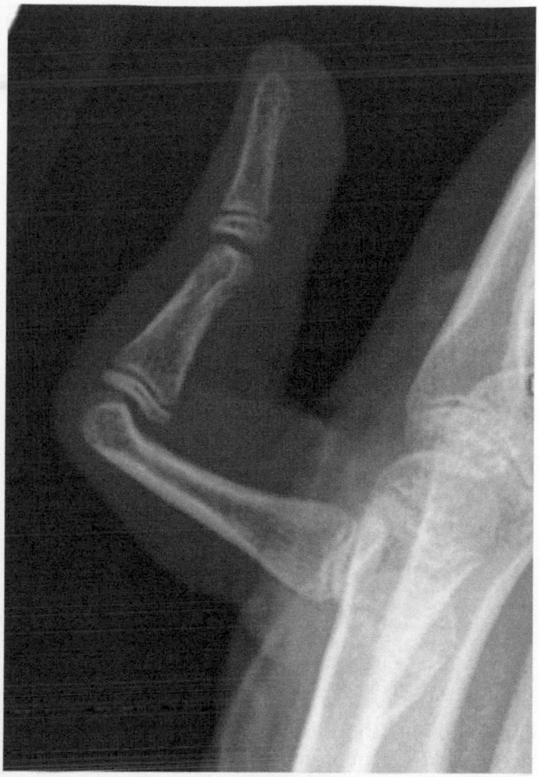

Fig. 5. Recurrence or worsening of preoperative flexion deformity is a common complication of the surgical treatment of camptodactyly, this one 8 years after deformity of 90° was corrected.

than preoperatively and only 33% regained full flexion.[25] In another series of 20 patients undergoing corrective operations, 13 patients were noted to be the same or worse after surgery.[20]

We have experienced the following common complications or incompletely addressed deformities as sources of treatment failure:

1. Progression of both PIP contracture and metacarpophalangeal (MP) hyperextension in nonoperative cases;
2. Progression or failed improvement of both PIP contracture and MP hyperextension in operative cases;
3. Isolated PIP postoperative residual stiffness; and
4. Bony remodeling of proximal phalanx head preventing full extension.

With failure of treatment ranging from 14% to 65%, surgical correction of camptodactyly remains an unsolved problem.[20,22] Our experience favors surgical correction, especially when compensatory posturing of MP hyperextension hampers function, such as with handwriting and playing ball sports. The MP hyperextension further aggravates PIP joint flexion, leading to a worsening of the deformity. Thus, surgical treatment is indicated to rebalance the tendon's forces when conservative measures such as stretching fail to correct both MP hyperextension and PIP flexion.

Authors' recommendations for avoiding deformity recurrence

1. Nonoperative splinting at night to include intrinsic plus position: MP flexion, PIP extension.
2. Surgical treatment at any age for progressive contractures after splinting failure.
3. Full palmar surgical exposure to reveal contributing pathology. Anomalous lumbricals or FDS are most commonly encountered. Additionally, we have encountered accessory contrahentes (anomalous, atavistic palmar muscles).[37] These anomalous muscles typically requires excision or release of tight/opposing structures.

Authors' preferred Method

If the FDS is present, we use this for an intrinsic balancing procedure. The FDS is split, 1 slip becomes an anticlaw force sutured to the A2 pulley, and the other is brought within the palm and transferred to the central tendon hood. The digit is then pinned and casted in the intrinsic plus position. If the fifth FDS is not available, then the adjacent fourth FDS tendon is used.

ULNAR POLYDACTYLY

Ulnar polydactyly is among the most common congenital hand anomalies with an incidence of 1 in 100 to 300 live births among African Americans and 1 in 1500 to 3000 live births among Caucasians.[38] It is often bilateral, found in isolation, and has an autosomal-dominant inheritance pattern. However, it may also be associated with chromosomal abnormalities or other associated syndromes.

The structural composition of the supernumerary digits ranges on a spectrum from rudimentary soft tissue appendages to fully formed digits. Several classification schemes have been utilized in the literature. Temtamy and McKusick[39] identified fully formed supernumerary digits as type A polydactyly and incompletely formed, nonfunctional supernumerary digits as type B polydactyly. Stelling and Turek[40] defined duplication of soft parts only as type 1, partial duplication involving osseous structures as type 2, and a fully duplicated ray, including the metacarpal as type 3.

Patients are frequently assessed in the newborn nursery and offices of pediatricians, family physicians, dermatologists, and hand surgeons. Evaluation of the patient should include x-rays of the affected hand if osseous structures are felt on examination, although we prefer to wait to obtain x-rays close to the time of surgery because perinatal x-rays show little in the way of osseous structures.

Treatment is based on the degree to which the supernumerary digit is formed. Soft tissue polydactyly may be excised, whereas more complex polydactyly may require reconstruction of the joint capsule, corrective osteotomy, and/or transfers of the hypothenar musculature. Traditionally and probably most commonplace is treating type 1 polydactyly in the newborn nursery or in the home with suture ligation. Suture material is tied snugly to the base of the supernumerary digit leading to necrosis of the digit, which eventually is easily removed or falls off on its own. Although reported as "simple, safe, and effective,"[41] our experience corresponds with others who report neuroma formation,[42,43] cyst formation,[44] aesthetically unacceptable residual stumps (**Fig. 6**),[45] and infection.[46] These previously underreported complications associated with this home treatment have led many authors to advocate for primary surgical excision.[43,46,47]

Singer and colleagues[38] reviewed 53 hands with Stelling and Turek types 1, 2, and 3 ulnar polydactyly treated with surgical excision with or without reconstruction. In short-term follow-up, 1 patient developed an infection and 3 developed a hypertrophic scar. Of 20 patients (30 polydactylies) available for long-term follow-up, 2 had a residual nubbin and 1 patient had a painful neuroma.

Authors' recommendations to prevent residual stumps and neuroma formation

1. For skin tag/free nubbins: If possible, primary removal is performed in the newborn nursery. The circumcision tray typically has most of the needed materials. We prefer instilling about 0.5 mL of 0.5% lidocaine with epinephrine into the base of the digit, excising the nerve and artery sufficiently proximally, and using a handheld cautery device such as is used in emergency departments for subungual hematomas. One absorbable suture and Dermabond (Ethicon, Somerville, NJ) sealing, with Coban (3M, Maplewood, MN) wrap typically suffices.
2. For bony deformity, we recommend applying Bone Wax (Ethicon, Somerville, NJ) over raw bony surfaces to reduce bony regrowth (**Fig. 7**).

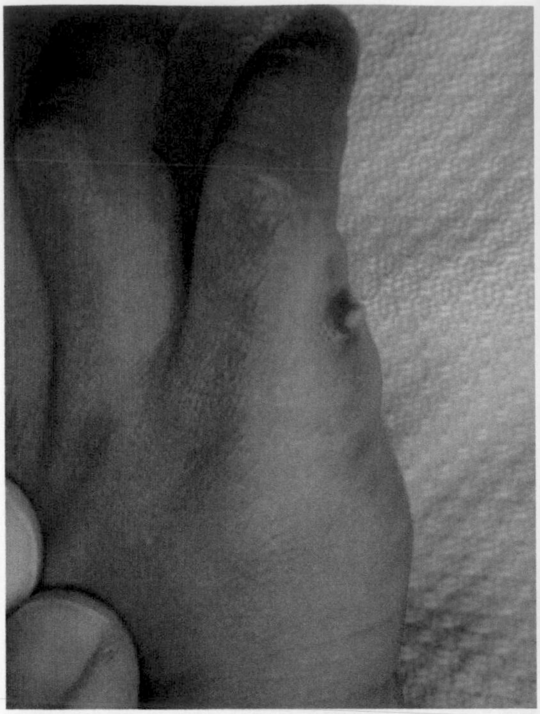

Fig. 6. Complications of suture ligation of ulnar polydactyly include neuroma formation, cyst formation, infection, and residual stumps as pictured here.

RADIAL POLYDACTYLY

Although ulnar polydactyly is relatively common, radial polydactyly is much more rare, with a reported incidence of 0.08 in 100,000 live births.[3] As with ulnar polydactyly, a spectrum of duplication is present with thumb polydactyly ranging from a bifid distal phalanx to an entirely duplicated ray and carpal bones. Importantly, radial polydactyly is not merely a duplication of a normal thumb, but 2 hypoplastic thumbs, and residual deformities after reconstruction are typically the rule.

The most widely utilized classification system is the Wassel classification.[48] This system progresses from the distal phalanx proximally starting with a bifid distal phalanx as type 1, duplicated distal phalanges as type 2, and so on. The pattern is interrupted with any triphalangeal thumb, which is classified as type 7. Several modifications have been proposed, including triphalangeal subtypes,[49] type IV subtypes,[50] and symphalangism, deviation, and triplication.[51] Nonetheless, the Wassel classification has persisted and continues to guide treatment.

Simple excision of the less developed digit, though commonly used historically, led to less optimal functional and aesthetic outcomes.[52,53] The MP and interphalangeal (IP) joints often developed a Z-deformity and joint instability with

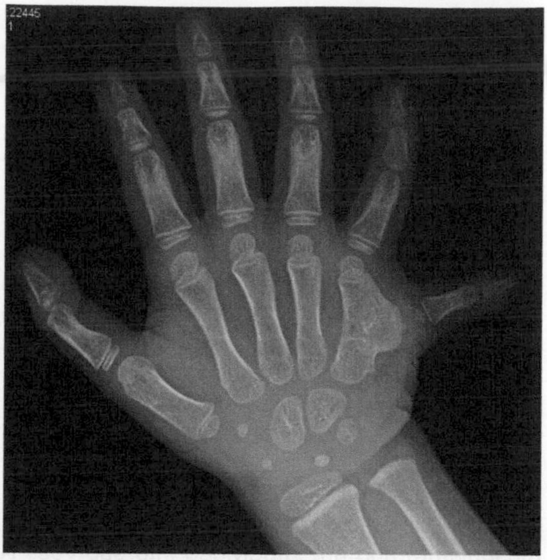

Fig. 7. A Stelling and Turek type 2 ulnar polydactyly that was treated with supernumerary digit resection with cleavage of the extra metacarpal portion from the fifth metacarpal shaft. Bone wax was applied to the raw bone surface to control hemorrhage and decrease bony regrowth.

off-axis pull of the tendons on the preserved phalanges and underlying bony deformity.[54,55] Currently, reconstructive procedures that are favored strive to rebalance the soft tissues and address bony alignment in conjunction with ablation.[55,56]

The goals of surgical treatment are to:

1. Align the joints and physes with the longitudinal axis of the thumb,
2. Provide joint stability in balance with functional motion,
3. Achieve balanced tendon pull,
4. Prevent nail deformity, and
5. Achieve appropriate length and bulk.

With these goals in mind, operative procedures aim to either reconstruct a single digit from the 2 hypoplastic digits or excise 1 digit and reconstruct the bony and soft tissue elements on the excised side. Currently, surgeons rarely perform the traditional Bilhaut procedure by combining 2 split nails into one for the distal phalanx duplication.[52,57,58] Although elegant in concept, it is almost impossible to combine 2 digits into an esthetically pleasing thumb because of the split nail and incongruent sizes of the 2 thumb parts. This author's preference is to remove the radial thumb nail at its natural split, and transpose the radial paronychial fold along with a retained ulnar bony portion of the discarded radial distal phalanx to provide breadth to the reconstructed thumb.

The most common approach to surgical treatment of thumb duplication at the level of the proximal phalanx (Wassel III/IV) is excision of the lesser or radial digit, tightening the radial collateral ligament, reattaching thenar and accessory thenar muscles distal to the MP joint to stabilize a deficiency, anomalous tendon repositioning (especially the flexor pollicis longus), and osteotomy as needed.[50,52,59]

Surgical results are reportedly inconsistent, and largely depend on the initial deformity. The greatest deformity, and thus incomplete correction, occurs with what we call the "diamond thumb" with significant angular deformity in Wassel IV (**Fig. 8**). An increasing need for reoperation exists as patients grow.[52,60–62] Common complications include stiffness, instability, malalignment that may worsen with growth, and undesirable cosmetic appearance (**Fig. 9**). Stutz and colleagues[60] reported the outcomes of 43 cases of radial polydactyly and noted a 19% long-term reoperation rate. The primary cause for revision surgery was instability with pain at the IP joint managed with arthrodesis. Larsen and Nicolai[62] reexamined 19 patients at an average of 22.5 years and noted 7 of the 19 patients were dissatisfied with the appearance of their thumb owing to the residual lateral deviation of the IP and MP joints; 14 thumbs demonstrated greater than 20° of malalignment. Similarly, Goldfarb and colleagues[63] noted angulation at the IP joint was the most commonly cited reason for decreased satisfaction with appearance in a series of 31 reconstructed thumbs. Surgery for radial polydactyly is challenging and requires precise reconstruction of bony and soft-tissue elements.

Authors' recommendations to prevent residual deformity and optimize function and appearance

1. Remove the radial nail but preserve part of radial distal phalanx to provide breadth for distal duplication (Wassel I/II).
2. Adequately expose the proximal and distal deforming structures, including conjoint extensors and flexors (all types).
3. Rebalance and reposition duplicated tendons with anomalous insertions.
4. Stabilize joints with collateral ligament advancement: IP (Wassel I/II) and MP (Wassel III/IV).

THUMB HYPOPLASIA

Thumb hypoplasia exists in a variety of presentations from an undersized thumb to complete absence of the thumb. It may occur as an isolated

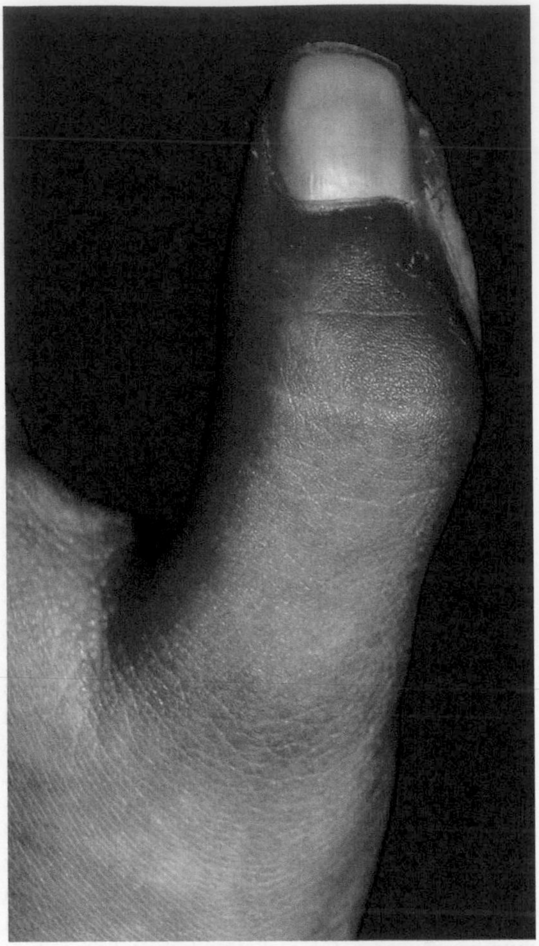

Fig. 8. Clinical appearance and radiographs of a Wassel IV radial polydactyly with significant angular "diamond thumb" deformity.

condition or associated with other congenital syndromes such as Holt-Oram syndrome, thrombocytopenia–absent-radius (TAR) syndrome, Fanconi's anemia and VACTERL (vertebral, anal atresia, cardiac, trachea, esophageal, renal, and limb defects) association.[3,64] As such, one should be suspicious for associated anomalies and perform a thorough multisystem evaluation of infants with thumb hypoplasia.

The modified Blauth classification characterizes disease severity and treatment.[65] A type 1 thumb is essentially normal with the exception of being undersized with mild thenar hypoplasia and thumb posture often in the plane of the fingers. A type 2 thumb is also undersized, but with a contracted web space, MP joint instability, and hypoplastic thenar musculature. Type 3 thumbs are characterized by both hypoplastic intrinsic and extrinsic musculature and are subdivided into subtypes A and B. Type 3A thumbs have stable carpometacarpal (CMC) joints, whereas 3B thumbs do not have stable CMC joints.[66] A type 4 thumb has no bony support and is termed the "floating thumb" (*pouce flottant*). Type 5 is complete aplasia.

The key distinction lies between types 3A and 3B, where CMC joint deficiency determines if the thumb is salvageable. In thumbs with a CMC joint, treatment includes reconstruction with first web space deepening, opponensplasty, MP joint ligamentous reconstruction or arthrodesis, and tendon transfer for extrinsic tendon deficiency.[66–68] However, when the CMC joint is not present, thumb amputation and index pollicization is indicated.[69,70]

Pollicization is a complex procedure that is the result of more than a century's worth of

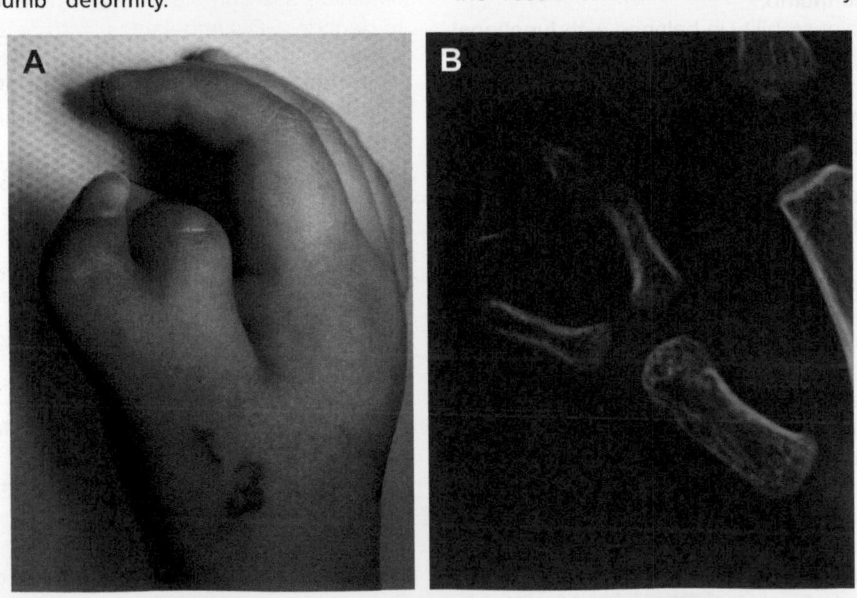

Fig. 9. (*A*) Complications of radial polydactyly reconstruction include nail deformity and angular deformity especially present at the interphalangeal joint. (*B*) Radiographic image.

contributions from many surgeons.[71] The basic principles of the operation were detailed by Buck-Gramcko.[65] Other authors have refined the procedure, but the basic concepts remain unchanged. The principles of the operation are as follows:

1. Incision that creates a first web space without scar and adequate skin coverage,
2. Ligation of the radial digital artery to the long finger and interfascicular dissection of the common digital nerve to isolate the neurovascular pedicle on the index finger,
3. Isolation of the flexor and extensor tendons and interosseous musculature from the index metacarpal and division of the intermetacarpal ligament,
4. Shortening of the index metacarpal through the proximal metaphysis and through the physis distally to prevent overgrowth,
5. Alignment of the index finger into the thumb position (abducted and pronated), and
6. Transfer the palmar and dorsal interossei to the ulnar and radial lateral bands, respectively to restore intrinsic function.

The surgical results of pollicization are generally favorable, although the outcome depends heavily on the preoperative degree of hypoplasia with patients with high-grade hypoplasias or radial deficiency fairing worse.[72–74] Percival and colleagues devised an assessment tool based on pinch, opposition, grasp, mobility, sensibility, and appearance and noted a 73% rate of excellent or good outcomes in 30 thumbs.[72] Utilizing Percival's criteria, Vekris noted 75% excellent and 19% good outcomes in 21 cases.[75] Long-term results have confirmed that the results of pollicization persist into adulthood.[76]

Potential surgical complications depend on the procedure and severity of hypoplasia. Mild hypoplasia procedures may involve recurrence of instability and first web contracture. For a type 2 or 3A thumb, the Huber transfer[77] repositions the abductor digiti minimi to mimic the absent abductor pollicis brevis. Known complications include devascularization of the pedicle about the pisiform,[78] carpal tunnel syndrome,[79] and ulnar nerve compression.[80]

For the challenging pollicization procedure, complications may be divided into early and late. Early complications include intraoperative neurovascular injury, arterial insufficiency, venous congestion, hematoma, infection, and marginal wound necrosis (**Fig. 10**). Late complications include scar contracture, stiffness, tendon adhesions, overgrowth or angular deformity owing to physeal problems, avascular necrosis, and instability of the new basilar thumb joint.[81–84]

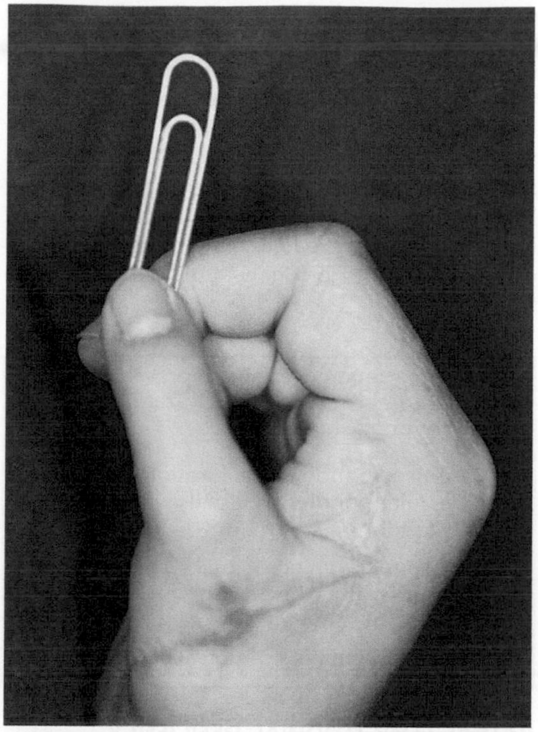

Fig. 10. Satisfactory functional result of index pollicization despite broad areas of scarring owing to secondary intention healing of areas marginal skin necrosis.

Buck-Gramcko[84] reported on the incidence of early complications in his series of 460 pollicizations. He reported 12 arterial injuries, complete digital necrosis in 1 case, and 2 cases of nerve injury with paralysis of the intrinsic muscles. Goldfarb and colleagues[82] reported on 73 pollicizations with 8 cases of perioperative complications. These were 4 cases of marginal skin necrosis, 3 cases of venous congestion, and 1 infection. These complications required 12 reoperations.

Several authors have reported long-term complications. Lochner and colleagues[83] reported on 85 pollicized digits at a minimum of 2 years after surgery. Long-term complications included 12 complete and 9 partial proximal phalangeal physeal arrests, 20 nonunions of the base of the index metacarpal, 10 unstable CMC joints, and 5 cases of metacarpal overgrowth. Three of the nonunions required subsequent operation, 1 unstable CMC joint was reconstructed, and 4 additional procedures were done in 2 patients owing to overgrowth. Goldfarb and colleagues[82] noted 7 cases of scar contracture, 1 case of redundant skin, 19 cases of limited opposition despite interosseous transfer, and 15 cases with limited thumb extension in a total of 73 pollicizations. There were 37 subsequent operations. Index pollicization leads to generally favorable outcomes with devastating complications being relatively rare. In our hands, the most common problem is contending with the bulk of the proximal muscles and relative shortage of overlying skin to cover the increased bulk, especially when a floating thumb is present (**Fig. 11**). This may lead to marginal flap necrosis, especially on the dorsum with the Buck-Gramcko technique.

Authors' recommendations to prevent early and late complications of pollicization for thumb hypoplasia

1. Careful attention to the location of the neurovascular bundles, especially when transferring tendons,
2. Generous trimming of bulky proximal muscles, especially when a hypoplastic thumb is removed at same time of pollicization, and
3. Generous trimming of dorsal skin.

RADIAL LONGITUDINAL DEFICIENCY

RLD is a relatively rare congenital anomaly that is commonly associated with other congenital malformations. It occurs in 0.5 per 10,000 live births.[85]

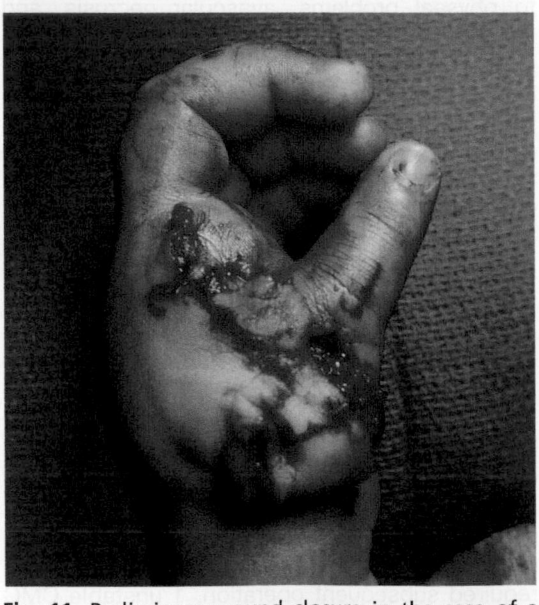

Fig. 11. Preliminary wound closure in the case of a pollicization performed in conjunction with hypoplastic thumb removal. A challenge exists with the flap creation and dealing with the relative mismatch of abundant new thenar muscles supporting a slender digit. This may lead to a tight closure, which predisposes to marginal wound necrosis (see **Fig. 10**).

RLD is frequently associated with Holt-Aram syndrome, thrombocytopenia–absent-radius (TAR) syndrome, and VACTERL syndromes. It presents with a spectrum of anomalies of the hand and forearm, ranging from mild hypoplasia of the radius to complete absence of the radius. Given the characteristic position of the hand in radial deviation owing to the absence of radial support, this condition has also been termed "radial club hand."

The initial evaluation of a patient with RLD begins with a thorough musculoskeletal evaluation with special attention paid to the spine because of the associated vertebral anomalies.[86] The initial workup should also include radiographs of the spine, renal ultrasound, echocardiogram, complete blood count, and chromosomal breakage test.

The phenotype of RLD displayed clinically depends on the degree of abnormal development of the fetus in utero. The upper limb first appears as an ectoderm-covered paddle in week 4 of gestation and limb development progresses thereafter under the control of several signaling molecules. The signaling molecule that is thought to have reduced function in RLD is fibroblast growth factor, which leads to decreased proximal-to-distal growth. Although longitudinal growth is disrupted, ulnar to radial growth continues via the zone of polarizing activity, leading to the spectrum of presentation from mild thumb hypoplasia to complete absence of the radius.[87]

Bayne and Klug[88] classified the radiographic appearance of the radius in RLD into types I through IV. Type I is a mildly shortened distal radius. Type II represents radii that are hypoplastic radius along the entire length of the radius. Partial absence of the radius is classified as type III, and complete absence is classified as type IV. With a deficient radius, the hand assumes a radially deviated and flexed position owing to the lack of radial support for the carpus. This deformity is exacerbated by pull of the radial-sided musculature. As such, treatment has been directed at maintaining a straight wrist, as well restoring any shortening of the extremity.

Treatment begins with splinting and stretching; however, based on the degree of deformity and functional deficit, surgical treatments including soft tissue distraction, centralization, and radial lengthening may be utilized. Centralization is indicated when there is a persistent radial deviation deformity. The procedure requires an ulnar-sided capsulotomy, release of the radial capsule and contracted radial-sided tendons, and reduction of the carpus onto the ulna, which may require an ulnar shortening osteotomy. A Kirschner wire is placed from the third metacarpal through the carpus and into the ulna, and the ulnar capsule and tendons are advanced as a checkrein against recurrent radial deviation.[88]

Recurrence of deformity is encountered frequently (**Fig. 12**). Shariatzadeh and associates[89] reported on 11 centralizations with a mean follow-up of 90 months. Although the immediate postoperative correction of the hand–forearm angle was 50°, 54% of this correction was lost at final follow-up. Similarly, Goldfarb and coworkers[90] reported long-term follow-up of 25 centralizations at 20 years follow-up and noted hand–forearm angles of 63° preoperatively, 16° immediately postoperatively, and 25° at final follow-up.

Several authors have proposed treatment options for the recurrent radial club hand deformity. Pike and colleagues[91] described 12 cases of ulnocarpal arthrodesis for recurrent deformities of 45°, inability to passively correct the wrist to within 25° of neutral, or both. Union was achieved in 11 cases within 4 months, and 1 patient required a revision arthrodesis. The authors note patient and parent satisfaction with function and appearance postoperatively and no cases of ulnar growth. Other options include flexor carpi radialis transfer to the dorsum of the carpus for deformity recurrence.[92]

Recurrence of deformity after centralization is common and expected. Our personal preference is to stabilize floppy wrists, with some element of radial positioning. In children with stiff elbows, bilateral involvement, absent thumbs, and stiff fingers, we no longer favor centralization because the radially deviated wrist and hand posture may contribute to hand-to-mouth function, similar to the role of the elbow. Traditional centralization with tendon transfers, wrist pinning, occasional removal of ulnar carpal bones, and removal of redundant skin has its set of complications, including growth plate arrest.

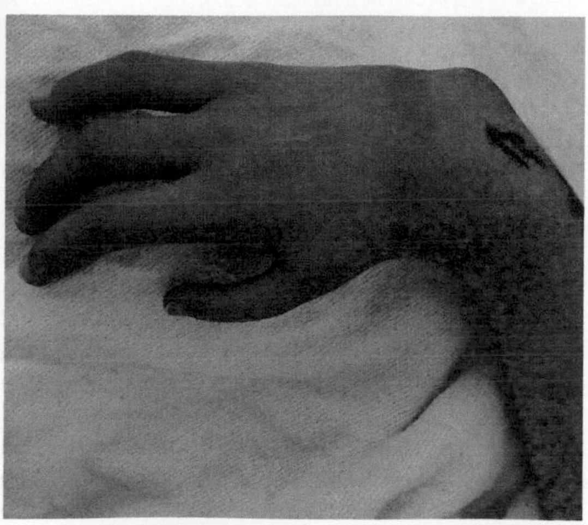

Fig. 12. Late recurrence of the radial "club hand" deformity after wrist centralization.

Authors' recommendations to decrease recurrence of deformity after the treatment of RLD

1. Release radial structures, taking care to protect the anomalous median nerve, and transfer tendons if they represent deforming structures.
2. Release joint structures cautiously, with centralizing or "radializing"[93] being attained without undue cartilage compression.
3. If centralization is deemed important, consider using a Steinman pin across the wrist joint, with no intention of removal, that is, let it break or back out so the soft tissues have time to adjust to the new position.
4. Be mindful of hardware complications, particularly in severely bowed ulna in the case of complete radial absence.

EPIDERMOLYSIS BULLOSA

EB refers to a group of disorders characterized by fragility of the skin and other epithelial-lined structures. This rare group of condition leads to blistering of the skin owing to abnormal adhesion between the various lamina of the skin. The classification of EB is based on the level of skin cleavage. EB simplex is a milder form that has an intradermal level of cleavage. Junctional EB is associated with skin cleavage at the lamina lucida in the basement membrane, and dystrophic EB has a level of cleavage within the papillary dermis secondary to abnormal collagen type VII.[94] The most severe form of EB is recessive dystrophic EB and patients frequently do not survive past age 30 owing to renal disease or squamous cell carcinoma associated with repeated scarring.[95]

Repeated shearing injuries to the skin produce blistering and scarring, which lead to progressive hand deformity. As a result of the cycles of injury, healing, and scar these patients develop pseudosyndactyly, digital and thumb adduction contracture, and loss of the fingernails. The end-stage appearance of these hands has been termed "cocoon hands" and "mitten hands."[96]

The goals of treatment are modest and include prevention of skin injury, activity modification, maintenance of nutrition, and restoration of hand function if compromised by contracture. Surgical goals include restoration of pinch and grasp by first web space and digital contracture release, independent finger movement by pseudosyndactyly

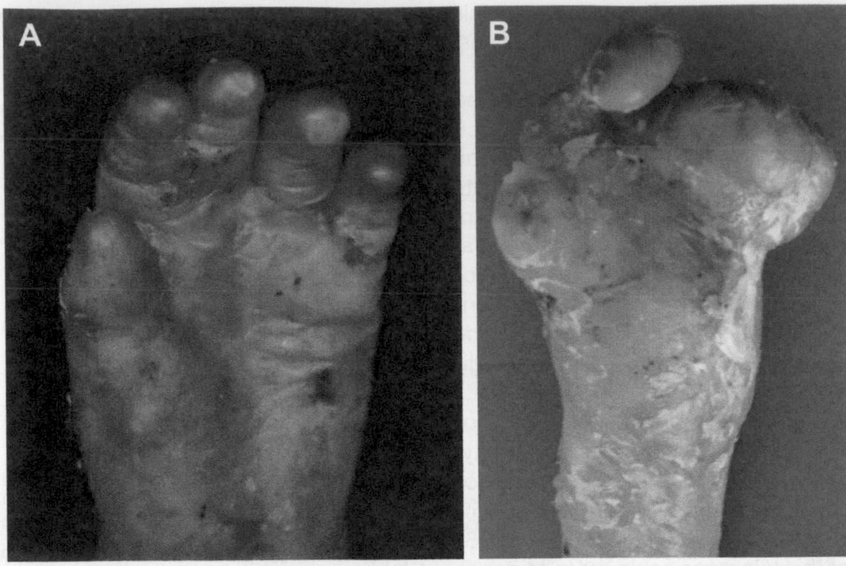

Fig. 13. (*A*) The hand of a young child after pseudosyndactyly release. (*B*) Years later, this hand demonstrates the seemingly inevitable progression of scar and contracture, even with judicious wound care.

release, and wrist flexion contracture release if present.[96,97] Surgical treatment requires multidisciplinary cooperation among many different specialists. Preoperatively dermatologic, dental, gastroenterologic, and pain management evaluation should be obtained. Perioperative considerations include type of anesthesia, intravenous access, patient positioning, and hemostasis. Postoperative issues include pain control, wound care, and, later, splinting and prevention of contracture recurrence.

The operative procedure begins with selective degloving of the epidermal cocoon over the volar epidermis tethering the wrist followed by release of the pseudosyndactyly of the digits. The first web space is released, which may require adductor fascial release in addition to the skin. Gentle manipulation of the digits and selective, sharp release of the sites of skin tension are utilized. Skin defects are then addressed with full-thickness or split-thickness skin grafts, allograft dermal matrix, and other skin substitute, or are left open.[98–101] Wounds are dressed with liberal use of antibiotic ointment and petrolatum gauze and well-padded long arm cast is applied. Patients typically return at 10 to 14 days for a dressing change and wound debridement under anesthesia.[97] Postoperatively, coordination care with a hand therapist is essential. The therapist fabricates splints with special attention directed at maintaining the web spaces and functional hand position.

Recurrence and progressive loss of function is the unfortunate norm in this disabling disease (**Fig. 13**). Recurrent contractures frequently recur within 2 to 5 years of surgery, although adulthood and splint wear do seem to confer decreased rate of recurrence.[96,97,102]

Authors' recommendations to minimize recurrence of deformity and contracture after surgical treatment of dystrophic EB

1. Faithful night splinting for maintaining wrist position and finger separation, and day wear of glove/bandages to separate digits.
2. Judicious wound care.
3. Multidisciplinary team of nutrition experts, dermatology, anesthesia, therapy, and hand surgeons convening to address complex decisions related to surgical intervention.

SUMMARY

The treatment of children with congenital hand differences is a challenging yet rewarding job. Although complications are inevitable, some can be avoided with attention paid to detail and implementing lessons learned from past experience.

REFERENCES

1. Percival NJ, Sykes PJ. Syndactyly: a review of the factors which influence surgical treatment. J Hand Surg Br 1989;14(2):196–200.
2. Barot LR, Caplan HS. Early surgical intervention in Apert's syndactyly. Plast Reconstr Surg 1986;77(2): 282–7.
3. Flynn JM, Lovell WW, Weinstein SL, editors. Lovell and Winter's pediatric orthopaedics. 7th edition.

Philadelphia: Wolters Kluwer Health/Lippincott Williams & Wilkins; 2014.
4. Mandarano-Filho LG, Bezuti MT, Akita R, et al. Análise casuística da sindactilia congênita: experiência com 47 pacientes. Acta Ortop Bras 2013; 21(6):333–5.
5. Toledo LC, Ger E. Evaluation of the operative treatment of syndactyly. J Hand Surg 1979;4(6):556–64.
6. Cronin TD. Syndactylism: results of zig-zag incision to prevent postoperative contracture. Plast Reconstr Surg 1956;18(6):460–8.
7. Brown P. Syndactyly—a review and long term results. Hand 1977;9(1):16–27.
8. McCarroll HR. Congenital anomalies: a 25-year overview. J Hand Surg 2000;25(6):1007–37.
9. Deunk J, Nicolai JP, Hamburg SM. Long-term results of syndactyly correction: full-thickness versus split-thickness skin grafts. J Hand Surg Br 2003;28(2):125–30.
10. Bauer TB, Tondra JM, Trusler HM. Technical modification in repair of syndactylism. Plast Reconstr Surg 1956;17(5):385–92.
11. De Smet L, Van Ransbeeck H, Deneef G. Syndactyly release: results of the Flatt technique. Acta Orthop Belg 1998;64(3):301–5.
12. Colville J. Syndactyly correction. Br J Plast Surg 1989;42(1):12–6.
13. Savaci N, Hoŝnuter M, Tosun Z. Use of reverse triangular V-Y flaps to create a web space in syndactyly. Ann Plast Surg 1999;42(5):540–1.
14. Niranjan NS, Azad SM, Fleming AN, et al. Long-term results of primary syndactyly correction by the trilobed flap technique. Br J Plast Surg 2005; 58(1):14–21.
15. Lumenta DB, Kitzinger HB, Beck H, et al. Long-term outcomes of web creep, scar quality, and function after simple syndactyly surgical treatment. J Hand Surg 2010;35(8):1323–9.
16. Vekris MD, Lykissas MG, Soucacos PN, et al. Congenital syndactyly: outcome of surgical treatment in 131 webs. Tech Hand Up Extrem Surg 2010;14(1):2–7.
17. Barabás AG, Pickford MA. Results of syndactyly release using a modification of the Flatt technique. J Hand Surg Eur Vol 2014;39:984–8.
18. Bulic K. Long-term aesthetic outcome of fingertip reconstruction in complete syndactyly release. J Hand Surg Eur Vol 2013;38(3):281–7.
19. Benson LS, Waters PM, Kamil NI, et al. Camptodactyly: classification and results of nonoperative treatment. J Pediatr Orthop 1994;14(6): 814–9.
20. Engber WD, Flatt AE. Camptodactyly: an analysis of sixty-six patients and twenty-four operations. J Hand Surg 1977;2(3):216–24.
21. Larner AJ. Camptodactyly: a 10-year series. Eur J Dermatol 2011;21(5):771–5.
22. Foucher G, Loréa P, Khouri RK, et al. Camptodactyly as a spectrum of congenital deficiencies: a treatment algorithm based on clinical examination. Plast Reconstr Surg 2006;117(6):1897–905.
23. O'Brien JP, Hodgson AR. Congenital abnormality of the flexor digitorum profundus, a cause of flexion deformity of the long and ring fingers. Clin Orthop Relat Res 1974;(104):206–8.
24. Miura T. Non-traumatic flexion deformity of the proximal interphalangeal joint-its pathogenesis and treatment. Hand 1983;15(1):25–34.
25. McFarlane RM, Curry GI, Evans HB. Anomalies of the intrinsic muscles in camptodactyly. J Hand Surg 1983;8(5 Pt 1):531–44.
26. Minami A, Sakai T. Camptodactyly caused by abnormal insertion and origin of lumbrical muscle. J Hand Surg Br 1993;18(3):310–1.
27. Siegert JJ, Cooney WP, Dobyns JH. Management of simple camptodactyly. J Hand Surg Br 1990; 15(2):181–9.
28. Goldfarb CA. Congenital hand differences. J Hand Surg 2009;34(7):1351–6.
29. Rhee SH, Oh W, Lee HJ, et al. Effect of passive stretching on simple camptodactyly in children younger than three years of age. J Hand Surg 2010;35(11):1768–73.
30. Goffin D, Lenoble E, Marin-Braun F, et al. Camptodactylie: classification et résultats thérapeutiques. A propos d'une série de 50 cas. Ann Chir Main Memb Super 1994;13(1):20–5.
31. Hori M, Nakamura R, Inoue G, et al. Nonoperative treatment of camptodactyly. J Hand Surg 1987; 12(6):1061–5.
32. Inoue G, Tamura Y. Camptodactyly resulting from paradoxical action of an anomalous lumbrical muscle. Scand J Plast Reconstr Surg Hand Surg 1994; 28(4):309–11.
33. Maeda M, Matsui T. Camptodactyly caused by an abnormal lumbrical muscle. J Hand Surg Br 1985;10(1):95–6.
34. Smith RJ, Kaplan EB. Camptodactyly and similar atraumatic flexion deformities of the proximal interphalangeal joints of the fingers. J Bone Joint Surg Am 1968;50(6):1187–249.
35. Ogino T, Kato H. Operative findings in camptodactyly of the little finger. J Hand Surg Br 1992;17(6): 661–4.
36. Steindler A. Congenital malformations and deformities of the hand. J Bone Joint Surg Am 1920; 2(12):639–68.
37. Stark HH, Otter TA, Boyes JH, et al. "Atavistic contrahentes digitorum" and associated muscle abnormalities of the hand: a cause of symptoms. Report of three cases. J Bone Joint Surg Am 1979;61(2):286–9.
38. Singer G, Kraus T, Petnehazy T, et al. Ulnar polydactyly - an analysis of appearance and postoperative outcome. J Pediatr Surg 2014;49(3):474–6.

39. Temtamy SA, McKusick VA. The genetics of hand malformations. Birth Defects Orig Artic Ser 1978; 14(3):i–xviii, 1–619.
40. Turek S. Orthopaedics: principles and their application. 2nd edition. Philadelphia: J.B. Lippincott; 1967.
41. Watson BT, Hennrikus WL. Postaxial type-B polydactyly. Prevalence and treatment. J Bone Joint Surg Am 1997;79(1):65–8.
42. Heras L, Barco J, Cohen A. Unusual complication of ligation of rudimentary ulnar digit. J Hand Surg Br 1999;24(6):750–1.
43. Leber GE. Surgical excision of pedunculated supernumerary digits prevents traumatic amputation neuromas. Pediatr Dermatol 2003; 20(2):108–12.
44. Dattner L. Complication after "home treatment" of polydactyly. J Pediatr 2010;156(3):504.
45. Mullick S. A selective approach to treatment of ulnar polydactyly: preventing painful neuroma and incomplete excision. Pediatr Dermatol 2010; 27(1):39–42.
46. Patillo D. Complications of suture ligation ablation for ulnar polydactyly: a report of two cases. Hand 2011;6(1):102–5.
47. Frieden IJ, Chang MW, Lee I. Suture ligation of supernumerary digits and "tags": an outmoded practice? Arch Pediatr Adolesc Med 1995;149(11): 1284.
48. Wassel HD. The results of surgery for polydactyly of the thumb. A review. Clin Orthop 1969;64:175–93.
49. Wood VE. Polydactyly and the triphalangeal thumb. J Hand Surg 1978;3(5):436–44.
50. Horii E, Hattori T, Koh S, et al. Reconstruction for Wassel type III radial polydactyly with two digits equal in size. J Hand Surg 2009;34(10):1802–7.
51. Zuidam JM, Selles RW, Ananta M, et al. A classification system of radial polydactyly: inclusion of triphalangeal thumb and triplication. J Hand Surg 2008;33(3):373–7.
52. Townsend DJ, Lipp EB Jr, Chun K, et al. Thumb duplication, 66 years' experience—a review of surgical complications. J Hand Surg 1994;19(6): 973–6.
53. Kelikian H, Doumanian A. Congenital anomalies of the hand. J Bone Joint Surg Am 1957;39-A(5): 1002–19.
54. Miura T. An appropriate treatment for postoperative Z-formed deformity of the duplicated thumb. J Hand Surg 1977;2(5):380–6.
55. Dobyns JH, Lipscomb PR, Cooney WP. Management of thumb duplication. Clin Orthop Relat Res 1985;(195):26–44.
56. Hartrampf CR, Vasconez LO, Mathes S. Construction of one good thumb from both parts of a congenitally bifid thumb. Plast Reconstr Surg 1974;54(2):148–52.
57. Tonkin MA, Rumball KM. The Bilhaut-Cloquet procedure revisited. Hand Surg 1997;2(1):67–74.
58. Naasan A, Page RE. Duplication of the thumb. A 20-year retrospective review. J Hand Surg Br 1994;19(3):355–60.
59. Tada K, Yonenobu K, Tsuyuguchi Y, et al. Duplication of the thumb. A retrospective review of two hundred and thirty-seven cases. J Bone Joint Surg Am 1983;65(5):584–98.
60. Stutz C, Mills J, Wheeler L, et al. Long-term outcomes following radial polydactyly reconstruction. J Hand Surg 2014;39(8):1549–52.
61. Mih AD. Complications of duplicate thumb reconstruction. Hand Clin 1998;14(1):143–9.
62. Larsen M, Nicolai JP. Long-term follow-up of surgical treatment for thumb duplication. J Hand Surg Br 2005;30(3):276–81.
63. Goldfarb CA, Patterson JM, Maender A, et al. Thumb size and appearance following reconstruction of radial polydactyly. J Hand Surg 2008;33(8): 1348–53.
64. Wolfe S, Pederson W, Hotchkiss R, et al. Green's operative hand surgery. 6th edition. Philadelphia: Churchill Livingstone; 2010.
65. Buck-Gramcko D. Pollicization of the index finger. Method and results in aplasia and hypoplasia of the thumb. J Bone Joint Surg Am 1971;53(8): 1605–17.
66. Manske PR, McCaroll HR. Index finger pollicization for a congenitally absent or nonfunctioning thumb. J Hand Surg 1985;10(5):606–13.
67. Kowalski MF, Manske PR. Arthrodesis of digital joints in children. J Hand Surg 1988;13(6):874–9.
68. Neviaser RJ. Congenital hypoplasia of the thumb with absence of the extrinsic extensors, abductor pollicis longus, and thenar muscles. J Hand Surg 1979;4(4):301–3.
69. Clark DI, Chell J, Davis TR. Pollicisation of the index finger. A 27-year follow-up study. J Bone Joint Surg Br 1998;80(4):631–5.
70. Kozin SH, Weiss AA, Webber JB, et al. Index finger pollicization for congenital aplasia or hypoplasia of the thumb. J Hand Surg 1992;17(5): 880–4.
71. Littler JW. On making a thumb: one hundred years of surgical effort. J Hand Surg 1976;1(1): 35–51.
72. Sykes PJ, Chandraprakasam T, Percival NJ. Pollicisation of the index finger in congenital anomalies. A retrospective analysis. J Hand Surg Br 1991;16(2): 144–7.
73. De Kraker M, Selles RW, van Vooren J, et al. Outcome after pollicization: comparison of patients with mild and severe longitudinal radial deficiency. Plast Reconstr Surg 2013;131(4):544e–51e.
74. Soldado F, Zlotolow DA, Kozin SH. Thumb hypoplasia. J Hand Surg 2013;38(7):1435–44.

75. Vekris MD, Beris AE, Lykissas MG, et al. Index finger pollicization in the treatment of congenitally deficient thumb. Ann Plast Surg 2011;66(2):137–42.
76. McDonald TJ, James MA, McCarroll HR, et al. Reconstruction of the type IIIA hypoplastic thumb. Tech Hand Up Extrem Surg 2008;12(2):79–84.
77. Huber E. Relief operation in the case of paralysis of the median nerve. 1921. J Hand Surg Br 2004; 29(1):35–7.
78. Manske PR, McCarroll HR Jr. Abductor digiti minimi opponensplasty in congenital radial dysplasia. J Hand Surg 1978;3(6):552–9.
79. Goldfarb CA, Leversedge FJ, Manske PR. Bilateral carpal tunnel syndrome after abductor digiti minimi opposition transfer: a case report. J Hand Surg 2003;28(4):681–4.
80. Cawrse NH, Sammut D. A modification in technique of abductor digiti minimi (Huber) opponensplasty. J Hand Surg Br 2003;28(3):233–7.
81. Foucher G, Medina J, Lorea P, et al. Principalization of pollicization of the index finger in congenital absence of the thumb. Tech Hand Up Extrem Surg 2005;9(2):96–104.
82. Goldfarb CA, Monroe E, Steffen J, et al. Incidence and treatment of complications, suboptimal outcomes, and functional deficiencies after pollicization. J Hand Surg 2009;34(7):1291–7.
83. Lochner HV, Oishi S, Ezaki M, et al. The fate of the index metacarpophalangeal joint following pollicization. J Hand Surg 2012;37(8):1672–6.
84. Buck-Gramcko D. Complications and bad results in pollicization of the index finger (in congenital cases). Ann Chir Main 1991;10(6):506–12.
85. Ekblom AG, Laurell T, Arner M. Epidemiology of congenital upper limb anomalies in 562 children born in 1997 to 2007: a total population study from Stockholm, Sweden. J Hand Surg 2010; 35(11):1742–54.
86. Goldfarb CA, Wall L, Manske PR. Radial longitudinal deficiency: the incidence of associated medical and musculoskeletal conditions. J Hand Surg 2006;31(7):1176–82.
87. Oberg KC, Feenstra JM, Manske PR, et al. Developmental biology and classification of congenital anomalies of the hand and upper extremity. J Hand Surg 2010;35(12):2066–76.
88. Bayne LG, Klug MS. Long-term review of the surgical treatment of radial deficiencies. J Hand Surg 1987;12(2):169–79.
89. Shariatzadeh H, Shariatzadeh H, Jafari D, et al. Recurrence rate after radial club hand surgery in long term follow up. J Res Med Sci 2009;14(3): 179–86.
90. Goldfarb CA, Klepps SJ, Dailey LA, et al. Functional outcome after centralization for radius dysplasia. J Hand Surg 2002;27(1):118–24.
91. Pike JM, Steffen JA, Goldfarb CA. Ulnocarpal epiphyseal arthrodesis for recurrent deformity after centralization for radial longitudinal deficiency. J Hand Surg 2010;35(11):1755–61.
92. Lamb DW. Radial club hand. A continuing study of sixty-eight patients with one hundred and seventeen club hands. J Bone Joint Surg Am 1977; 59(1):1–13.
93. Buck-Gramcko D. Radialization as a new treatment for radial club hand. J Hand Surg 1985;10(6 Pt 2): 964–8.
94. Intong LR, Murrell DF. Inherited epidermolysis bullosa: new diagnostic criteria and classification. Clin Dermatol 2012;30(1):70–7.
95. Fine JD, Mellerio JE. Extracutaneous manifestations and complications of inherited epidermolysis bullosa. J Am Acad Dermatol 2009;61(3):387–402.
96. Bernardis C, Box R. Surgery of the hand in recessive dystrophic epidermolysis bullosa. Dermatol Clin 2010;28(2):335–41, xi.
97. Ladd AL, Kibele A, Gibbons S. Surgical treatment and postoperative splinting of recessive dystrophic epidermolysis bullosa. J Hand Surg 1996;21(5): 888–97.
98. Fivenson D, Scherschun L, Cohen LV. Apligraf in the treatment of severe mitten deformity associated with recessive dystrophic epidermolysis bullosa. Plast Reconstr Surg 2003;112(2):584–8.
99. Jutkiewicz J, Noszczyk BH, Wrobel M. The use of biobrane for hand surgery in Epidermolysis bullosa. J Plast Reconstr Aesthet Surg 2010;63(8): 1305–11.
100. Campiglio GL, Pajardi G, Rafanelli G. A new protocol for the treatment of hand deformities in recessive dystrophic epidermolysis bullosa (13 cases). Ann Chir Main Memb Super 1997;16(2):91–100.
101. Marín Bertolín S, Amaya Valero JV, Neira Giménez C, et al. Surgical management of hand contractures and pseudosyndactyly in dystrophic epidermolysis bullosa. Ann Plast Surg 1999;43(5): 555–9.
102. Terrill PJ, Mayou BJ, Pemberton J. Experience in the surgical management of the hand in dystrophic epidermolysis bullosa. Br J Plast Surg 1992;45(6): 435–42.

Index

Note: Page numbers of article titles are in **boldface** type.

Hand Clin 31 (2015) 377–380
http://dx.doi.org/10.1016/S0749-0712(15)00023-2
0749-0712/15/$ – see front matter

J

L

M

N

P

R